DOCTOR OF NURSING PRACTICE

Enhancing Professional Development

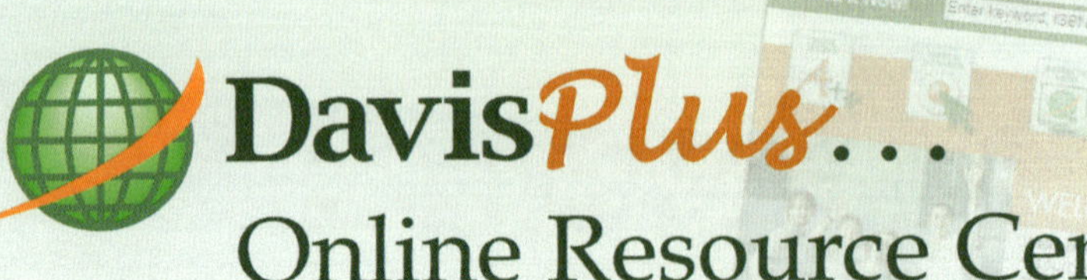

Online Resource Center

Davis*Plus* is your online source for a wealth of learning resources and teaching tools, as well as electronic and mobile versions of our products.

STUDENTS

Unlimited FREE access.
No password.
No registration.
No fee.

INSTRUCTORS

Upon Adoption.
Password-protected library of title-specific, online course content.

Visit http://davisplus.fadavis.com

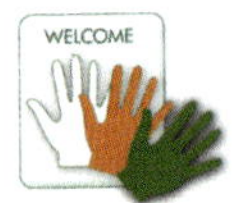

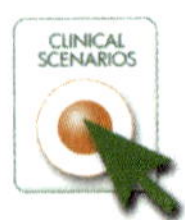

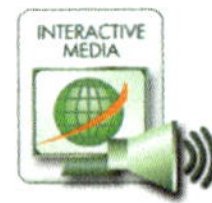

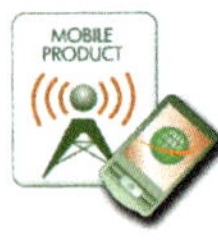

Explore more online resources from F.A.Davis...

DAVIS'S DRUG GUIDE.com
powered by
Unbound Medicine®

www.drugguide.com

is Davis's Drug Guide Online, the complete Davis's Drug Guide for Nurses® database of over 1,100 monographs on the web.

Taber's Online
powered by
Unbound Medicine®

www.tabers.com

delivers the power of Taber's Cyclopedic Medical Dictionary on the web. Find more than 60,000 terms, 1,000 images, and more.

DAVIS'S Laboratory and Diagnostic Tests with Nursing Implications
powered by
Unbound Medicine®

www.LabDxTest.com

is the complete database for Davis's Comprehensive Handbook of Laboratory and Diagnostic Tests with Nursing Implications online. Access hundreds of detailed monographs.

www.FADavis.com

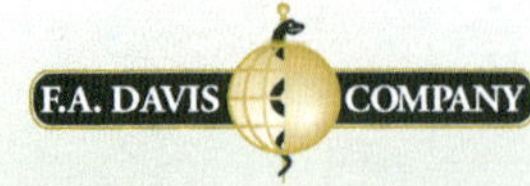

DOCTOR OF NURSING PRACTICE

Enhancing Professional Development

Ruth McCaffrey, DNP, ARNP, FNP-BC, GNP-BC

Professor
Florida Atlantic University
Boca Raton, Florida

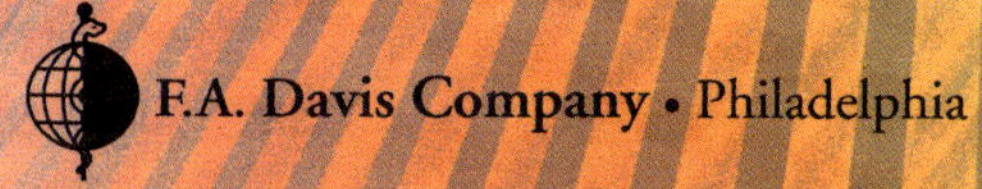
F.A. Davis Company • Philadelphia

F. A. Davis Company
1915 Arch Street
Philadelphia, PA 19103
www.fadavis.com

Last digit indicates print number: 10 9 8 7 6 5 4 3 2 1

Printed in the United States of America

Publisher, Nursing: Joanne Patzek DaCunha, RN, MSN
Director of Content Development: Darlene D. Pedersen
Project Editor: Jamie M. Elfrank
Design & Illustration Manager: Carolyn O'Brien

Library of Congress

ISBN10: 0-8036-2736-X
ISBN13: 978-0-8036-2736-9

Dedication

I would like to dedicate this book to three people who inspired and supported me in my nursing career. First, my husband Bill McCaffrey, who is always there for me, always positive, and always loving. The second is my mother-in-law Grace McCaffrey, who is gone now but who was a nurse and an inspiration for my nursing career. Grace loved nursing as an honored and respected profession throughout her life. After 9/11, Grace, age 85, wanted to volunteer in the emergency rooms of New York City to help survivors of the World Trade Center tragedy. Her life was spent in caring for others. Finally, I want to dedicate this book to Ellis Youngkin, PhD, ARNP, who was and is my mentor in all things related to advanced practice nursing and teaching. Her patience and support can never be measured and continue to sustain me as I move through my life.

Epigraph

"Nursing is an art: and if it is to be made an art, it requires an exclusive devotion as hard a preparation, as any painter's or sculptor's work; for what is the having to do with dead canvas or dead marble, compared with having to do with the living body, the temple of God's spirit? It is one of the Fine Arts: I had almost said, the finest of Fine Arts."

—*Florence Nightingale*

"The illiterate of the future will not be those who cannot read. It will be the person who does not know how to learn, unlearn and relearn."

—*Alvin Toffler*

Contributors

Mary Bishop, DNP, RN, NEA, BC, FACHE
Adjunct Faculty
Florida Atlantic University
Boca Raton, Florida

Kenneth Lowrance, DNP, APRN, FNP-BC
Vice President, Clinical Services
Goodall-Witcher Healthcare Foundation
Clifton, Texas

Kelly J. McCaffrey, PhD
Assistant Professor
Gwinnett College
Atlanta, Georgia

Jamie M. Elfrank, candidate for MA in Publishing

JoAnn Franklin, DNP, RN, FNP, GNP, and Psychiatric NP
Great Mines Health Center FQHC
Potosi, Missouri

Eve Holzemer, DNP, ANP-BC
Adult Nurse Practitioner
Instructor, Department of Neurology & Psychiatry
Administrative Director Clinical Research Unit
Saint Louis University
St. Louis, Missouri

Rose Sherman, EdD, RN, FAAN
Associate Professor
Christine E. Lynn College of Nursing
Florida Atlantic University
Boca Raton, Florida

Todd Swinderman, PhD, RN
Coordinator Quality Management
North Florida Regional Medical Center
Gainesville, Florida

Reviewers

Martha Raile Alligood, PhD, RN, ANEF
(Academy of Nursing Education Fellow)
Professor
East Carolina University
Greenville, North Carolina

E. Faye Anderson, DNS, RN, NEA-BC
Associate Professor and DNP Coordinator
University of Alabama Huntsville College of Nursing
Huntsville, Alabama

Janet Baker, DNP, APRN, ACNS-BC, CPHQ
Director of Graduate Nursing
Urusline College
Pepper Pike, Ohio

Beverly Baliko, PhD, RN
Assistant Professor
University of South Carolina
Columbia, South Carolina

Laura S. Bonanno, DNP, CRNA
Assistant Professor/Program Director of Nurse Anesthesia Program
Louisiana State University Health Sciences Center School of Nursing
New Orleans, Louisiana

Patricia M. Burbank, DNSc, RN
Professor
University of Rhode Island
Kingston, Rhode Island

Maria A. Connolly, PhD, APN/CNS,CNE, FCCM, ANEF
Professor of Nursing; Director of Research & Grantsmanship
College of Nursing University of St. Francis
Joliet, Illinois

Linda Carman Copel, PhD, RN, PMHCNS, BC, CNE, NCC, FAPA
Professor of Nursing
Villanova University
Villanova, Pennsylvania

Mary Katherine Crabtree, DNSc, FAAN, APRN-BC
Professor, DNP Faculty
Oregon Health & Science University
Portland, Oregon

Bernadette D. Curry, PhD, RN
Dean Emerita and Professor
Molloy College
Rockville Centre, New York

Catherine Dearman, RN, PhD
Professor of Nursing
University of South Alabama College of Nursing
Mobile, Alabama

Jean E. DeMartinis, PhD, FNP-BC
Associate Professor
University of Massachusetts Amherst, School of Nursing
Amherst, Massachusetts

Mary Enzman-Hines, RN, PhD, CNS, CPNP, AHN-BC
Professor and DNP Program Coordinator
Beth El College of Nursing and Health Sciences at the University of Colorado, Colorado Springs
Colorado Springs, Colorado

Frances A. Freitas, PhD, MSN, CME
Director
Kent State University
Kent, Ohio

Phyllis S. Hansell, EdD, RN, FAAN
Dean and Professor
Seton Hall University
College of Nursing
South Orange, New Jersey

Donna R. Hodnicki, PhD, FNP-BC, FAAN
Professor, Chair
Georgia Southern University
School of Nursing
Statesboro, Georgia

Gretchen S. McDaniel, DSN, RN
Professor of Nursing
Ida V. Moffett School of Nursing
Samford University
Birmingham, Alabama

Carrie J. Merkle, PhD, RN, FAAN
Associate Professor, Nursing
The University of Arizona College of Nursing
Tucson, Arizona

Joan M. Nelson, DNP, APRN-BC
Associate Professor
University of Colorado, College of Nursing
Aurora, Colorado

Anita C. Reinhardt, PhD, RN
New Mexico State University
Assistant Professor, School of Nursing
Las Cruces, New Mexico

Rebecca F. Wiseman, PhD, RN
University of Maryland School of Nursing
Assistant Dean, Shady Grove Campus
Rockville, Maryland

Acknowledgments

I would like to acknowledge Donna Hathaway, PhD, RN, Dean of the College of Nursing at University of Tennessee Health Science Center. Dr. Hathaway has been a mentor in assisting me to understand the disruptive innovation that is the doctor of nursing practice degree. She has been essential to my understanding of the AACN essentials. I would also like to acknowledge the students in the DNP program at Florida Atlantic University for providing insight into their own practice issues and for important discussions regarding the need for the DNP and ideas concerning the best way forward for advanced practice nursing.

Also, thank you to Caryn Abramhovitz, who so patiently edited each chapter. I would like to acknowledge two very special people from F. A. Davis, Joanne DeCuhna and Jamie Elfrank, who were always supportive and who helped guide the unfolding of this book in a way that makes sense and will be helpful to students.

Special thanks to the DNP LLC for the assistance in reaching out to DNP graduates, and thanks to all the graduates who allowed their exemplars to be included with this text.

Table of Contents

Introduction

Welcome to the *Doctor of Nursing Practice: Enhancing Professional Development.* This book is designed to provide students with an introduction to the essential elements of Doctor of Nursing Practice education as developed by the American Association of Colleges of Nursing (AACN). Each of the eight essentials may be taught separately in a DNP program or several may be combined in one course; this book is intended to provide an overview and discuss some of the most important issues in each of the essentials to develop a basic understanding and perspective on the importance of each essential element. Beyond the essentials, two other chapters are included. One presents some essential issues and important information in the areas of writing and publishing. For nurses educated at the doctoral level, writing becomes an essential element of practice that must be studied and learned. Publishing is critical to disseminate findings of excellence in practice and translational research so that others may benefit from these examples and is important to the future of advanced practice nursing and health care in general. The final chapter discusses residency, portfolio development, and the final or capstone project. Creating a meaningful final project that may help to guide advanced nursing practice is an important aspect of the DNP program, and this book provides some guidelines for the creation of these meaningful projects. Health care in the United States is rapidly changing in an attempt to decrease cost while increasing access and focusing on health promotion and disease prevention. As changes in health care unfold, there will be an increased need for advanced practice nurses. Advanced practice nurses will require increased knowledge and education in population-based care, health policy, economics, informatics, evidence-based practice, and leadership to influence health care in order to improve care and reduce the high cost of health care. The Doctor of Nursing Practice (DNP) is a doctoral degree for nurses at the highest level of nursing practice. The AACN has proposed that the DNP degree will be the level of entry for all advanced practice nurses by 2015. Although this goal may not be reached, nurses with the advanced education and knowledge provided by the DNP will certainly be leaders in the advanced practice nursing movement.

The DNP has been described as a disruptive innovation in nursing education (Hathaway, Jacob, Stegbauer, Thompson, & Graff, 2006). This book discusses the concepts and elements necessary to propel this innovative disruption into the mainstream of nursing education and provide the discipline with knowledgeable professionals who will sustain and promote nursing now and in the future. Even before the DNP was firmly established, nursing leaders were discussing the need for a practice focus for doctoral nursing education. Lash (1987) stated that nursing cannot thrive unless there is a concerted effort to connect the intellectual activities within the nursing profession with the realities of patient care. Practice is the foundation for theory, and theories are developed in practice to inform or be tested. According to Lash, a doctoral program having "nursing" in its title is guilty of misrepresentation if it ignores the importance of patient care.

As you read each chapter in this book, reflect on the growth and advancement of the nursing profession and how the DNP could promote and use theoretical, research, and practice knowledge to change the face of health care in the United States.

Some of the questions that still remain unanswered or only partially answered regarding DNP education and outcomes of obtaining a DNP degree include the following:

a. Will the DNP become the entry-level degree for advanced practice?
b. Will DNP graduates be eligible for tenure-earning positions at colleges and universities?
c. Will the DNP be accepted as a member of research teams or be able to apply for and receive research funding? What types of research are most appropriate for the DNP graduate?
d. How will the DNP graduate and the PhD or DNS graduate work together to further the profession and discipline of nursing?
e. How will the DNP lead advanced practice nurses as changes occur in the health care system? Will these graduates be able to provide leadership in entrepreneurship, health policy, and population-based care in the complex health system of the United States.

As DNP-prepared nurses grow in number, these decisions will be influenced by those who have attained the highest level of education in nursing practice.

Making the decision to begin a doctoral program has many implications for students and their families. The path toward the DNP degree is a journey that will bring you to the highest level of understanding regarding the nursing discipline and profession. This understanding is historical, theoretical, and practical in nature and leads to new levels of knowledge and experience in the field. Many groups, both inside and outside nursing, are pressing for evidenced-based practice to enhance clinical effectiveness. According to Downs (1989), adequate preparation of doctoral candidates is among the most important and pressing educational issues facing the nursing profession today, and this group of nurses must develop critical and creative studies within the science of nursing, including nursing theories and their evaluation. Doctoral scholarship will also benefit the users of nursing services who depend on nursing advocacy, caring, and competence to enhance health and well-being.

To meet the needs of society, nursing graduate education strives to create professional nurses who are comfortable working in both an interprofessional and an intraprofessional work environment, to be leaders and work within the profession, and to work as members of a multidisciplinary team. This level of skill and knowledge promotes the foundational nursing paradigm that includes effective, efficient disease management; health promotion; disease prevention; and a focus on holistic, client-centered care (AACN, 2006). To accomplish these goals and position advanced practice nurses better to work within a professional multidisciplinary team, the AACN has advocated that advanced practice nurses obtain a terminal clinical degree in the discipline of nursing. The title of this terminal clinical degree has been designed by the AACN as the *Doctor of Nursing Practice (DNP).* The need for advanced practice nurses to advance their knowledge as clinical experts and nursing leaders becomes more apparent yearly as the United States seeks ways to increase access to health care and to make health care safe, efficient, and effective. Advanced practice nurses will continue to be fundamentally important to health care in the United States and in other countries around the world.

For many years, nursing leaders and educators lamented the gap between nursing research and nursing practice. Collins and Robinson (1996) listed three areas that are needed in creating nursing practice based on evidence, developing practitioner research, integrating research into practice, and disseminating research to inform practice. These authors proposed a "link" nurse be educated to develop practice guidelines based on evidence and experience. Over the next decade, as evidence-based practice and practice guidelines replaced habit and usual practice as the best method for developing nursing practice, the need for this "link" nurse became more important. When considering the creation of a practice doctorate for clinically focused advanced practice nurses, educators referred to Boyer's (1990) model for educating and creating nursing scholars. In this model, scholarship is redefined from the narrow focus on research and theory development to a broader focus, which includes practice-based processes in teaching that involve excellence in both classroom presentation of skills and knowledge and research and application. To accomplish excellence in nursing practice, Boyer believed that a new model was needed that calls for nurse scholars to embrace the process of knowledge application and the scholarship of practice.

The DNP is excellently positioned to become the "link" nurse within practice. DNPs are leaders in the field of nursing practice who are educated to translate research findings into practice guidelines and create innovative practice settings to meet the health-care needs of a diverse population. Although the nurse scientist with a PhD or DNS and the advanced practice nurse with a DNP differ in education and knowledge, they are complementary and exemplify the need for multiple layers of education in the preparation of nurses.

Providers of primary health care are in short supply in the United States. According to the Institute of Medicine (IOM) at the National Institutes of Health (NIH): "Primary care is the provision of integrated, accessible healthcare services by clinicians who are accountable for addressing a large majority of personal healthcare needs, developing a sustained partnership with patients, and practicing in the context of family and community" (Institute of Medicine Committee on the Future of Primary Care, 1996).

Providing this type of comprehensive care will be the challenge as health care continues to be at the forefront of national debate. Mundinger (2005) asked the following questions:

- Who will provide this type of comprehensive primary care?
- Who are the expert practitioners needed to manage chronic illness?
- Who can work with patients to change health behaviors and adopt a healthy lifestyle for health promotion and disease prevention?
- Who will ensure timely and knowledgeable translation of science into practice?
- Who will generate new evidence for continuous improvement in practice and health-care outcomes?

Mundinger answered these questions by proposing the DNP as uniquely educated and positioned to provide this type of care. She stated that as advanced practice nurses adopt the DNP as entry into practice, they will foster increased confidence, develop more assertive accountability and responsibility, and create roles not considered in the past (Mundinger, 2005). The most important goal of the DNP according to Mundinger is to provide "exquisitely sensitive and knowledgeable care to patients who desperately need this resource" (Mundinger, 2005, p. 176). A further consequence is for the public to see DNPs in care settings increasing awareness of the broad scope of nursing practice and in general increasing the public's idea of nursing as a discipline. Creating teams of healthcare providers that include DNPs, doctors of medicine, doctors of pharmacy, and others will provide patients with the best possible care and outcomes.

As you begin this journey into advanced practice or as you begin to extend your knowledge in a post-master's DNP program, it is important to open your mind to new ideas and an expanded notion of what is required to be an effective advanced practice nurse. I hope you will embrace your journey and strive to lead the nursing profession into a new era of practice-based excellence at all levels.

—Ruth McCaffrey

References

American Association of Colleges of Nursing. (2006). The essentials of doctoral education for advanced nursing practice Retrieved from http://www.aacn.nche.edu/publications/position/DNPEssentials.pdf

Boyer, E. (1990). *Scholarship reconsidered: Priorities for the professoriate.* Princeton, NJ: The Carnegie Foundation for the Advancement of Teaching.

Collins, C., & Robinson, T. (1996). Bridging the research-practice gap: The role of the link nurse. *Nursing Standard (Royal College of Nursing (Great Britain), 10*(25), 44–46.

Downs, F. (1989). Differences between the professional doctorate and the academic/research doctorate. *Journal of Professional Nursing, 5*(5), 261–265.

Hathaway, D., Jacob, S., Stegbauer, C., Thompson, C., & Graff, C. (2006). The practice doctorate: Perspectives of early adopters. *Journal of Nursing Education, 45*(12), 487–495.

Institute of Medicine Committee on the Future of Primary Care. (1996). *America's health in a new era.* Washington, DC: National Academy Press.

Lash, A. A. (1987). The nature of the doctor of philosophy: Evolving conceptions. *Journal of Professional Nursing, 3*(2), 92–101.

Mundinger, M. (2005). Who's who in nursing: Bringing clarity to the doctor of nursing practice. *Nursing Outlook, 53,* 173–176.

CHAPTER

1

DOCTOR OF NURSING PRACTICE: EVOLUTION, EDUCATION, AND PRACTICE

Objectives:

By the end of the chapter, students should be able to:

1. Provide a brief history of doctoral studies in the United States and an overview of advanced practice nursing, and analyze the history of doctoral preparation for nurses specifically.
2. Describe the underlying principles, foundation, evolution, and groups involved in the creation of the doctor of nursing practice (DNP) degree.
3. Argue both for and against the DNP degree as entry into advanced nursing practice.
4. Define "primary care" as an important aspect of the U.S. health-care system in its approach to health promotion, disease prevention, and reduced cost.
5. Analyze the shortage of primary care providers and the creation of the DNP as appropriate to fill that gap.
6. Explain the differences in preparation and expectations between the DNP and PhD or doctor of nursing science (DNS) programs, and discuss the requirements needed to enter and complete a DNP program.
7. Provide examples of successful DNP graduates in practice and leadership, and provide helpful online resources for students in DNP programs.

This chapter presents the foundational ideas and philosophy for the doctor of nursing practice (DNP) as a terminal—or highest possible—degree in nursing. The DNP, a practice-focused doctorate, creates knowledgeable experts in advanced nursing practice, person-centered care, and clinical leadership. In the interprofessional health-care settings of today, the DNP establishes nursing values as essential to the health and well-being of patients, families, communities, and the nation. Because policy makers and health-care leaders have stated that the future of health care in the United States will be focused on interprofessional teams of experts in a group environment (Institute of Medicine, 2001), the DNP will be a valuable member of the team of experts, promoting nursing values and focusing on providing quality health care that includes health promotion and disease prevention.

Until more recently, the doctorate of philosophy degree (PhD) in nursing has been the traditional option for all students who want to achieve a terminal nursing degree. The PhD prepares nurses who have interests in the areas of research and teaching at the university level. A PhD-prepared nurse conducts research to extend nursing knowledge and tests nursing theories to strengthen the discipline. PhD-prepared nurses who teach in university settings are able to ground new nurses and nurses at the graduate level in disciplinary knowledge and nursing values.

In contrast to the research and teaching focus of the PhD, the DNP has a practice orientation. The DNP prepares nurses to assume responsibility for practice, leadership, and health policy and to focus on population-based and individual care. Students in DNP programs have course work in interdisciplinary collaboration, health-care engineering, systems approaches to managing care, and other areas of practice leadership that prepare them to work effectively within the complex health-care system. PhD programs usually have several courses on nursing theory, qualitative and quantitative research methods, and the role of nursing scholars; the programs end with a formal dissertation research study.

The DNP is the natural outgrowth of a larger innovation begun in the late 1960s with the advent of nurse practitioner (NP) programs, according to Donna Hathaway, PhD, Professor and Dean at the University of Tennessee Health Science Center College of Nursing, a school where the DNP has flourished for more than 10 years. In other words, the DNP, as a clinical doctorate, is the natural evolution for advanced practice nurses in their desire to create a health-care system that is consistent with nursing ideas and values.

Other nursing leaders (Mundinger, Starck, Hathaway, Shaver, & Woods, 2009) describe the need for the DNP as entry to advanced practice to provide a solution for the increasing need for a large number of well-qualified clinicians to provide coordinated, comprehensive, safe, accessible, and high-quality care across a continuum of community, hospital, and long-term health-care settings. The National Academy of Science (NAS) at the National Institutes for Health (NIH) has endorsed the DNP as a nonresearch doctorate that prepares expert practitioners who can also serve as clinical faculty. The American Association of Colleges of Nursing (2010a) has provided the following reasons for the DNP as entry into advanced practice in the same way that the Doctor of Pharmacy (PharmD) for pharmacists, Medical Doctorate (MD) for physicians, or Juris Doctorate (JD) for attorneys is the entry into practice:

- The movement to the DNP is about producing the most competent nursing clinicians possible to meet the health-care needs in the United States.
- Raising educational expectations is common across professions striving for excellence (p. 1).

Advancing Your Knowledge

F.W. has been a nurse practitioner for 5 years. During that time, his knowledge has expanded, and he is comfortable in his role as health-care provider. He has a base of patients who are loyal to him and have complete confidence in his ability to manage their health. F.W. would like to expand his role as an advanced practice nurse and become involved in community and state health-care policy planning for health care. In addition, he has thought about teaching in an advanced practice program. Although he has a clinical preceptor, he would like to try teaching a didactic class for advanced practice nurses and believes he has much to add to the knowledge nurses receive both in the classroom and in practice. At some point in his career, F.W. hopes to open his own practice and work with the underserved while preparing new nurse practitioners for practice in a setting that he can control. He strongly believes that helping patients navigate the complex health-care system is the role of the primary care provider. Although he has many good ideas of how to accomplish his goals, F.W. realizes that there is a lot he does not know and that he would have a better opportunity to reach his goals with a doctoral education. Because his area of interest is firmly grounded in clinical practice and the application of new knowledge in patient care, he decides to apply to a DNP program.

1. What are the pros and cons that F.W. should consider when determining how to further his education (DNP, PhD, or other advanced education)?
2. How would a terminal degree in nursing practice benefit F.W.'s patients and his community?
3. In his book, *The Seven Habits of Highly Effective People,* Steven Covey gives students an assignment of writing their personal mission statement. He asks them to write a document that identifies the most important aspects of their lives. A personal mission statement can be written for one's professional life as well. Write a mission statement that describes your personal mission in obtaining a DNP degree. What is important about the DNP for you? Why did you choose this doctorate rather than the PhD or DNS?

This chapter provides the DNP student with an overview of doctoral education in nursing. It describes the underlying principles and evolution of the DNP degree and explains the differences in preparation and expectations between the DNP and PhD or DNS. The chapter continues by arguing both the barriers to and the positives of the DNP degree as a terminal degree in nursing and as entry into advanced nursing practice. The chapter discusses primary care in the United States in the context of advanced practice nursing. This chapter ends by offering examples of successful DNP graduates in practice and leadership.

Overview of Doctoral Education in the United States

As nursing explores the adoption of the DNP as a terminal doctoral degree for advanced practice, a general understanding of doctoral education in the United States may be valuable. The broad purpose of doctoral education is to provide preparation in leadership and broader system thinking and to prepare students to be innovators and move a discipline forward. The word *doctor* comes from the Latin word *doctus,* which means "teacher." The criteria and curriculum in doctor preparation for professionals have advanced over the years, changing from a loosely arranged individual plan of study to rigorous and scholarly programs that use both classroom and mentorship to advance knowledge and provide experiences in research and practice.

The Carnegie Institute supported work outlining the future of all levels of education in the United States (Walker, Gold, Jones, Bueschal, & Hutching, 2008). The group described a definition of the position of individuals prepared with doctoral degrees as "stewards of the discipline" (p. 161). They posited that a steward is a scholar in the fullest sense because he or she can generate new knowledge imaginatively and critically conserve valuable and useful ideas. It is the responsibility of these stewards to transmit what they know to others through writing, teaching, and application. Stewardship also has an ethical and moral dimension. A steward does not simply collect accomplishments but is someone to whom the integrity of the discipline can be trusted, and who will ensure quality and vitality in the discipline now and in the future.

When universities were established in the late 19th century in the United States, they awarded doctorates primarily in the sciences and later the arts. By the early 20th century, universities began to offer doctoral degrees in the social sciences, which included education. Today's doctoral graduates are not only teachers but also scholars, professionals, and practitioners who lead society forward. As society becomes more specialized in technology and more diverse and complex in knowledge and expectations, individuals educated at the doctoral level in all disciplines can understand and assist in the creation of advances and innovations.

The first PhD degrees in the United States were awarded by Yale University in 1861. Before that time, only baccalaureate degrees were awarded at American universities. Master's degrees were awarded not for graduate academic work but rather as honorary degrees based on monetary contributions to the school. By the late 1800s, professional doctorates were awarded in medicine (MD) and dentistry (DDS). These were not considered to be terminal degrees and were conferred on students who were clinically prepared as professional clinicians. To keep in step with the need for research and advanced knowledge, many medical doctors and dentists began to obtain more education and become prepared as PhDs in addition to having clinical degrees. Most PhD-prepared physicians and dentists continue to be involved in both research and practice (Association of Medical Colleges, 2007).

Brief History of Doctoral Education in Nursing

Nursing is late in adopting formal doctoral education as the entry into leadership and professional practice; this may be due partly to the fact that nurses were originally educated outside the mainstream of higher education, in hospital settings. Also, the medical profession spoke out against advanced education for nursing. When Adelaide Nutting became the first professor of nursing at Columbia Teachers College in 1907, she was rebuked in the *Journal of the American Medical Association*:

> Every attempt at initiative on the part of nurses should be reproved by the physician. The professional instruction for nurses should be entrusted exclusively to the physician, who can only judge what is necessary for them to know. There is a need for large numbers of trained nurses who will perform simple duties and attend to the sick. The work she has to do is ordinary service and does not require a high school education nor three years of hospital training. Nurses are helpers and agents for the physician not co-workers or colleagues. The training of nurses should be simplified and take no more than learning simple tasks at the hands of the physician *(Morimer & McGann, 2005, pp. 123–126)*.

Despite these disheartening remarks from medicine, with the help of nursing leaders who had a very different view of the importance of the discipline in 1924, Teachers College at Columbia University established a nursing-focused doctoral degree. Individuals who completed the program were awarded an educational doctorate degree (EdD). This program focused on the preparation of teachers of nursing and the preparation of nursing leaders. The first PhD in nursing was offered at New York University in 1934. The focus of this first PhD program was the science of unitary human beings (Malinski, 1986). In the 1950s, the University of Pittsburgh began a nursing PhD program in maternal and child nursing, which emphasized the importance of clinical research to advance nursing knowledge and the profession of nursing.

Boston University subsequently created a unique nursing doctoral model, the DNS. The degree was the first to focus on the nurse as a professional practitioner in the role of providing nursing care. Over time, the DNS degree was adopted by many universities as an alternative to the PhD. Nevertheless, over time, the DNS became more research-focused and now has much of the same content and emphasis on research as the PhD. Few DNS programs are available today because most schools offering nursing doctoral programs offer the PhD.

Early Controversy—Defining the Science of Nursing

One of the issues that confronted the first group of nursing programs at the doctoral level was that nursing science was not well defined or well described. Science is "to know," and the goal of scientific inquiry is to uncover truth. Scientific knowledge is typically logical and orderly. Because nursing science is embedded in practice, however, it requires knowledge of humans as individually unique and different—the counterpoint to logic and order. Truths in nursing science may be different at different times and for different groups of people.

To illustrate this point, much of nursing research has been qualitative in design, with an emphasis on understanding experience better and uncovering individual and cultural ideas (Miller, 2010). Nurse researchers must often begin to understand a problem by "coming to know" the person or persons and their individual situations before they can begin outcomes-oriented research and manipulate situations to define best practices. Most nursing research is focused on understanding the human response to disease and on developing theories and interventions to (1) mitigate the negative impact of disease and (2) create interventions to prevent disease and improve health and well-being (Cordeau, 2009). For example, nursing research attempts to understand the experience of a cancer diagnosis and how the disease affects the overall quality of life (Tobin & Begley, 2008).

In many scientific disciplines, such as chemistry, biology, and physics, empirical research has been the only method for gaining knowledge in the discipline. Empirical science is only one mode of inquiry in nursing. Philosophical and nonempirical methodologies are gaining increasing importance as modes of scientific inquiry (Winters & Balleau, 2003). In the area of health and well-being, the ability to influence health behaviors and understand the experience of disease and disability has become more accepted as nursing science has advanced (Barrett, 2010). Different people may have different feelings because of gender, ethnicity, race, religious beliefs, family situation, and social support. Nursing science is also connected to social science, physical science, and psychology, adding to its diversity and complexity and making its definition even more nebulous. Nonetheless, nursing did ultimately arrive at its own definition. The International Council of Nurses provides the following definition of nursing:

> Nursing encompasses autonomous and collaborative care of individuals of all ages, families, groups and communities, sick or well and in all settings. Nursing includes the promotion of health, prevention of illness, and the care of ill, disabled and dying people. Advocacy, promotion of a safe environment, research, participation in shaping health policy and in patient and health systems management, and education are also key nursing roles *(International Council of Nurses, 2010).*

Growing Demand for Clinical Leaders

In an attempt to begin to develop a body of knowledge for nursing, early nurse scholars and leaders obtained doctoral degrees in other disciplines, such as anthropology, education, and the social sciences, because the body of knowledge in these areas was well established and focused on aspects of human care that nurses could embrace (Grace, 1989). Between 1955 and 1970, the U.S. Public Health Service funded 156 nurses in doctoral study through a Pre-doctoral Research Fellowship Program. Almost none of these nurses received doctoral degrees in nursing. In 1959, the Division of Nursing within the Health Resources and Services Administration created a Faculty

Research Development Grant program to increase the capacity of nursing faculty in the area of nursing research.

Since that time, the number of nursing programs offering the research doctorate has increased, from 70 in 1998 to 176 in 2008. PhD programs continue to proliferate in an effort to meet the growing demand for nursing researchers and nursing faculty. The focus of these programs remains research and teaching, which is desirable in the effort to continue to build disciplinary knowledge and prepare the next generation of nursing scholars.

Dividing Doctoral Education in Nursing

Although nursing is constructed as a traditional discipline seeking knowledge through research, it is also a practical discipline that uses research to guide practice and support the primary mission of the profession of providing compassionate quality care to individuals in need (Ponte et al., 2007). Evidence exists that one level of doctoral education cannot fulfill the two needs: (1) to create nursing scientists who focus on the generation of new nursing knowledge through research and (2) to develop clinical nurse leaders who translate and educate nurses in the use of this knowledge in practice (AACN, 2004). Rather, two doctoral level programs—differently oriented—better fulfill the needs of the advanced practice nursing community.

In the late 1970s, the College of Nursing at Case Western Reserve University began the first clinical nursing doctoral program and awarded graduates a doctor of nursing (ND) degree. As originally conceptualized by Dr. Rozella Schlotfeldt, dean of the Francis Payne Bolton College of Nursing at Case Western Reserve University, the ND would be the entry into nursing practice as the MD is the entry into medical practice (Schlotfeldt, 1964). Dr. Schlotfeldt based this perception on the premise that medical and nursing leadership should work together to solve problems and promote health and well-being in patients. She believed that the ND would prepare nurses to collaborate with their medical partners as equals to promote the welfare of patients. In order for nurses and physicians to work as colleagues, Dr. Schlotfeldt outlined four assumptions:

1. That both physicians and nurses take responsibility for helping patients experiencing stress caused by microbial invasion, physiologic malfunction, psychological trauma, and social deprivation: the patient is the focus of all medical and professional nursing practice.
2. That physicians and nurses communicate and collaborate in relation to the needs of the patients they serve.
3. That both physicians and nurses participating in the investigation have the requisite scientific knowledge for decisions each is called on to make independently in the interest of the patient's welfare.
4. That the system in which services are delivered to patients can be altered (p. 775).

Finally, Dr. Schlotfeldt posited that this type of patient care would rely on cooperative planning between the MD and the ND. She found nothing in the ethical codes of either profession to preclude realignment of functions carried out by the physician and nurse, and she believed that as scientific understanding and technology advanced, the roles would naturally require such realignment.

Although the ND never evolved into a practice entry degree because of the need for larger numbers of nurses than could be produced in ND programs, many ND graduates became leaders in the nursing field and used the knowledge gained in the ND program to enrich and further their careers. ND degree programs were started at several other universities around the United States, including the University of Colorado, Rush University, and the University of South Carolina. All of these schools continue to offer a clinical doctorate in nursing, but the ND title has been eliminated, and the DNP title has been adopted as proposed by the American Association of Colleges of Nursing for practice-oriented doctorate degrees.

Education of Advanced Practice Nurses

In 2004, the AACN began to discuss how advanced practice nurses should be educated and what level of education would best meet the needs of students and of the public. Although this discussion is ongoing, the AACN did adopt the position that the doctoral level was appropriate for entry into advanced practice. This group also developed a timeline that marks 2015 as the year when this change to doctoral-level preparation for advanced practice nurses will be in place (AACN, 2004). The AACN DNP Task Force developed a document that identifies reasons why the DNP is appropriate for entry into advanced practice (Box 1-1). In October 2005, the Commission on Collegiate Nursing Education (CCNE), the accrediting body responsible for nurse credentialing examinations and designations, stated that the DNP was the only type of practice doctorate it would consider for accreditation. This statement provides impetus to maintain consistent titling for the clinical doctorate in nursing.

The American Nursing Credentialing Center (2010) completed a survey to which 4284 advanced practice nurses responded. Demographic information for respondents indicated that most were white non-Hispanic (92%) and female (94.3%). Of respondents, 71% indicated that they were currently practicing in an advanced practice role. The roles were divided into 76.7% nurse practitioners, 11.9% midwives, 10.8% clinical nurse specialists, and less than 1% nurse anesthetists. The educational levels of respondents were 70.3% master's level and 22.6% doctoral level (7% were DNP graduates). In answer to the survey's major question—"What do you envision as the desired future for certification of nursing holding the DNP degree in the year 2010?"—59.7% indicated a preference for single comprehensive endpoint certification, with the DNP degree required for entry into advanced practice. A tiered certification system, with advanced practice first being certified at the master's level and later certified at a higher level for the DNP, was preferred by 40%.

Box 1-1

Reasons for Developing the DNP as Entry Into Advanced Practice

1. In 1995, the Pew Health Professions Commission called for new approaches to health care and the education of health-care professionals (Pew Health Professions Commission, 2003).
2. The IOM Quality Initiative (2001) identified serious health-care safety issues and called for a reallocation of health-care resources to ensure optimal standards of care and the basic safety of U.S. consumers.
3. Many other health-care disciplines require professional or practice doctorates as entry into practice, including pharmacy, physical therapy, occupational therapy, and medicine. The DNP would provide parity for nursing to be viewed as an equal partner at the health-care discussion table.
4. PhD and DNS programs in nursing have only 500 graduates per year despite the increase in number of programs. In addition, the average age of a doctoral graduate in nursing has increased from 45 years old in 1997 to 49 years old in 2009. The implication is that nurses continue to enter doctoral programs later in life and that many doctorate-prepared nurses will retire in the next 10 years (National Center for Health Statistics, United States, 2007).
5. The nursing and health-care professions are experiencing increasing complexity and diversity that require additional education to prepare nurse clinicians and leaders. These changes call for the development of new skills in management, education, and organizational systems and a population-based approach to health-care management.
6. Committee for Monitoring the Nation's Changing Needs for Biomedical, Behavioral, and Clinical Personnel, Board on Higher Education and Workforce, National Research Council. (2005) has stated that nursing could meet the need for clinical faculty if a nonresearch clinical doctorate could be developed similar to the MD and PharmD.

Source: From AACN DNP Task Force (Rhodes, 2011).

Although the issue of entry into advanced practice is not settled, and discussion both in favor of and against the DNP degree continues, more than 100 universities have begun DNP programs, and the number of DNP graduates is steadily increasing. DNP programs can begin at the post–master's level for individuals already prepared as advanced practice nurses, and baccalaureate-to-DNP programs have been developed for individuals who are newly entering advanced practice education. DNP programs are accredited by the CCNE, with accreditation focused on the ability of the DNP program to educate students in accordance with the AACN "Essentials of Doctoral Education for Advanced Nursing Practice" (2006) (Box 1-2).

A post–master's program for nurses already in advanced practice who want to return to school and undertake a DNP degree incorporates the eight essentials outlined by the AACN and focuses on meeting the needs of an increasingly complex and changing health-care system. Many of the post–master's degree programs have fewer credit hours than the PhD because students have already completed a larger number of master's credits to become advanced practice nurses. The Bachelor of Science in nursing–to–DNP curriculum includes all of the elements necessary to be credentialed as an NP, clinical nurse specialist (CNS), midwife, nurse anesthetist, or nurse executive as well as the advanced elements related to the DNP.

Box 1-2

AACN DNP Essentials

1. **Scientific underpinning of practice:** The DNP provides the terminal academic preparation for nursing practice. The scientific underpinnings of this education reflect the complexity of practice at the doctoral level and the rich heritage that is the conceptual foundation of nursing.
2. **Organizational and system leadership for quality improvement and systems thinking:** To improve patient and health-care outcomes, eliminate health disparities, and promote patient safety and excellence in practice, the DNP focuses on the needs of sets of populations or a broad community.
3. **Clinical scholarship and analytical methods for evidence-based practice:** Scholarship and research are the hallmarks of doctoral education. A scholar applies knowledge to solve a problem via the scholarship of application. Nursing practice epitomizes the scholarship of application through its position where the sciences, human caring, human needs, and new understandings emerge.
4. **Information systems/technology and patient care technology for the improvement and transformation of health care:** The DNP supports and improves patient care and health-care systems and provides leadership within health-care systems and academic settings.
5. **Health-care policy and advocacy:** Political activism and a commitment to policy development are central elements of professional nursing practice, and the DNP graduate has the ability to assume a broad leadership role on behalf of the public as well as the nursing profession.
6. **Interprofessional collaboration for improving patient and population health outcomes:** The current complex, multitiered health-care environment depends on the contributions of highly skilled and knowledgeable individuals from multiple professions. DNP members of these teams have advanced preparation in the interprofessional dimension of health care that enables them to facilitate collaborative team functioning and overcome impediments to interprofessional practice.
7. **Clinical prevention and population health for improving health in the United States:** DNP graduates will be leaders in health promotion and risk reduction and illness prevention for individuals and families.
8. **Advanced nursing practice:** All DNP graduates are expected to demonstrate refined assessment skills and base practice on the application of biophysical, psychosocial, behavioral, sociopolitical, cultural, economic, and nursing science as appropriate to their area of specialization.

Source: American Association of Colleges of Nursing, 2006.

Advancing Your Knowledge

M.W. is an RN–to–BSN student who will graduate this year. She is interested in becoming a nurse practitioner and is confused by the choices available and does not know whether to pursue a master's degree program in advanced practice or apply to a DNP program. She has heard about the AACN proposal for the DNP to be the entry level into advanced practice but is unsure if that will truly be the requirement. M.W. has heard arguments from friends, program advisors, and local advanced practice nurses on both sides of this issue. Some say to go ahead and get the DNP because it would position her better for advanced practice. Others question why take the extra semesters of work when an NP can be obtained at the master's level? Still others say that physicians may not like the DNP, which may make it more difficult to get a job.

1. Based on your knowledge of doctoral education in nursing and the essential elements that are mandated for DNP education and the increased complexity that exists in health care, how would you advise M.W.?
2. Make a list of pros and cons for the DNP as entry into advanced practice, and provide a response to each telling whether you agree or disagree and why. Discuss your personal reasons for starting the DNP program.

Overview of Advanced Practice Nursing

In 1992, the National Councils of State Boards of Nursing (NCSBN) and the American Nurses Association (ANA) promoted the designation of the advanced practice nurse. This was an important step for nursing because the ANA declared that specialization—including the advanced practice nurse designation—is a mark of the advancement of the nursing profession. The term *advanced* can be defined as "ahead of or further along in progress, complexity, knowledge and skill or pertaining to or embodying ideas, practices, attitudes, taken as being more enlightened or liberal than the standardized, established, or traditional" (http://dictionary.reference.com/browse/advanced). This definition is enlightening in the case of advanced practice nursing. Nurses in advanced practice develop complex thinking skills and knowledge that focuses on whole persons, communities, and the entire health-care system. *Advanced practice nurse* is a broad term that typically applies to the following five specialty nursing roles:

- Certified nurse midwife
- Certified registered nurse anesthetist
- Clinical nurse specialist
- Nurse executive
- Nurse practitioner

Each specialty practice group addresses health-care problems in different groups of patients in varied health-care settings, and each is recognized differently within the health-care sector. Midwives are independent practitioners who specialize in women's health and obstetrics. Nurse anesthetists are involved in working with surgical patients to monitor and administer anesthesia. CNSs are experts in one area of nursing, such as cardiovascular, mental health, or urological care. These nurses work in health-care settings as educators, leaders, and patient advocates. Nurse executives are leaders in nursing management and are often responsible for development and implementation of large budgets and groups of personnel to provide patient care in different settings. NPs provide care to individuals in many settings and are responsible for assessment, diagnosis, and treatment of disease and health promotion and disease prevention activities.

In 2006, the NCSBN created a draft vision paper entitled *The Future Regulation of Advanced Practice Nursing* (2006). In this document, the NCSBN states that the diversity among state regulations for advanced practice is confusing to nurses and other stakeholders. This group recommends that there be increased uniformity in education for advanced practice and that all advanced practice nurses be independent practitioners who do not require supervision. A consensus model for advanced practice registered nurse (APRN) education (NCSBN, 2008) has been developed by a group of nursing leaders and the NCSBN that identifies four components of adequate preparation for APRNs: licensure, accreditation, credentialing, and education (LACE).

1. Licensure is receiving authority to practice.
2. Accreditation is a process whereby educational programs are reviewed and, if approved, are recognized as meeting the standards to provide APRN education.
3. Certification is the process whereby a student demonstrates achievement, knowledge, and skills within a specific practice area.
4. Education is the method of preparation for APRN graduates.

Midwives

The original idea for advanced practice nursing started early in the 19th century with midwives and nurse anesthetists. Lay midwives trace their history back to ancient Greece and Egypt. In early Western civilization, midwives were respected members of the community, but in the 1800s this group fell into disfavor because of the advent of physicians in the specialty. In a revival during the 20th century, Mary Breckenridge (Rooks, 1997) founded the Frontier Nursing Service School of Midwifery and Family Nursing in 1925 as a private charitable organization serving an area of about 700 square miles in southeastern Kentucky.

The number of midwives practicing in the United States is increasing, with 50% directly involved in patient care (Gray, Ratliff, & Mawyer, 2000). A midwife is recognized as a responsible and accountable professional who works in partnership with women to give the necessary support, care, and advice during pregnancy, labor, and the postpartum period; to conduct births; and to provide care for the infant. This care includes instituting preventive measures, promoting normal birth, detecting complications in mother and child, accessing medical or other appropriate assistance, and carrying out emergency measures. Certified nurse midwives are educated as advanced practice nurses specifically in the care of pregnant women and the delivery and care of infants. Completing a DNP would provide education for midwives in the areas of leadership, practice management, and health policy that would enable them to be stronger advocates for pregnant women and newborns.

Nurse Anesthetists

Nurse anesthetists were the first formally accredited advanced practice nurses in the United States and were the first professional group to provide anesthesia services. Established in the late 1800s, nurse anesthesia developed in response to the requests of surgeons seeking a solution to the high morbidity and mortality rates attributed to anesthesia at that time. Surgeons saw nurses as a cadre of professionals who could give their undivided attention to patient care during surgical procedures. Serving as pioneers in anesthesia, nurse anesthetists became involved in the full range of specialty surgical procedures and in the refinement of anesthesia techniques and equipment. The earliest existing records documenting the anesthetic care of patients by nurses are those of Sister Mary Bernard at St. Vincent's Hospital in Erie, Pennsylvania, in 1877. The most famous nurse anesthetist of the 19th century was Alice Magaw, who worked at St. Mary's Hospital in Rochester, Minnesota. That hospital, established by the Sisters of St. Francis and operated by Dr. William Worrell Mayo, later became internationally recognized as the Mayo Clinic.

The first formal educational programs preparing nurse anesthetists were established in 1909. Founded in 1931, the American Anesthesia Nurses Association (AANA) is the professional association for this group, representing more than 37,000 nurse anesthetists nationwide. The AANA developed and implemented a certification program in 1945 and instituted mandatory recertification in 1978. There is much debate among anesthesiologists and nurse anesthetists regarding the role of each professional in health care. Although this debate has been contentious at times, nurse anesthetists remain a mainstay in the provision of safe and effective anesthesia services. Nurse anesthetists educated at the practice doctorate level would use the knowledge in areas such as leadership, health policy, and population care to advocate for patients and solidify their ability to provide safe and quality care in the area of anesthesia services.

Clinical Nurse Specialists

A CNS is an advanced practice nurse whose care focuses on a specific patient population. Five general areas make up the duties of a CNS: clinical practice, teaching, research, consulting, and management of patient care (Sparacino, Cooper, & Minirak, 2005). The CNS role began to evolve in 1900 when Katherine DeWitt called for the development of nursing specialties. In 1943, Frances Reiter outlined the role of the CNS as consisting of three spheres. The first sphere was clinical competence, including caring, curing, and counseling. The second sphere was coordination and continuity of patient care. The third sphere was labeled "professional maturity," and in this role the CNS was to work with the physician and share "mutual responsibility for the welfare of the patient" (Reiter, 1966, p. 277).

Another leader in the CNS evolution was Hildegard Peplau, who developed the master's degree program in psychiatric nursing for graduate psychiatric CNSs at Rutgers University in 1948. Also pivotal to the CNS role as it exists today was the program developed in the 1950s at Cornell University's School of Nursing. In this program, CNSs became experts in clinical care for a defined population of patients, such as oncology, nephrology, and intensive care. In 1976, the role of the CNS was outlined by the ANA in the following position statement:

> The clinical nurse specialist (CNS) is a practitioner holding a master's degree with a concentration in specific areas of clinical nursing. The role of the CNS is defined by the needs of a select client population, the expectation of the larger society and the clinical expertise of the nurse *(American Nurses Association Congress for Nursing Practice, 1976).*

The CNS was prepared to care directly for a specific population of patients by exercising leadership ability and judgment. In 1995, the role of the CNS was adopted by the AACN, which supported merging the CNS/NP role in the curricula of graduate education; this has been adopted in varying degrees by different states and in different academic settings.

The functional areas in which the CNS focuses include direct clinical practice, expert coaching, collaboration, consultation, research, clinical and professional leadership, and ethical decision making (Fitzpatrick & Wallace, 2009). CNSs work in a wide variety of practice settings and specialties to provide effective and efficient patient care. In 2009, the National Association of Clinical Nurse Specialists developed a list of CNS competencies for the DNP that reflect the additional knowledge, skills, and abilities that should be achieved through practice doctorate education.

Advanced Nurse Executives

Nurses who are certified as advanced nurse executives are also designated as advanced practice nurses and are eligible for DNP education, according to the AACN. The term *nurse executive* as a level of certification for nursing leaders is new and replaces the designation of nurse administrator. Nurses with this level of administrative responsibility require knowledge of systems, organizational and health policy, informatics, and population. The American Organization of Nurse Executives (AONE) supports the DNP but believes that master's degree options should remain for nurse administrators, especially options at the nurse manager level. AONE cites financial and time constraints as reasons to have master's degree options as well as the DNP degree for nurse administrators.

However, nurse executives have been graduating from DNP programs in high numbers (Waxman & Maxworthy, 2010). The reason for this trend may be that the DNP serves the purpose of advancing knowledge of health-care delivery and health-care policy in the United States, including trends in payment, nursing, and reimbursement. Nurse executives need extensive knowledge in these areas.

Many nurse executives prepare and manage budgets that far exceed the budgets of chief executive officers of many U.S. companies, yet they have little formal education in the areas of finance and budgeting. Nurse executives require skills in leadership and systems thinking that go beyond the level of a master's-prepared nurse and that only the DNP can offer. Nurse executives feel that the doctoral designation and an increased understanding of scientific and research methods allows them to work more collegially with MDs, PharmDs, and others educated at the doctoral level (Waxman & Maxworthy, 2010).

Nurse Practitioners

The final and perhaps largest group of nurses included as potential students in DNP programs are NPs. An NP is a registered nurse (RN) who has completed advanced education and training in the diagnosis and management of common medical conditions, including chronic illnesses. Nurse practitioners provide a broad range of health-care services. They provide many of the same services provided by physicians and maintain close working relationships with physicians. An NP can serve as a patient's regular health-care provider. NPs are prepared to do the following:

- Take health histories and provide complete physical examinations;
- Diagnose and treat many common acute and chronic problems;
- Interpret laboratory results and x-rays;
- Prescribe and manage medications and other therapies;
- Provide health teaching and supportive counseling with an emphasis on prevention of illness and health maintenance; and
- Refer patients to other health professionals as needed.

In 1948, the ANA campaigned for direct reimbursement for nursing services, which paved the way 40 years later for direct reimbursement to NPs.

Evolution of the Nurse Practitioner Role

The concept of the NP, as it is known today, was first described by Dr. Loretta Ford in the 1960s, who helped create the first training program for pediatric NPs. As part of the graduate nursing program, the pediatric NP program graduated students who provided pediatric general care to rural children in Colorado. Because the NP was a new concept with few leaders and champions in the early years, programs were haphazardly developed at different levels and even included certificates without graduate standing.

Some physician groups were very supportive of the advanced practice nurse concept at first. In 1964, Dr. Duncan Reid proposed a family NP role to replace the general family physician because of the rise of the specialist physician and lack of interest for general practice among students. Similarly, the American Congress of Obstetricians and Gynecologists supported the development of an OB/GYN NP. The American Association of Family Practice supported the NP role for primary care in rural areas.

In recent years, however, physicians have seen NPs thrive in urban settings as well, which has sparked debate in the American Medical Association (AMA) and other groups regarding the need for supervision and collaboration restrictions for NP practice. Depending on the state, this debate often creates an impediment to the autonomy and ability of the NP to practice independently. In response to this debate, the ANA (1993) published a pamphlet entitled *Primary Health Care: The Nurse Solution,* in which it specified the following parameters of the NP role:

- Performing physical examinations and taking health histories;
- Assessing and evaluating common symptoms of acute illnesses, such as colds, infections, and asthma;
- Prescribing and managing medication regimens for common or acute conditions;
- Managing chronic health problems, such as diabetes, hypertension, and depression;
- Providing screening and preventive services, such as blood pressure screening, nutrition counseling, immunizations, and smoking cessation programs;
- Providing prenatal care, family care, and delivery of normal pregnancies; and
- Identifying health needs that require referral for more specialized care.

In the United States, the board of nursing of each state determines licensure regulations for advanced practice nurses. There are significant differences between requirements of licensure and relicensure among states. Some of the differences involve continuing education requirements, need for certification, supervisory requirements, and prescriptive authority. The NCSBN (1993) has published a position paper on advanced practice (Box 1-3).

At the present time, there are about 160,000 NPs in the United States (American College of Nurse Practitioners, 2008). That number is expected to grow rapidly over the next decade as health care in the United States expands to cover more people, and health promotion and disease prevention play a larger role in health-care provision.

Nurse Practitioners as Independent Health-Care Providers

Although the scope of practice and authority of NPs has been established, some question the preparedness and competency of the NP. NPs perceive themselves as having a unique area of expertise that complements the area of expertise of physicians, whereas the medical profession generally perceives the NP as a "physician extender" who needs supervision, rather than as an independent practitioner (Flanagan, 2000).

Research supports the NP perception as more accurate and effective. In a meta-analysis of 35 studies, Horrocks, Anderson, and Salisbury (2002) found that patients were more satisfied with care from an independent NP than with care provided by an MD. When compared, outcomes of services and treatments

Box 1-3

NCSBN Definition of Advanced Practice Nursing

The advanced practice of nursing by NPs, nurse anesthetists, nurse midwives, and CNSs is based on the following:

1. Knowledge and skills acquired in basic nursing education.
2. Demonstration of minimal competency in basic nursing as evidenced by licensure as an RN.
3. A graduate degree with a major in nursing or a graduate degree with a concentration in an advanced nursing practice category, which includes both didactic and clinical components; advanced knowledge in nursing theory, physical and psychosocial assessment, appropriate interventions, and management of health care.

Skills and abilities essential for an advanced practice RN within the designated area of practice include:

1. Assessing clients, synthesizing and analyzing data, and understanding and applying nursing principles at an advanced level.
2. Providing expert guidance and teaching.
3. Working effectively with clients, families, and other members of the health-care team.
4. Managing clients' physical and psychosocial health–illness status.
5. Using research skills.
6. Analyzing multiple sources of data, identifying alternative possibilities regarding the nature of a health-care problem, and selecting appropriate treatment.
7. Making independent decisions in solving complex client care problems.
8. Performing diagnostic actions and prescribing therapeutic measures consistent with the area of practice and recognizing limits of knowledge and experience, planning for situations beyond expertise and consulting with or referring clients to other health-care providers as appropriate.

Source: National Council of State Boards of Nursing, 1993; National Organization of Nurse Practitioner Faculty National Panel for NP Practice Doctorate Competencies, 2006.

provided by NPs and MDs, including prescriptions, return consultations, and referrals, were the same. The researchers stated that "quality of care was in some ways better for nurse practitioner consultations" (p. 820).

Other studies have compared NP and MD practice in emergency departments, pediatric and neonatal care, nursing homes, and intensive care units. In each case, NPs were found to be as effective and efficient as MDs in treating patients, and patients were more satisfied with NP care than they were with care provided by the MD (Hooker & McCaig, 1996; Miller, 1997; Mitchell-Dicenso et al., 1996; Rhee & Dermyer, 1996). Another study revealed that when physicians work as colleagues with NPs, medical care is enhanced, and patient outcomes improve (McCaffrey, Hayes, & Farrell, 2011). With this kind of success, why do we need to prepare advanced practice nurses at the doctoral level? By advancing

NP education, NPs will enhance their knowledge in the areas needed to serve an expanding and diverse community, including population-based approaches to care, health-care policy, and health-care management.

Advancing Your Knowledge

A group of advanced practice nurses is meeting for its first class in the DNP program. Each type of advanced practice nurse is represented in this group—midwives, nurse anesthetists, clinical nurse specialists, nurse executives, and nurse practitioners. As the nurses review the essentials of DNP education (see Box 1-2) and look at the learning objectives for each of the essentials, they discuss how these essential elements will assist them in advancing their own practices.

1. Take each advanced practice role and discuss how each of the essentials might benefit nurses in that role as they complete the DNP program.
2. How could these different groups of advanced practice nurses work together to create a more seamless health-care system across the continuum of care?
3. Why is it important for each advanced practice nurse to understand other types of advanced practice nursing? How could legislative and health policy goals be more attainable if all of these different groups of advanced practice nurses worked together?

Brief History and Overview of the DNP

The health-care delivery system in the United States has been described as "broken," with escalating costs, inadequate access to services, and wasteful spending policies (AACN, 2006; IOM, 2001). The Institute of Medicine (IOM) at the National Institutes of Health (NIH) has called for restructuring of all health-care professions, with increased education to reduce health errors and improve the financial burden caused by fragmentation and failures within the health-care system. The DNP is the nursing response to this call. It is intended to prepare advanced practice nurses to play a role in resolving some of the existing problems in health care. The DNP program does so by creating models of care to meet the current needs of individuals who are underserved (Wall, Novak, & Wilkerson, 2005).

Creating and Defining the DNP

The first four universities to initiate DNP programs were Columbia University, the University of Kentucky, the University of Tennessee at Memphis, and the University of Colorado. Several other schools, including Rush University, the University of South Carolina, and Case Western Reserve University, converted nursing doctoral programs to DNP programs over the course of several years.

Over time, as more universities began clinical doctoral programs in nursing, the name of the degree was changed for consistency to *doctor of nursing practice*. In 2002, the AACN officially adopted this name. There are more than 100 DNP programs in the United States at the present time, with more in the planning stages (Kaplan & Brown, 2009). The rapid growth in the number of and attendance in DNP programs is due to the knowledge that health care is becoming more complex as patient needs become more complex. Health-care providers of today and tomorrow will need to manage not only the health of patients but also their families and communities. The American Association of Medical Colleges (2000) defines *population health* as encompassing the ability to (1) assess the health needs of a specific population; (2) implement and evaluate interventions to improve the health of that population; and (3) provide care for individual patients in the context of the culture, health status, and health needs of that population. Boland (1996) further stated that population-based care involves a new way of seeing individuals seeking health care. It is a way of seeing the patient not as an individual but as a member of a group with shared health-care needs. This approach does not detract from individuality but rather adds another dimension to treatment, as individuals benefit from the guidelines developed for the populations to which they belong (Boland, 1996). A population-based approach to health care requires a different skill set than that possessed by most advanced practice nurses. The DNP graduate is envisioned as the professional who will earn this skill set, understand population-based care across the continuum of health-related services, and be able to advocate for patients and provide leadership in health policy.

The DNP promotes and implements a higher level of education for the advanced practice nurse to meet the essentials proposed by the AACN (2006). Increased knowledge is required to navigate the health-care system, learn about new technologies, develop a systems approach to population-based health-care delivery, and master leadership principles. The advanced knowledge and experience required for the DNP, such as that related to population-based care, cannot be adequately crammed into the number of semesters allotted for master's study, and a terminal doctoral degree is more appropriate for the objectives each student must master.

Planning and Evaluating DNP Programs

The rapid growth of the number of DNP programs has not allowed time for appropriate program evaluations to take place. DNP program adequacy and quality and the accomplishments of nurses who graduate with a DNP degree should receive intense scrutiny through formative and summative evaluations to review the program delivery and quality and the program outcomes. Some formative evaluation of DNP programs takes place when universities obtain CCNE accreditation. The CCNE uses a standardized method for evaluating program content, teaching, appropriate faculty, and clinical sites as well as success in placing students in appropriate clinical areas for practice experience.

Because the DNP degree is relatively new, summative evaluation is just beginning to emerge. Because outcome measures of DNP education have not been established, evaluating the impact of DNP graduates on the health-care system will take some time.

One proposed type of summative evaluation is an exit examination for DNP students. Passing the examination and receiving certification is an earned credential that demonstrates an individual's specialized knowledge, skills, and decision-making ability. The intent of the competency-based DNP certification examination, created by the Council for the Advancement of Comprehensive Care (CACC), is to assess the knowledge and skills necessary to support advanced clinical practice. The DNP certification examination is comparable in content and similar in format, measures the same set of competencies, and applies similar performance standards as step 3 of the United States Medical Licensing Examination (USMLE). The step 3 examination is the final step for licensure for MD candidates; the CACC examination is used only for certification for graduates of DNP programs. In 2009, 19 DNP students took the examination, with a 57% pass rate.

Many universities and DNP groups have not accepted the CACC examination as necessary or beneficial for DNP certification. One reason for this lack of acceptance is that the examination is primarily a medical examination rather than a nursing-focused examination. The underlying paradigm of nursing (person, environment, health, and care) is not the central basis for the test. Most NPs already take a board certification examination from either the AACN or the American Academy of Nurse Practitioners to become credentialed as advanced practice nurses for state licensure. Many in the field think the advanced practice board examinations are sufficient and should be taken at the end of the DNP programs as they become entry into advanced practice. The AANC and Academy examinations are written by nurses and have a nursing focus and nursing content. The idea is that DNP graduates practice from a different framework than new medical school graduates, and so competency for advanced nursing practice should be measured differently. Physician groups are also unhappy with the idea of using this test for DNP certification because it seems to make a statement that DNPs who pass this examination have the same types and levels of knowledge as physicians. Whether or not some of the knowledge between medicine and nursing is shared, the professions have two different approaches to patient care and two distinct bodies of knowledge.

Before beginning a DNP program, most schools conduct a needs survey to determine whether advanced practice nurses in the area are interested in returning to school for a DNP degree and, if so, the type of program format that would be most attractive to them. Because most DNP students continue to work while attending school, many programs are conducted completely online or are Web-assisted with some in-person class meetings. Students considering application for a DNP program should determine which type of program format they prefer and whether a program has been accredited before applying. Attending an accredited program provides students with assurances that they will be receiving a quality and well-designed educational experience.

Purpose and Intent of DNP Programs

In 2002, the AACN Task Force on the Practice Doctorate met to consider the need for and to develop an initial outline for the nursing clinical doctorate. In 2004, the group adopted a position statement calling for a "transformational change" in the level of education required for professional advanced practice nurses, recommending that advanced practice nurses receive doctoral-level preparation. This position statement emerged from multiple factors, including the expansion of scientific knowledge required for safe nursing practice and growing concerns regarding the quality of patient care delivery and outcomes.

The IOM created a report entitled "Future of Nursing, Leading Change Advancing Health" (IOM, 2010). In this report, the IOM made four key statements about the use of nurses in health care for Americans:

- Nurses should practice to the full extent of their education and training. Related to the DNP, this would mean that the advanced practice nurse educated with a DNP should be a leader in health-care provision and provide care to patients based on his or her education and experience.
- Nurses should achieve higher levels of education and training through an improved education system that promotes seamless academic progression. As DNP-prepared nurses who wish to be involved in education move into clinical education positions, it could help to reduce the faculty shortage and realize greater opportunities for further education in nursing.
- Nurses should be full partners with physicians and other health-care professionals in redesigning health care in the United States. For the DNP graduate, this means that as health care becomes more and more a team effort, the DNP is an equal member of the team with others at the same education level, including physicians, pharmacists, and physical therapists.
- Effective workforce planning and policy making require better data collection and improved information infrastructures. Preparing DNP graduates with an advanced understanding of informatics will enable them to assume leadership positions in workforce planning and policy making.

In its DNP position statement of 2004, the AACN identified the following benefits of practice-focused doctoral programs:

- Development of needed advanced competencies for increasingly complex practice, faculty, and leadership roles. Areas of advanced competencies include leadership, informatics, research, theory, and evidence-based practice.
- Enhanced knowledge to improve nursing practice and patient outcomes. Areas of advanced competencies are areas that strengthen the scientific understanding of DNP-prepared nursing including the ability to translate research findings into the practice arena.
- Enhanced leadership skills to strengthen practice and health-care delivery. The DNP-prepared nurse has been exposed to knowledge regarding the principles of leadership and management, the need for team work, and

collegiality and positive communications in nursing and throughout the health-care field.

- Better match of program requirements and credits and time with the credential earned. Most master's programs are around 30 credits, whereas the advanced practice nurse master's programs range from 40 to 60 credits. When advanced practice nurses receive a master's degree, they have already gone far beyond the expectations of this degree and are close to the level of a doctoral degree. Making the DNP the entry into practice would allow these nurses to earn a terminal degree and have parity with other health-care professionals of their level while earning the appropriate number of credits for the degree.
- Provision of an advanced educational credential for nurses who require advanced practice knowledge but do not need or want a strong research focus (e.g., practice faculty). The DNP allows nurses who have a passion for nursing practice and are not as interested in research as the primary focus of their career to earn a terminal degree in the discipline and teach clinical nursing if they so desire.
- Enhanced ability to attract individuals to nursing from non-nursing backgrounds. Individuals who return to school for a baccalaureate nursing degree after obtaining baccalaureate degrees in other disciplines often desire to go on to advanced degrees as well. The DNP would allow and encourage these new nurses with two baccalaureate degrees to pursue a terminal degree in nursing practice.
- Increased supply of faculty for practice instruction. As clinical-focused faculty, the DNP could help to reduce the faculty shortage in nursing (AACN, 2004, p. 5).

Although the AACN has indicated that as of 2015 the DNP will be the degree necessary for advanced practice, complete consensus on this has not been reached among the state boards of nursing or credentialing bodies such as the American Nurses Credentialing Center or the American Academy of Nurse Practitioners. The CCNE is continuing to accredit master's NP programs as well as DNP programs.

Advancing Your Knowledge

K.S. is contemplating beginning a DNP program at a local university. She has reviewed the program objectives, the course work, and the outcome requirements of the program and feels that they will increase her knowledge and prepare her to be a leader in nursing practice, especially as the health-care system continues to change. She and several others who are planning to begin the DNP program are discussing how the DNP degree will be meaningful to their future practice and how the DNP will affect their roles as advanced practice nurses. As they review the outcomes that Kaplan and Brown (2009) have outlined and the AACN benefits of a practice-focused doctorate, it becomes more obvious how the DNP will affect their practices individually and health care as a whole.

1. Review the Kaplan and Brown outline and the AACN benefits statements, and describe the benefits to advanced practice from furthering education and obtaining a DNP.
2. How do you think you can enhance your personal self-concept of advanced practice? How will it help you as an advanced practice nurse?
3. The DNP is a degree, not a role; how will this degree strengthen you personally as an advanced practice nurse? How can nursing in general benefit from an increased number of doctorate-prepared nurses who are practice experts?

Reasons the DNP Degree Should Be the Entry into Advanced Practice Nursing

Many believe that requiring a doctoral degree as entry into advanced practice nursing would increase the visibility and creditability of advanced practice nurses as health-care providers in their own right and not "physician extenders." Advanced practice nurses provide care based on a nursing framework, and the doctoral designation creates an opportunity to be on a level with other health-care providers, including physicians, pharmacists, and physical therapists. Advances for Nurse Practitioners (2010) surveyed advanced practice nurses to determine their feelings about the DNP. Although not all of the responses were favorable, the following quotes help to explain the need for advanced practice nurses to have parity with other health-care providers:

> "The DNP degree will be the beginning of the end for the 'glass ceiling' that has separated MDs and NPs that perform nearly identical roles. Esoterically it will rewrite the 'see your doctor' mentality that permeates health care in the mind of the average consumer, and on a more practical note it will level the 'mental playing field' that has historically kept nurses from aspiring to greater heights and allowing them to be key players in health care. We will look back on this in 20 years and smile."

> "This degree will allow NPs a seat at many tables where we have been excluded. We need to sit at every table where decisions are made about the health of our patients and the tools we use to provide care. This degree will allow our voice to be heard."

DNP programs, as entry into the profession, have the potential to transform nursing to meet the needs of society better. Kaplan and Brown (2009) outlined the following potential outcomes from this transformative process:

- Creating and adopting new roles in health care and policy development
- Increasing the influence of advanced practice nurses in health care and policy development
- Promoting leadership of advanced practice nurses in their workplaces and health-care organizations
- Enhancing the self-concept of advanced practice nurses
- Strengthening interprofessional relationships and collaborations

The DNP as a terminal degree is now supported by many nursing organizations, including the American Association of Colleges of Nursing, National Organization of Nurse Practitioner Faculty, American Organization of Nurse Executives, and the National Association of Clinical Specialists.

One of the most important reasons for creating the DNP as the entry into advanced practice is to prepare advanced practice nurses to practice in the increasingly complex health-care system with an emphasis on community and primary health care. The clinical doctorate is a way to provide nurses with a terminal degree and acknowledge their expertise while including additional course work that focuses on population-based care, leadership, application of research to practice, evidence-based practice, finance, and emerging scientific innovations. These additional competencies are critical in the changing and increasingly complex health-care climate. The health-care system is increasing in complexity in several contexts:

- Navigating the system to secure the required care for patients;
- Offering patient education and counseling to increase quality and satisfaction; and
- Managing more and more complex chronic diseases.

Treating and monitoring chronic diseases, educating patients, and updating the treatment plan take extended time and teamwork. In addition, the health-care system is and will continue to become more complicated as the focus shifts from disease management to health promotion and disease prevention. In settings where patient education and working to change health behaviors are priorities, nurses are essential, and their knowledge and skills directly affect the quality of care that patients receive. As complexity of health-care expands and the population ages and becomes more diverse, the burden of providing person-centered care and the ethics of providing that care will also expand, increasing the necessity for qualified advance practice nurses to manage the need. These educational objectives are contained within DNP education programs. The programs provide expanded knowledge not currently found in master's programs for advanced practice nurses and include population-based care; leadership; informatics; practice management; health-care policy; and an expansion on the link between theory, research, and practice to promote evidence-based practice. With this expanded education, the advanced practice nurse with a DNP will be able to provide quality primary health care that is patient-centered, culturally competent, and safe to an ever-growing number of Americans.

DNP as Resolution to the Primary Care Shortage

The Institute of Medicine Committee on the Future of Primary Care (1996) redefined primary care. Within this new definition are the following assumptions:

1. Primary care will be the logical foundation of an effective health-care system because primary care can address most health problems present in the population.

2. Primary care will be essential to achieving the objectives that together constitute value in health care—quality of care (including achievement of desired health outcomes), patient satisfaction, and efficient use of resources.
3. Personal interactions that include trust and partnership between patients and clinicians will remain central to primary care (p. 6).

Primary care will be an important instrument for achieving stronger emphasis on (a) health promotion and disease prevention and (b) care of chronically ill patients, especially elderly patients with multiple problems. The trend toward integrated health-care delivery systems will continue and will provide both opportunities and challenges for primary care.

The projections for the future in terms of adequate numbers of primary care providers are worrisome. There is a severe shortage of general practitioners or primary care physicians, and that shortage is predicted to continue for years to come (Pear, 2009). One of the most pressing practice needs within the U.S. health-care system is additional primary care providers (Epperly, 2010). Primary health-care providers continue to be in short supply, and the number of medical students who go into primary care or family medicine residencies continues to decline. The American Academy of Family Physicians (2007) predicts a shortage of 40,000 primary care physicians (including family practice, internal medicine, pediatrics, and obstetrics/gynecology) by 2020. The number of medical students choosing the primary care specialty has declined by 52% since 1997. At the present time, only 2% of medical school graduates choose primary care as a career.

The DNP is uniquely positioned to work with others to assist in the resolution of the shortage of primary health-care providers (Mundinger et al., 2000). Advanced practice nurses have already demonstrated an ability to provide quality health care within a primary care setting (Fletcher, Baker, Copeland, Reeves, & Lowery, 2008). With the additional education DNPs receive in the areas of leadership, practice management, and health-care policy, these nurses are well positioned to become leaders in providing primary care, in creating positive patient outcomes and patient-centered care to improve patient satisfaction, and in using resources efficiently. As mentioned earlier in the chapter, because the DNP is well educated in population-based health, he or she is able to care for larger groups of patients with chronic diseases and create programs that influence disease prevention and health promotion. Another aspect that is central to the education of the DNP is teamwork, collegiality, and positive communications. These skills make the DNP a leader in integrated health-care delivery systems that are cost-effective and provide quality care that is culturally aware and person-centered (Table 1-1).

The primary health-care provider is the first line of defense for patients in the United States to promote health and prevent illness and cares for patients who have chronic health problems. As the backbone of the health-care system, primary care providers educate consumers in health promotion and disease prevention, treat common acute problems, monitor and educate patients regarding

Table 1-1

CNS Competencies for the DNP

On completion of a practice doctorate CNS program, the graduate will possess the CNS competencies listed in the "Core practice doctorate clinical nurse specialist (CNS) competencies" (National Association of Clinical Nurse Specialists, 2009) and the following:

Sphere of Influence	Description
Client sphere	**1.** Conducts evidence-based, comprehensive assessment of client health-care needs, integrating data from multiple sources that could include the client and interprofessional team members. **2.** Implements client assessment strategies based on analysis of psychometric properties, clinical fit, feasibility, and utility. **3.** Uses advanced clinical judgment to diagnose client conditions related to disease, health, and illness within cultural, ethnic, behavioral, and other contexts. **4.** Designs, implements, and evaluates a broad range of evidence-based interventions for clients, which may include prescribing and administering pharmacological and other therapeutic interventions. **5.** Directs the analysis and dissemination of outcomes of client care programs based on multiple considerations, including socioeconomic, cultural, and environmental factors; epidemiology; symptoms; cost and clinical effectiveness; satisfaction; safety; and quality. **6.** Advocates for integration of client preferences and rights in health-care decision making among the interprofessional team. **7.** Applies principles of teaching and learning and health literacy to design, provide, and evaluate client education. **8.** Participates as a practice specialist in the translation and generation of knowledge. **9.** Provides expert consultation for clients with complex health-care needs using a broad range of scientific and humanistic theories.
Nurse and nursing practice	**1.** Provides leadership to the interprofessional team to incorporate ethical principles in health-care planning and delivery. **2.** Facilitates interprofessional collaboration in the achievement of practice outcomes. **3.** Provides leadership to the interprofessional team in translating knowledge into practice. **4.** Promotes development of competencies of health-care team members related to care delivery and evaluation, professional growth, and effective team functioning. **5.** Promotes improvements in health-care team processes as they impact clinical and fiscal outcomes.

Continued from page 26 Table 1-1

CNS Competencies for the DNP

Sphere of Influence	Description
Organization/system	**1.** Uses organizational and system theory to facilitate and create clinical environments that promote care delivery that is evidence-based, outcome-focused, collaborative, cost-effective, and ethical. **2.** Leads the development, management, and evaluation of information technology to promote safety, quality, and resource management. **3.** Evaluates and improves system-level programs and outcomes based on the analysis of information from relevant sources, such as databases, benchmarks, and epidemiologic data. **4.** Develops and disseminates synthesis and application of evidence to advance client care and health-care delivery. **5.** Designs entrepreneurial programs of care that improve delivery and outcomes of health care. **6.** Secures fiscal and other resources for system-level programs and for evaluation of interventions, products, and services. **7.** Shapes health-care policy at local, regional, and national levels to optimize client health and health-care system delivery. **8.** Demonstrates leadership by advocating for the profession of nursing through participating in professional organizations, boards, and task forces at the institutional, local, state, national, and international levels.

Source: National Association of Clinical Nurse Specialists (2009).

chronic disease, and guide patients to the correct specialist when specialty care is required. In addition, the role of the primary care provider has expanded to include aspects of social medicine, intergenerational care, and culturally competent care. Countries around the world with appropriate primary care resources score well when it comes to health outcomes and cost.

The National Organization of Nurse Practitioner Faculty (2006) prepared the first national list of competencies for advanced practice nurses. The organization has since added additional competencies that apply only to DNP graduates (Table 1-2). These competencies are measurable outcomes for students in DNP programs. They illustrate that advanced practice nurses with a DNP degree have higher levels of knowledge and skill than advanced practice nurses educated at the master's level. In addition, the competencies address the complexity and challenges facing health care in the United States now and in the future and position the DNP to be a leader in health-care discussions

Table 1-2

National Organization of Nurse Practitioner Faculty DNP Competencies (2006)

Competency Area	Description
Independent practice	**1.** Practices independently by assessing, diagnosing, treating, and managing undifferentiated patients. **2.** Assumes full accountability for actions as a licensed independent practitioner.
Scientific foundation	**1.** Critically analyzes data for practice by integrating knowledge from arts and sciences within the context of nursing's philosophical framework and scientific foundation. **2.** Translates research and data to anticipate, predict, and explain variations in practice.
Leadership	**1.** Assumes increasingly complex leadership roles. **2.** Provides leadership to foster interprofessional collaboration. **3.** Demonstrates a leadership style that uses critical and reflective thinking.
Quality	**1.** Uses best available evidence to enhance quality in clinical practice. **2.** Evaluates how organizational, structural, financial, marketing, and policy decisions impact cost, quality, and accessibility of health care. **3.** Demonstrates skills in peer review that promote a culture of excellence.
Practice inquiry	**1.** Applies clinical investigative skills for evaluation of health outcomes at the patient, family, population, clinical unit, systems, and community levels. **2.** Provides leadership in the translation of new knowledge into practice. **3.** Disseminates evidence from inquiry to diverse audiences using multiple methods.
Technology and information literacy	**1.** Demonstrates information literacy in complex decision making. **2.** Translates technical and scientific health information appropriate for user need. **3.** Participates in development of clinical information systems.
Policy	**1.** Analyzes ethical, legal, and social factors in policy development. **2.** Influences health-care policy. **3.** Evaluates impact of globalization on health-care policy development.
Health delivery system	**1.** Applies knowledge of organizational behavior and systems. **2.** Demonstrates skills in negotiating, consensus building, and partnering. **3.** Manages risks to individuals, families, populations, and health-care systems. **4.** Facilitates development of culturally competent health-care systems.
Ethics	**1.** Applies ethically sound solutions to complex issues.

and autonomous providers of health care to communities and individuals. DNP programs prepare nurses who wish to practice in one of the five areas of advanced nursing practice with expanded levels of scientific knowledge placing an increased emphasis of quality, safety, and patient outcomes. Advanced practice nurses who are prepared at the doctoral level are better prepared to address issues in an increasingly complex health-care delivery system and have a title that creates a more level playing field with other health-care disciplines (AACN, 2004). All individuals who wish to become advanced practice nurses should be educated to the level of the DNP. Adding the DNP essentials to the competencies from master's programs completes the educational preparation and prepares advanced practice nurses to provide health care to populations and communities across the United States.

Advancing Your Knowledge

A group of nurse practitioners has decided to open an independent primary care practice. The group has obtained a collaborating physician and has met all of the conditions that are required by the state. One of the advanced practice nurses in the group has completed a post–master's DNP and based on the course work and experiences obtained in her program has many good suggestions concerning how to start the practice, what services to provide, and how to attract a population of patients that the advanced practice nurses can manage competently. The local medical society is disturbed by this practice and has urged its member physicians not to refer to this practice and not to support these advanced practice nurses in any way. The DNP has been able to set up a meeting with the medical society board to discuss the issues regarding primary care practice by advanced practice nurses.

1. If you were the DNP, how would you approach this meeting?
2. How would you present the need for increased access to primary care?
3. How could you convince the medical society board that opening a primary care practice could benefit the physicians in the area?
4. What services could you cite as being offered within the practice that would benefit patients in the community and improve physician job satisfaction?
5. How could a multidisciplinary method of health care in the community benefit patients and families and possibly reduce the overall cost of care? How could systems be designed to assist people who currently lack access to basic care?

Barriers to the DNP

Since the inception of the practice doctorate in nursing, some have felt that dividing doctoral education into practice and research might be detrimental to the study of nursing and the advancement of nursing in society (Fulton & Lyon,

2005; Meleis & Dracup, 2005; Silva & Ludwick, 2006). Others feel that the master's degree is sufficient for advanced practice nursing and that requiring the DNP as entry into advanced practice will reduce the numbers of advance practice nurses and the number of colleges and universities that offer these programs. Physicians are concerned about the DNP and feel that using the term *doctor* to identify doctors of nursing practice in the practice setting will confuse patients as to whether they are seeing a physician or nurse practitioner; they feel that the term should be reserved for medical doctors alone. Still others feel that creating the DNP to increase nurses' ability to influence policy and decision making will prove to be frustrating because Americans are not interested in health-care reform.

As with any change in paradigm, the nursing profession and society struggle with role identity, creating enough workers to meet societal demands, and maintaining quality within the educational structure at each level in the profession. Olshansky (2005) suggested that a DNP is necessary if nurses are "to 'be at the table' in an equal capacity with other healthcare providers and policymakers, providing input into and leadership for major decisions that affect the health and health care of our citizens."

Although many universities have begun DNP programs, smaller liberal arts colleges that have nurse practitioner and other advanced practice master's degrees are unable to open doctoral programs and would be left out of advanced practice education if the entry level is the DNP. Other issues in the area of entry into advanced practice include the extra cost for a DNP versus a master's degree and decreased numbers of advanced practice nurses as need for these providers increases (Vogel, 2007). Silva and Ludwick (2006) voiced a concern about the lack of social policy discussion in the DNP documents from AACN. These authors believe that any improvement in the provision of health care should include social policy, such as access to care, navigation of the health-care system, and creation of systems that provide the right amount of care at the right time for the right price. Other reasons for opposition to the DNP exist, as does uncertainty regarding the DNP's place in the health-care system and how these expert nurses will be used.

Concerns From PhD-Prepared Nurses

PhD-prepared nurses have also voiced some concerns. PhD-prepared nurses worry that the DNP may reduce the number of students in PhD programs. With a shortage of nursing faculty in nursing programs and the increased need for PhD-prepared nurses to conduct research in hospital and larger health-care settings, a reduction in PhD graduates would be detrimental to the discipline. Despite this fear, the number of PhD programs within U.S. universities is increasing, as is enrollment in PhD programs, and the DNP drain on the PhD does not seem to be evident (AACN, 2009). Some DNP graduates may become involved in teaching within nursing programs at colleges and universities and relieve the faculty shortage that currently exists and is forecast to remain problematic for the next several decades (AACN, 2010b). The role of the DNP graduate in nursing education is new, and each college and university must decide whether DNPs will be on a tenure track or a clinical track in their teaching roles. Adding practice specialists to nursing education programs fits within the Boyer (1990) model for scholastic excellence, expanding nursing education from the current classroom-oriented focus to a more practice-focused and experiential model. Including DNP-prepared educators moves nursing education from a pure focus on knowledge generation to a more diverse focus that includes knowledge application or the scholarship of practice (AACN, 2006).

Effect of DNP on Nursing Faculty Shortage

Fulton and Lyons (2005) voiced concern that DNP programs would track students away from PhD programs where research to strengthen the discipline is taught. However, the DNP does not appear to be attracting nurses who might otherwise enroll in PhD programs. The AACN found no evidence that practice doctorates reduce the number of PhD-prepared nurses in schools or those graduating. The AACN found that most individuals who are entering DNP programs would not have contemplated doctoral education in research and education; these nurses are focused on practice to meet their personal educational goals (AACN, 2010b).

The faculty shortage in nursing may be improved by adding the DNP to the terminal degrees offered in nursing. As a practice discipline, nursing requires that faculty, instructors, and teachers be clinically competent experts in the current and latest aspects of nursing practice. Many colleges of nursing are creating clinical faculty to meet the needs of students in this area. DNPs are well situated to become clinical faculty members and to guide students at all educational levels in nursing practice, clinical expertise, and patient safety.

Concerns by Physicians

Physician groups are concerned that there is role confusion between the MD and the DNP. Resolution 211, passed by the AMA House of Delegates (2006), accused nurses and other "nonphysicians" with doctoral degrees of misleading patients to believe that they are receiving care from a physician. The resolution states further that the AMA resolves to work with individual states to identify and prosecute individuals who misrepresent themselves as physicians to their patients. This resolution has resulted in seven states (Georgia, Illinois, Maine, Missouri, Ohio, Oklahoma, and Oregon) having statutes or regulations prohibiting NPs and other doctorate-prepared health professionals from using the title "doctor." There is no documentation that using the title "doctor" is confusing to patients or misrepresents the level of education and ability of the provider. Nevertheless, advanced practice nurses with a doctorate degree are advised to state clearly that they are a doctor of nursing practice to avoid this type of confusion. Although both groups provide health care to different types of patients, there are fundamental differences in the approach to patient care between the DNP and the MD. The DNP is a nurse who provides care using a nursing framework in which person, caring, environment, and health are overriding aspects within the discipline, whereas the MD practices using the framework of medicine, which focuses on physiology, diagnosis, and cure. The DNP is focused on health, health promotion, and disease prevention as well as treatment and cure. The physician is more focused on treating each individual patient for the problems that currently exist, diagnosing those problems, and, if possible, providing curative therapies. One reason that NPs have become a stronger group in the area of primary care is that they are more interested in coordinating care, educating patients, and providing transitional care when patients go from one care setting to another. In a society where chronic diseases are the most common problems in health care, these attributes allow the NP to have improved patient outcomes compared with physicians (Gambino, Planavsky, & Gaudette, 2009).

Title Encroachment

How do advanced practice nurses currently introduce themselves to patients: "Nurse Sally," "Nurse Practitioner Tom," or "CNS Terri"? Patients often call the NP or CNS or other advance practice nurse "doctor" because they are used to calling a health-care provider by that name. Titling is important to demonstrate collegiality and respect for the disciplines providing health care. With the DNP as entry into advanced practice, the term *doctor* should be used to identify individuals who have completed the terminal degree. It is important, however, to identify the fact that the doctorate is in nursing rather than medical practice. For example, the DNP can say, "Hello, I am Dr. Smith, a doctor of nursing practice, and I will be seeing you today."

Other professions such as medicine and dentistry have been identified with the professional doctorate and have used the term *doctor* to identify their level of expertise and knowledge. Other disciplines have moved to the doctorate as the entry into advanced practice or are currently moving their entry into practice to the doctoral level. Pharmacists are now required to hold a doctor of pharmacy (PharmD) degree to practice. Other disciplines moving in the same direction include physical therapy, occupational therapy, optometry, and audiology. Consumers of health-care services will be acquainted with their health-care providers as "doctor" in different specialties rather than simply medical doctors.

As mentioned previously, the AMA has passed resolution 211, which supports a prohibition of the use of the professional title of "doctor" to any group except medical doctors and osteopaths (Klein, 2007). The AMA has drafted a resolution that the term *residency* should be used only by medical doctors and dentists. The resolution reasons that patients would be confused when the title of *resident* is applied to nonphysicians in training. These resolutions are not binding, but, as mentioned, seven states (Georgia, Illinois, Maine, Missouri,

Ohio, Oklahoma, and Oregon) have passed laws supporting resolution 211. Other states have laws that allow nonphysicians to use the term *doctor* as long as they also include their title of licensure. An example of an appropriate use of the title for nonphysicians would be "Dr. Susan Smith, DNP," or "Dr. Sam Smith, NP." DNPs and individuals with a PhD in nursing can and should use their academic degree credentials in all settings. Using the term *doctor* in conjunction with the appropriate licensure title is acceptable in most states.

The AACN has answered this resolution from the AMA by stating that the title of "doctor" is common to many disciplines and is not the domain of any one group of health professionals. Many advanced practice RNs currently hold doctoral degrees and are addressed as "doctors," which is similar to how other expert practitioners in clinical areas are addressed, including clinical psychologists, dentists, and podiatrists. In all likelihood, advanced practice RNs will retain their specialist titles after completing a doctoral program.

In December 2009, a letter to the AMA signed by 26 national professional nursing organizations chastised the AMA for numerous factual misrepresentations and misleading conclusions when discussing advanced nursing practice and the role of advanced practice nurses in health care. These groups stated that the AMA was inappropriate in its attempt to discredit the quality of education, credentialing, and practice of members of another profession. These groups further stated that a thorough and objective review of the comprehensive data would have found overwhelming evidence of the high quality of care provided by NPs. Not only is it inappropriate for one profession to try to regulate another, but also the use of terms such as *limited license provider* is misleading and creates more confusion among patients. Finally, these nursing groups stated that during a time when the United States faces a failing health-care delivery system with so many unmet health-care needs, individual health-care professions should evaluate their own disciplinary knowledge and practice for improvement and ways to enhance, not further restrict, patients' access to health care. Health-care teams that include many different providers are needed to care adequately for patients in the current complex health-care arena. Actions to marginalize other health-care professions do not achieve this objective and ultimately fail the patients who should be the focus of our professional efforts (AACN, 2010a).

Bridging the Gap Between Academic and Clinical Nursing

Meleis and Dracup (2005) believed that adopting the DNP in nursing might further separate practice, theory, and research and diminish the interaction of the three that are needed to establish the evidence for quality and safe health-care practice. These authors believed that the DNP might enlarge the gap that already exists between academic and clinical nursing and increase discord within the profession. Nevertheless, research findings from studies conducted by PhD-prepared nurses currently take at least 10 years to become standard practice, proving that there is an inefficient connection between research and practice. The DNP-prepared nurse may increase efficiency in the transition from research to practice. The DNP-prepared nurse understands the need for evidence-based practice and is a leader and change agent in the field. In the hands of a DNP-prepared nurse, research findings may more easily become integrated into practice, bridging the gap between academic and clinical nursing.

In addition, in some cases, DNP-prepared nurses may work with PhD-prepared nurses to carry out research. The PhD could design the framework and research methodology and apply for funding, and the DNP partner could provide the entrance into the clinical setting and carry out the research and data collection in the practice setting. This collaboration may prove especially important in rural areas that do not have access to an academic medical center where research is the norm. Table 1-3 provides some useful Web sites for students who want to determine how each of the advanced practice roles views the DNP.

Table 1-3

Web Sites of Interest to DNP Students

Web Site Name	URL	Useful Features
National Association of Clinical Nurse Specialists	*http://www.nacns.org/*	Includes information for clinical nurse specialists regarding the association's stance on education, licensure, title, and other topics
American Association of Colleges of Nursing	*http://www.aacn.nche.edu/dnp/index.htm*	Provides information on advance practice issues and regulation of practice
American Association of Nurse Anesthetists	*http://www.aana.com/*	Provides information for nurse anesthetists regarding the association's stance on education, licensure, title, and other topics
American College of Nurse Midwives	*http://www.midwife.org/*	Provides information for nurse midwives regarding the association's stance on education, licensure, title, and other topics
American Nurses Association	*http://www.nursingworld.org/*	Provides access to the *American Journal of Nursing,* responses to legislative and governmental issues. Responds to other professional group resolutions

Continued from page 34 Table 1-3

Web Sites of Interest to DNP Students

Web Site Name	URL	Useful Features
American Organization of Nurse Executives	*http://www.aone.org*	Provides information for nurse executives regarding the association's stance on education, licensure, title, and other topics. Provides access to the AONE journal
Commission on Collegiate Nursing Education	*http://www.aacn.nche.edu/ccne/reports/accprog.asp*	Provides information on nursing program requirements, credentialing, and accreditation
Doctors of Nursing Practice	*http://doctorsofnursingpractice.ning.com/*	Includes blogs and articles; offers the chance to participate in other students' capstone projects; includes a link to the group's annual conference
National Organization of Nurse Practitioner Faculty	*http://www.nursingworld.org/*	Provides information about nurse practitioner programs and innovations in advance practice education and responds to issues in the area of advanced practice nursing.

Program Change From Master's to DNP

Some nurse leaders are concerned that the adoption of the DNP, with its extended length compared with the master's degree, may diminish the number of programs available in the United States. This debate appears to be similar to the debate about whether the RN should be educated at the bachelor of science in nursing level or at the associate's degree level as entry into practice. The main argument on behalf of the associate's degree was that such programs could produce nurses at a faster rate to meet the needs of society. In advanced practice, however, the additional DNP classes, including the residency hours required in DNP programs, are essential to providing advanced practice nurses with the credentials and knowledge they need to perform the duties of the advanced practice nurse successfully. There is a concern among educators that all universities that currently have master's level nursing programs would not be given approval by their administration and academic senates to offer a doctoral degree. Although there are many programs, the need for advanced practice nurses has grown and will continue to grow as health-care policy changes; reducing the number of advanced practice nursing programs could reduce the number of advanced practice nursing graduates for the workforce.

DNP programs are increasing at top speed, and many colleges have complete online programs. There are currently more than 100 DNP programs with more in the planning stages. The AACN (2010b) completed a survey that shows 72% of colleges and universities that offer a master's level advanced practice degree have instituted or are planning to institute a DNP program. Some programs are post–master's degrees where advanced practice nurses are able to go back to school and obtain the DNP. Many programs are moving to the BS-to-DNP format. This format allows nurses who wish to go into advanced practice to start the doctoral program early and usually complete the program in a streamlined manner.

Prescriptive Authority and Oversight

Another barrier to practice is the constraint many states place on prescriptive authority for nurses in advanced practice. Although advanced practice nurses have been shown to provide care that is as safe as that of their physician counterparts, oversight of NP practice by physicians is still required in many states. Advanced practice nurses lose autonomy when physician oversight is required to prescribe medication, to refer a patient for hospice and home health services, or to sign death certificates. In the 12 states where there is no required physician oversight for prescriptive authority, advanced practice nurses are very independent (Plager & Conger, 2007).

Although many states have removed this barrier to practice, many others still require written protocols of oversight for NP practice. In some cases, advanced practice nurses have had to hire physicians simply to sign this protocol, and this places them at an unfair disadvantage in terms of financial viability. The IOM (2001) stated that to improve health-care services in the United States, barriers to practice such as protocols and the need for physician oversight should be eliminated to stimulate interest among advanced practice nurses to fill the vacancies that exist in primary care. The AMA (Sorrell, 2009) is opposed to removing barriers for fear of diminished power in health care.

Credentialing and Reimbursement

Credentialing of advanced practice nurses by insurers to be able to bill and receive payment for services can be a barrier to all advanced practice, including the DNP. In states where physician oversight of NP practice is required, only 17% of managed care organizations credential NPs compared with 78% of managed care organizations in states where oversight is not required (Hanson-Turton, Ritter, Rothman, & Valdez, 2006). Inability to be recognized as an NP in practice on an insurer's provider list or panel is a barrier to autonomous practice. As DNPs explore independent practice through advanced knowledge in health-care policy and leadership, they will advocate for inclusion on insurance panels and be better placed to obtain this recognition and be able to become independent providers.

Along with credentialing NPs on an insurance panel, levels of reimbursement for NPs are a barrier to practice. Medicare regulations reimburse NPs at 85% of the amount allowed for physicians. This practice fails to recognize the true contributions of NPs, especially in the areas of health promotion and disease prevention, which are essential to cost-effective care. In addition, Medicare billing codes are based on medical diagnoses and do not include any codes for nursing care, further tilting practice toward a medical model of care. Not providing codes for nursing care and other nonmedical diagnostic and therapeutic requirements also motivates both physicians and NPs to be less than truthful on billing statements.

Advancing Your Knowledge

S.B. is the chief nursing officer in a hospital. She has completed her DNP and is working with physicians and other staff at the hospital to accept her new title as Dr. S.B.

J.T. is a CNS who works in the same hospital and also has completed her DNP. She would like to use her title as well. Both of these nurses are receiving some "push back" not only from the physicians but also from the hospital administration and the hospital staff who want to know how these two nurses can effectively, and without causing confusion, designate themselves as doctors of nursing practice.

F.M. is an NP who has a DNP and is running for the legislature. Physicians are upset that she uses the title Dr. F.M. in her campaign even though she is careful to note that she is a doctor of nursing practice.

1. How would you go about claiming your education title while not creating an adversarial working relationship with others if you were one of the three nurses in the scenarios?
2. Why is it important for DNP-prepared nurses to use their title in the practice setting?
3. Discuss the other barriers to the DNP and frame a response to each either in agreement or in disagreement, and explain why you feel the way you do.

Advancing Your Knowledge

Two students at the same university (one a PhD student and one a DNP student) decide to do a research project together. The PhD student has ideas about research methodology and a theoretical framework on which to base the research. The DNP student has ideas about what population would be best to study, how to initiate the intervention, and what outcomes to measure. They work together and complete the research project and afterward have a better understanding of each other's strengths.

1. Describe how research-focused PhD nurses and clinically focused DNP nurses could work together to improve the health and well-being of people around the world.

Continued on page 38

Advancing Your Knowledge *Continued from page 37*

2. Why are both types of nursing experts necessary in the discipline? How are they complementary; how are they distinctly different?
3. Interview a PhD student to get his or her answers to these questions and see how these answers might differ from your answers.

Role of DNPs in Practice Today

Nurses who have earned a DNP degree are currently in positions of leadership and have entrepreneurial knowledge that positions them well for the future of health care. DNPs likewise are becoming faculty members at many colleges and universities. In these positions, DNPs are able to prepare expert clinical nurses, participate in research, and guide schools of nursing toward new and innovative knowledge regarding health-care delivery.

DNP graduates are taking their knowledge of finance, health-care policy, and leadership to become entrepreneurs and opening practices as independent practitioners (Zagury, 2009). Although such practices have been successful under the leadership of advanced practice nurses without a doctoral degree, the current group of DNP-educated NPs may be more successful in negotiating with insurers and government agencies for reimbursement; many NPs are finding that physicians are more willing partners or employees in practices led by DNPs. Other entrepreneurial opportunities exist for DNPs in the areas of consulting in health-care informatics and compliance with state and federal legislation. This type of entrepreneurship is essential to the future of the nursing profession.

With advanced education in leadership and a clear understanding of health-care policy, DNPs are also positioned to take on leadership positions within existing institutions such as hospitals, home health agencies, or community agencies. As health care becomes more focused on community health, there will be an ever-expanding role for the DNP in the area of health-care leadership and innovation.

Finally, for DNP graduates who are interested in health policy and legislation of health-care issues, working with legislators to achieve goals in the areas of access to care, payment for health care, and division of health-care resources may be interesting. With advanced knowledge regarding health-care policy, finance, and leadership, a DNP is well situated to be an advisor or run for office.

Things to Consider Before Starting a DNP Program

As noted at the beginning of this chapter, the decision to undertake doctoral education is an important one and should be considered carefully. Whether courses are delivered live or via the Internet, students should expect to spend many hours outside the classroom completing assignments and advancing their knowledge in areas important to them. Doctoral study prepares students to be leaders and experts in an area of nursing. Much of the work assigned or expected will be to prepare for this level of activity, responsibility, and leadership.

Although doctoral work is usually an exciting and positive experience, it requires commitment and time. Doctoral students generally report being pushed and challenged to grow personally and intellectually in positive directions. Creating an intellectual community in doctoral education is essential for high-quality learning. Knowledge-centered, multigenerational communities of scholars foster the development of new ideas and encourage intellectual risk taking. Classmates in nursing doctoral programs are often colleagues and friends long after graduation, and fellow graduates often assist each other in projects, job searches, and furthering career goals.

Online Resources

Many online resources are available to assist in the quest for the DNP degree (Table 1-4). The Web site Doctors of Nursing Practice found at http://www.doctorsofnursingpractice.org/privacypolicy.html was the capstone project of a

Table 1-4

Requirements for Advanced Practice Registered Nurses

The definition of an advanced practice registered nurse (APRN) is a nurse:

1. Who has completed an accredited graduate-level education program preparing him or her for one of the four recognized APRN roles;
2. Who has passed a national certification examination that measures APRN, role, and population-focused competencies and who maintains continued competence as evidenced by recertification in the role and population through the national certification program;
3. Who has acquired advanced clinical knowledge and skills preparing him or her to provide direct care to patients as well as a component of indirect care; however, the defining factor for *all* APRNs is that a significant component of the education and practice focuses on direct care of individuals;
4. Whose practice builds on the competencies of registered nurses (RNs) by demonstrating a greater depth and breadth of knowledge, a greater synthesis of data, increased complexity of skills and interventions, and greater role autonomy;
5. Who is educationally prepared to assume responsibility and accountability for health promotion and/or maintenance as well as the assessment, diagnosis, and management of patient problems, which include the use and prescription of pharmacological and nonpharmacological interventions;
6. Who has clinical experience of sufficient depth and breadth to reflect the intended license; *and*
7. Who has obtained a license to practice as an APRN in one of the four APRN roles: certified registered nurse anesthetist (CRNA), certified nurse midwife (CNM), clinical nurse specialist (CNS), or certified nurse practitioner (CNP).

Source: Consensus Model for APRN Regulation. (2008). Retrieved from http://www.nursingworld.org/EspeciallyForYou/AdvancedPracticeNurses/Scope-of-Practice/Consensus-Model-for-APRN-Regulation.aspx

group of students at University of Tennessee Health Science Center in Memphis. This Web site contains a host of information and areas for discussion. It also provides different blogs for student and graduate DNPs on numerous DNP-related topics, including jobs, legal issues, practice issues, policy and legislative issues, salaries, and other concerns. Special groups can be established to discuss other issues to create a blog by specialty, such as psychiatric or nurse executives, or by area, such as California.

The Doctors of Nursing Practice Web site also provides a list of DNP student capstone projects; this allows students who are contemplating their capstone project to view what others have done and the outcomes of their work. The Web site provides the name of the student, an e-mail link to that person, the title of the capstone project, the school where the student is enrolled in the DNP program, and an abstract of the project. This information can be very helpful to students who are at the beginning of a DNP program and anxious to identify a capstone project for themselves that is meaningful and interesting as part of their professional development.

The Web site allows viewers to see many of the seminal articles regarding the beginnings of the DNP, articles on health policy, and articles on other issues that are important to DNP students and graduates. There are opportunities to be participants in DNP capstone projects through completing surveys or providing information.

Doctors of Nursing Practice, LLC, also hosts a yearly DNP conference where students and graduates are able to present their capstone project findings and other issues regarding advanced practice. The Web site includes a direct link to the conference and allows students to submit abstracts for conference presentations and posters.

Conclusion

Nursing is a late adopter of doctoral education in general and is still evolving as a distinct discipline. Uncovering and delineating the body of knowledge that is uniquely nursing is the role of the PhD-prepared nurse scientist. PhD-prepared nurse scientists identify and comprehend this body of knowledge through research, theory development, and testing. It is often a lengthy process for research findings to become standards of practice in nursing, however, and sometimes these findings are never fully implemented in routine nursing practice. Some nursing leaders have identified the need for a clinical expert in nursing who is educated at the doctoral level. The new degree of DNP allows nurses who are focused on practice rather than on research to obtain a terminal degree in their discipline and continue to maintain their focus.

The DNP degree is still being debated by nurses and individuals in other professions outside nursing. Some of the benefits of the degree are as follows:

- The DNP prepares expert clinicians.
- The DNP compares with other professions where the entrance into advanced practice is at the doctoral level (e.g., MD, PharmD).

- The DNP allows clinically focused experts to obtain a terminal degree in clinical practice rather than research.
- The DNP improves opportunities for doctorate-prepared nurses to participate in health-care decision making.

Concerns about the DNP degree include the following:

- The DNP decreases the number of PhD-prepared nurses to fill academic vacancies.
- The DNP redirects the discipline away from research.
- The DNP creates two divergent terminal degrees in the discipline.

Although the AACN has made a statement that the entry into advanced practice will be the educational level of the DNP, the CCNE has stated that it will continue to accredit master's programs for NPs. While controversy continues over the role of the DNP, many universities are opening DNP programs, and enrollment is increasing. Advanced practice nurses have indicated that they are ready for doctoral education that focuses on clinical issues rather than the traditional doctoral preparation in research.

Nurses entering DNP programs today have the opportunity to establish the DNP as a viable and important part of nursing education. As you learn and grow in the next phase of your professional education, you will assist in the determination of the future of nursing and the future of health care in the United States.

References

Advances for Nurse Practitioners. (2010). DNP survey results: What do NPs really think about the DNP? Retrieved from http://www.doctorsofnursingpractice.org/cmsAdmin/uploads/DNPSurveyResults_001.pdf

American Association of Colleges of Nursing. (2004). Position statement on the practice doctorate in nursing. Retrieved from http://www.aacn.nche.edu/publications/position/DNPpositionstatement.pdf

American Association of Colleges of Nursing. (2006). Essentials of doctoral education for advanced nursing practice. Retrieved from http://www.aacn.nche.edu/publications/position/DNPEssentials.pdf

American Association of Colleges of Nursing. (2009). Amid calls for more highly educated nurses, new AACN data show impressive growth in doctoral nursing programs. Retrieved from http://doctorsofnursingpractice.ning.com/forum/topics/amid-calls-for-more-highly

American Association of Colleges of Nursing. (2010a). AACN joins the nursing community in response to AMA report. Retrieved from http://www.aacn.nche.edu/publications/annual-reports/ar2001.pdf

American Association of Colleges of Nursing. (2010b). Nursing faculty shortage facts sheet. Retrieved from http://www.aacn.nche.edu/Media/Factsheets/facultyshortage.htm

American Association of Medical Colleges. (2000). Population based care: Definitions and application. Retrieved from http://www.thci.org/downloads/topic11_00.pdf

American College of Nurse Practitioners. (2008). National survey of nurse practitioners. Retrieved from http://www.acnpweb.org/i4a/pages/index.cfm?pageid=3353

American Medical Association House of Delegates, Resolution 211 (A-06), June 12, 2006. Retrieved from http://www.acnpweb.org/files/public/ama_resolution_904_11_06.pdf

American Nurses Association. (1993). Nursing facts from the American Nurses Association. In *Primary healthcare: The nursing solution*. New York, NY: ANA.

American Nurses Association. (1976). Congress for Nursing Practice. Definition: Nurse practitioner, nurse clinician, and clinical nurse specialist. Pamphlet: American Nurses Association, Kansas City, MO.

American Nurses Credentialing Center (2010). ANCC DNP survey released. Retrieved from http://nursing.advanceweb.com/Article/ANCC-Issues-Statement-on-Doctor-of-Nursing-Practice.aspx

Association of American Medical Colleges. (2007). MD/PhD dual degree training. Retrieved from https://www.aamc.org/students/considering/exploring_medical/research/61032/mdphd/

Barrett, R. (2010). Strategies for promoting the scientific integrity of nursing research in clinical settings. *Journal for Nurses in Staff Development, 26*(5), 200–205.

Boland, P. (Ed.). (1996). *Redesigning health care delivery* (159–163). Berkeley, CA: Boland Health Care.

Boyer, E. (1990). *Scholarship reconsidered: Priorities for the professoriate*. Princeton, NJ: The Carnegie Foundation for the Advancement of Teaching.

Committee for Monitoring the Nation's Changing Needs for Biomedical, Behavioral, and Clinical Personnel, Board on Higher Education and Workforce, National Research Council. (2005). Monitoring the nation's health education needs. The National Academies Press.

Cordeau, M. (2009). A method for historicizing the lived experience. *Advances in Nursing Science. History of Nursing, 32*(1), 75–90.

Epperly, T. (2010). AAFP statement: 2009 resident match results sharpen focus on family physician shortage, health system reform american association of family physicians. Retrieved from http://www.aafp.org/online/en/home/media/releases/newsreleases-statements-2009/2009-resident-match-results-sharpen-focus-on-family-physician-shortage.html

Fitzpatrick, J., & Wallace, M. (2009). *The doctor of nursing practice and clinical nurse leader: Essentials of program development and implementation for clinical practice.* New York, NY: Springer Publishing.

Flanagan, L. (2000). Nurse practitioners: Growing competition for family physicians. *American Family Practice Journal, 322*, 432–435.

Fletcher, C. E., Baker, S. J., Copeland, L., Reeves, P. J., & Lowery, J. C. (2008). Nurse practitioners' and physicians' views of NPs as providers of primary care to veterans. *Urologic Nursing, 28*(5), 397.

Fulton, J. S., & Lyon, B. L. (2005). The need for some sense making: Doctor of nursing practice. *Online Journal of Issues in Nursing, 10*(3), 4.

Gambino, K., Planavsky, L., & Gaudette, H. (2009). Transition toward nurse practitioner managed clinic. *Journal of Cardiovascular Nursing, 24*(2), 132–139.

Grace, H. K. (1989). Issues in doctoral education in nursing. *Journal of Professional Nursing, 5*(5), 266–270.

Gray, M., Ratliff, C., & Mawyer, R. (2000). A brief history of advanced practice nursing and its implications for WOC advanced practice. *Journal of Wound, Ostomy, and Continence Nurses, 27,* 48–54.

Hanson-Turton, T., Ritter, A., Rothman, N., & Valdez, B. (2006). Insurer policies create barriers to healthcare access and consumer choice. *Nurse Economist, 24*(4), 204–211.

Hooker, R. S., & McCaig, L. (1996). Emergency department uses of physician assistants and nurse practitioners: A national survey. *American Journal of Emergency Medicine, 14,* 245–249.

Horrocks, S., Anderson, E., & Salisbury, C. (2002). Systematic review of whether nurse practitioners working in primary care can provide equivalent care to doctors. *British Medical Journal, 324*(7341), 819–823.

Institute of Medicine. (2001). *Crossing the quality chasm.* Washington, DC: National Academies Press.

Institute of Medicine. (2010). The Future of Nursing: Leading Change, Advancing Health. Retrieved from http://www.iom.edu/Reports/2010/The-Future-of-Nursing-Leading-Change-Advancing-Health.aspx

Institute of Medicine Committee on the Future of Primary Care. (1996). *America's health in a new era.* Washington, DC: National Academy Press.

International Council of Nurses. (2010). Definition of nursing. Retrieved from http://www.icn.ch/about-icn/icn-definition-of-nursing/

Kaplan, L., & Brown, M. A. (2009). Doctor of nursing practice program evaluation and beyond: Capturing the profession's transition to the DNP. *Nursing Education Research, 30*(6), 362–366.

Klein, T. (2007). Are nurses with a doctor of nursing practice degree called doctor? *Medscape Nurses.* Retrieved from http://www.medscape.com/viewarticle/563176

Malinski, V. M. (1986). *Explorations on Martha Rogers' science of unitary human beings.* Norwalk, CT: Appleton-Century-Crofts.

McCaffrey, R., Hayes, R., & Farrell, S. (2011). An educational program to promote positive communication and collaboration between nurses and medical staff. *Journal of Nursing in Staff Development, 27*(3), 121–127.

Meleis, A. F., & Dracup, K. (2005). The case against the DNP: History, timing, substance, and marginalization. *Issues in Nursing, 10*(3).

Miller, S. (1997). Impact of a gerontological nurse practitioner on the nursing home elderly in the acute care setting. *AACN Clinical Issues, 8,* 609–615.

Miller, W. (2010). Qualitative research as evidence: Utility in nursing practice. *Clinical Nurse Specialist 24*(4), 291–297.

Mitchell-Dicenso, A., Guyatt, G., Marrin, M., et al. (1996). A controlled trial of nurse practitioners in neonatal intensive care. *Pediatrics, 98,* 1143–1148.

Morimer, B., & McGann, S. (2005). *New directions in nursing history: International perspectives.* New York, NY: Rutledge Press.

Mundinger, M., Kane, R., Lenz, E., Totten, A., Tsai, W., Cleary, P., Friedewald, W., Siu, A., & Shelanski, M. (2000). Primary care outcomes in patients treated by nurse practitioners or physicians: A randomized trial. *JAMA, 283*(1), 59–68.

Mundinger, M. O., Starck, P., Hathaway, D., Shaver, J., & Woods, N. F. (2009). The ABCs of the doctor of nursing practice: Assessing recourses, building a culture of clinical scholarship and curricular models. *Journal of Professional nursing, 252,* 69–74.

National Association of Clinical Nurse Specialists. (2009). Core practice doctorate clinical nurse specialist (CNS) competencies. Retrieved from http://www.nacns.org/docs/CorePracticeDoctorate.pdf

National Center for Health Statistics, United States. (2007). *Online Health United States*. Hyattsville, MD: Public Health Service; Table 27, p. 133.

National Council of State Boards of Nursing. (1993). Regulation of advanced practice: NCSBN position paper. Retrieved from https://www.ncsbn.org

National Council of State Boards of Nursing (2006). Vision Paper: Future Regulation of Advanced Practice Nursing. Retrieved from https://www.ncsbn.org/Draft_APRN_Vision_Paper.pdf.

National Organization of Nurse Practitioner Faculty National Panel for NP Practice Doctorate Competencies. (2006). Practice doctorate nurse practitioner entry-level competencies. Retrieved from http://www.nonpf.com/displaycommon.cfm?an=1&subarticlenbr=14

Olshansky, E. (2005). Are nurses at the table? A new nursing degree could help. *Journal of Professional Nursing, 20,* 211–212.

Pear, R. (2009). Shortage of doctors an obstacle to Obama's goals. New York Times. April 26, 2009. Retrieved from http://www.nytimes.com/2009/04/27/health/policy/27care.html

Pew Charitable Trust (2003) Health professionals education: A bridge to quality. Board of Health Care Services, National Academies Press.

Plager, K., & Conger, M. (2007). Advanced practice nursing: Constraints to role fulfillment. *The Internet Journal of Advanced Practice. 9*(1) 19-25.

Ponte, P. R., Glazer, G., Dann, E., McCollum, K., Gross, A., Tyreell, R., Washington, D. (2007). The power of professional nursing practice: An essential element of patient and family centered care. *Online Journal of Issues in Nursing, 12*(1) Manuscript 3. http://nursingworld.org/MainMenuCategories/ANAMarketplace/ANAPeriodicals/OJIN.aspx

Reiter, F. (1966). The nurse clinician. *American Journal of Nursing, 66*(2), 274–279.

Rhee, K. J., Dermyer A. L. (1995). Patient satisfaction with a nurse practitioner in a university emergency service. *Annals of Emergency Medicine,* (2), 130–132.

Rhodes, M. (2011). Using effects based reasoning the examine the DNP as the single entry degree for advanced practice nursing. *Online Journal of Issues in Nursing 16*(3).

Rooks, J. (1997). *Midwifery and childbirth in America*. Philadelphia, PA:Temple University Press.

Schlotfeldt, R. M. (1964). Schlotfeldt Papers, Center for the Study of the History of Nursing, School of Nursing, University of Pennsylvania.

Silva, M. C., & Ludwick, R. (2006). Is the doctor of nursing practice ethical? *Online Journal of Issues in Nursing*. Retrieved from http://nursingworld.org/MainMenuCategories/ANAMarketplace/ANAPeriodicals/OJIN.aspx

Sorrell, A. L. (2009). AMA meeting: Physicians supervision of nurses sought in all practice agreements. *American Medical News*. Retrieved from http://www.ama-assn.org/amednews/2009/06/29/prsj0629.htm

Sparacino, P., Cooper, P., & Minirak, P. (2005). *The clinical nurse specialist: Implementation and impact.* Norwalk, CT: Appleton & Lange.

Tobin, G., & Begley, C. (2008). Receiving bad news: A phenomenological exploration of the lived experience of receiving a cancer diagnosis. *Cancer Nursing, 31*(5), E31–E39.

Vogel, W. (2007) Author's reply to readers' responses to "Advanced Practice Nurses Say 'No' to a Mandatory Doctor of Nursing Practice Degree." Retreived from http://www.ncbi.nlm.nih.gov/pmc/articles/PMC1924977/

Walker, G., Gold, C., Jones, L., Bueschal, A., & Hutching, P. (2008). Carnegie Foundation rethinks the future of doctoral education. Retrieved from http://www.carnegiefoundation.org/print/6618

Wall, B., Novak, J., & Wilkerson, S. (2005). The doctor of nursing practice development: Reengineering healthcare. *Journal of Nursing Education, 44*(9), 396–402.

Waxman, K., & Maxworthy, J. (2010). The doctorate of nursing practice degree and the nurse executive: The perfect combination. *Nurse Leader, 8*(2), 31–33.

Winters, J., & Ballou, K. (2003). The idea of nursing science. *Journal of Advanced Nursing, 45*(5), 533–535.

Zagury, C. (2009). Nurse entrepreneur: Expanding career alternatives. *Nursing Spectrum.*

CHAPTER

2

SCIENTIFIC UNDERPINNINGS FOR PRACTICE

Objectives:

By the end of the chapter, students should be able to:

1. Identify and analyze the progression of philosophical and scientific thought through the ages.
2. Analyze the components of nursing theory and the need for theory, theory testing through research, and practice to be closely linked.
3. Relate the foundation of nursing practice to theoretical thought.
4. Describe different types and levels of theories and the application of each.
5. Reconstruct the development of nursing theory from Nightingale through the middle range theory.
6. Formulate the ability to use middle range theory in the practice setting, and test theoretical concepts in these settings.
7. Evaluate the ethical responsibilities of advanced practice nurses.
8. Examine the concept of social justice as it relates to advanced practice nursing.
9. Recognize the ability of organizational systems thinking to benefit health-care settings, and provide examples.
10. Evaluate the essence of nursing practice as it relates to theoretical, practice-based, ethical, and systems thinking.

In the American Association of Colleges of Nursing (AACN) *Essentials of Doctoral Education for Advanced Nursing Practice* (2006), the scientific underpinnings for practice include integrating nursing science with ethics and biophysical, psychosocial, and organizational sciences as the basis for advanced nursing practice and synthesizing nursing theories with theories from other disciplines to develop new approaches to practice. The impetus for this essential material for doctor of nursing practice (DNP) education came from the idea that theory is meant to guide practice. Understanding theory and its application to practice will allow the DNP graduate to lead the nursing profession by formulating and implementing theoretical frameworks for practice.

The DNP is challenged with using scientific knowledge to change practice patterns in ways that benefit patients, families, communities, and the nation. The DNP graduate must be prepared with a solid understanding of science and theory to be successful in implementing domain-specific knowledge and perspectives into practice. The DNP as a practice expert can develop new nursing practice models using a theoretical base that has been tested and shown to be effective. Nursing scientists have expanded nursing knowledge, and the DNP is challenged to take that knowledge and apply it to practice situations. Although an advanced practice nurse educated at the master's level has theoretical knowledge and may use that knowledge in individual practice settings, the DNP has knowledge regarding theory integration into practice on a systems level and is a leader in the effort to infuse theoretical knowledge into nursing practice. In the *Essentials of Doctoral Education for Advanced Nursing Practice,* the AACN (2006) has proposed the following outcomes from DNP education in the area of science and theory.

The DNP program prepares the graduate to:

1. Integrate nursing science with knowledge from ethics and the biophysical, psychosocial, analytical, and organizational sciences as the basis for the highest level of nursing practice.
2. Use science-based theories and concepts to:
   - Determine the nature and significance of health and health-care delivery phenomena;
   - Describe the actions and advanced strategies to enhance, alleviate, and ameliorate health and health care delivery phenomena as appropriate; and
   - Evaluate outcomes.
3. Develop and evaluate new practice approaches based on nursing theories and theories from other disciplines (AACN, 2006, p. 9).

Theoretical ideas within any profession, including nursing, form a paradigm under which the profession operates. A paradigm is a framework containing all of the commonly accepted views about a subject, framing how we view the world and each other. The nursing paradigm provides a structure for what direction research should take and how services and research within the discipline should be performed.

To understand paradigmatic thinking over the course of history and the development of the scientific process, the advancement of theoretical knowledge, and changes in patterns of thought throughout the ages, it is helpful to review the progression of the philosophy of science. Appreciating how scientific thought has developed and the shifts in scientific paradigms over time helps to provide an understanding of the way scientific knowledge has been acquired and how the theories that drive knowledge have developed.

History of the Philosophy of Science

How do we know what we know? How do we understand the world around us? How do we embrace new knowledge when it refutes old knowledge? Before Columbus and Newton, most people in the world were absolutely sure the world was flat. In this paradigm, scientists believed that if you sailed away from Europe you would eventually fall off the edge of the earth into oblivion. Now that we are absolutely certain the world is round, we hold true the paradigm that gravity will not allow us to "fall off" of the world.

One way in which we develop knowledge and come to comprehend the world around us is through scientific inquiry. This inquiry comprises the scientific method for testing facts: theory development and theory testing. When Columbus searched for a new route to the West Indies, he was also testing the theory that the world was flat. When he discovered the New World, he did not sail "over the edge" of the earth, as many people thought he would. Columbus tested a scientific theory and found it to be false. In doing so, another theory was created, one that posited that the world was round. This theory has been tested and has led to other scientific theories, such as Newton's theory of gravity. Theory development and testing occurs in all disciplines, and it is what makes disciplinary knowledge important and useful.

To understand the way knowledge changes, we must first understand the history of knowing and where knowledge comes from. *Science* (from the Latin word *scientia,* meaning "knowledge") is, in its broadest sense, any systematic knowledge base or prescriptive practice that is capable of resulting in a prediction or predictable type of outcome. In this sense, science may refer to a highly skilled technique or practice. The philosophy of science essentially refers to epistemology (the study of the nature of knowledge) as it is applied to science. Table 2-1 lists the different eras of scientific thought that are discussed in this chapter.

Greek Philosophers

The best way to understand current scientific theory is to understand the history of science and knowing through the ages. The history of science in Western civilization began with Socrates (470–399 BCE). Before the time of Socrates and other Greek philosophers, it was believed that the gods regulated all of nature,

Table 2-1

Eras of Scientific Thought

Era	Dates
Greek philosophers	470 BCE–322 BCE
Middle Ages	476 AD–1550 AD
Age of Enlightenment	1550–1800
Industrial Revolution	1750–1850
Modern philosophy	1950–Current

and things happened as the gods willed rather than by any natural force. Socrates changed this way of thinking.

Greek philosophers set up a method of thinking that is still prevalent today. The Greek philosophers spurred humans to feel as though they had some control over the world and could learn about the workings of the natural world in an effort to control it. Many authors concede today that Greek philosophy, with its focus on the role of reason and logic, has shaped all of Western thought since its inception (Lampert, 2010). The following cursory review of ancient Greek philosophers shows how thought shifted in the scientific world from a dependence on the gods who guided all life events to the idea that individuals had the ability to understand, create, and shape their destiny.

Socrates

Socrates used a teaching method for his students that did not present facts but asked questions to spur students to find answers and uncover truth for themselves. The phrase "the unexamined life is not worth living" comes from the philosophy of Socrates because he believed that if you did not examine every aspect of life, you did not grow. Many teachers today use the Socratic method of teaching to enable students to find answers on their own through personal inquiry and self-examination.

Socrates was the first philosopher who believed that right actions were not dictated by the gods but rather came through human intellectual independence and self-examination. He suggested that what is to be considered a good act is not good because gods say it is but because it is useful to humans in our effort to be better, more fulfilled, and happier. Ethics was no longer a matter of surveying the gods or scripture for what was good or bad. Rather, ethics consisted of the findings of what was good and just, as found through self-examination and reflection on fairness in life.

Plato

Plato (437–347 BCE) was Socrates' student and was responsible for putting many of his teacher's thoughts in writing for posterity. Plato believed in justice and equality and allowed both men and women to attend his lectures. A hotbed of philosophical and scientific discussion, Plato's academy would become the center of Greek learning for almost a millennium. It is regarded by many as the first known university in the world.

Plato's philosophy divides reality into two categories: *ontos,* or *ideal* (that which is true, permanent, spiritual, and eternal), and *phenomena* (the manifestations or expressions of the ideal). The ideal is available to us only through thought, whereas phenomena are available to us through our senses. In Plato's paradigm, thought was vastly superior to the senses as a means of getting to the truth.

Plato believed that although the soul would always choose to do good, the challenge lay in the soul recognizing what was good. In Plato's philosophy, someone who does something bad requires education, not punishment; he needs to be shown the correct or better definition of what is good so that the soul can embrace the true good. Plato was interested in justice as an extension of good and evil. To describe the concepts of justice and honor, Plato wrote a dialogue called *The Republic* in which he describes how to live a good and just life.

Aristotle

Aristotle (384–322 BCE) was a student of Plato and is considered the father of modern logic. Aristotle identified two powers in the soul—desire and reason—that appear to be moving forces. Desire may prompt actions in violation of reason, which often leads to wrong actions. By identifying that individuals can act against reason based on their desires, Aristotle was the first to identify the idea of the human ego.

Aristotle believed the world could be understood through detailed observation and cataloging of phenomena. He wrote that scientific knowledge is fundamentally empirical or measurable. Aristotle described his thoughts as teleological, meaning that everything is always changing and moving and has some goal, aim, or purpose. Aristotle was the first to conclude that ethics were required to fit an individual situation rather than one rule for all. Every action needs to be judged according to all relevant circumstances and situations. Equity or fairness is the foundation of modern law and justice.

Advancing Your Knowledge

The discipline of nursing takes a holistic view of humans, health, and the environment. Before the Greek philosophers, people believed that the gods directed all aspects of life and that an individual did not have self-will or the ability to influence his or her own destiny. In the progression of thought from Socrates to Aristotle, there was a philosophical shift to the idea that there were two equal influences on life—*ontos* and *phenomena*. The perception was that thought was more important in understanding humans than what could be gathered through the senses. This perception led to Aristotle's ideas about cause and effect, which are consistent with much of scientific theory today.

1. How have these philosophies shaped the history of humankind? How have they connected us to each other as humans, to the environment in which we live, and to the spiritual aspects of human nature?
2. How might nursing theorists disagree with Plato and point out that the knowledge derived from the senses and the spiritual might greatly influence a person's way of being and interaction with the world?
3. Research and review Aristotle's four causes of matter. How do each of these relate to caring for persons, to nursing practice, or to the idea that persons are more than the sum of their anatomical parts?

Philosophy in the Middle Ages

The era known as the Middle Ages began in Europe during the fifth century, following the fall of the Roman Empire. During the Middle Ages, monastic life was idealized by the Church, and the epitome of life was to withdraw from society and science. The people of the Middle Ages believed that the center of all truth and the understanding of experience was in knowing God's will and that a preoccupation with material phenomena was a serious neglect of one's soul and one's dependence on God. Life and health were not concerns of the church; the church was more focused on the ability to have a good life after death. The church became the center of religious, moral, scientific, and sociological thought. The church taught that rather than a vehicle for truth, the material world was put in place to distract humans from the real task—living the sort of life that would get you into heaven. As knowledge about the natural world grew, the absolute power of the church began to be seen as incomplete. When evidence that many of the church's antiscience teachings were erroneous became stronger, the paradigm of scientific thought shifted again.

Philosophy in the Age of Enlightenment

The paradigm shift that occurred in opposition to the beliefs held during the Middle Ages created an era of rapid growth in the areas of scientific knowledge, art, and culture. This time of knowledge expansion in history has been labeled the Age of Enlightenment and occurred from 1550 to 1800. The Age of Enlightenment was focused on humanism or the idea that human intellect and creativity were trustworthy and human experience was, to some extent, a reliable foundation on which to base thought and knowledge. With its intellectual, scientific, and cultural emphasis, the Age of Enlightenment advocated reason as the primary source for authority. Experience was believed to be the central concern of humans and the best method for increasing knowledge. During this time, scientists and philosophers posited that human sensory experience was a valid way of understanding the universe.

The Enlightenment was less a set of ideas than it was a set of values. At its core was a critical questioning of traditional institutions, customs, and morals. As with all great scientific movements, the Age of Enlightenment pushed the envelope to increase knowledge and provide answers to questions based on scientific theory. During the Age of Enlightenment, scientists began to develop the idea that it was unwise to abandon theories whenever a conflict arose between the theory and observational data. Rather, scientists of the time looked for ways to eliminate the conflict without having to give up their theories. This attitude developed because virtually every theory conflicts with some observational data, and observed data may not be completely understood in and of itself.

Descartes

One of the most influential thinkers during the Age of Enlightenment was René Descartes (1596–1650). Descartes is called the Father of Modern Philosophy because he theorized that no one can know anything as true without a doubt and that all truth was relative to man's understanding. Descartes constructed a system of knowledge discarding perception as unreliable and instead admitting only deduction as a method for determining truth. He theorized that the thinking mind is more real than the body in which it is housed (this is often called the Cartesian mind-body split—where the mind and body operate separately from each other, and the mind is superior to the workings of the body). Descartes' most famous statement is "Cogito ergo sum," which means "I think, therefore I am." The simple meaning of this phrase is that if someone is wondering whether or not he or she exists, that is in and of itself proof that the person does exist.

Pascal, Bacon, Da Vinci, and Copernicus

Two other important philosophers of this period were Blaise Pascal (1623–1662) and Sir Francis Bacon (1561–1626). Pascal invented the microscope and telescope, which advanced the scientific revolution of the time and caused an epistemological transformation. These instruments provided the scientists of the time with empirical and sensory verification of the existence of matter smaller and farther away than could be viewed by the naked eye. Bacon devised the trial and error method of determining facts and defining knowledge. During this time, knowledge was separated into different types of science, such as botany, biology, physiology, and chemistry. Scientists began to view the world as a well-functioning machine.

During this era, Leonardo da Vinci (1452–1519) began experiments in machine design and the makeup of the human body from the inside. He believed that the entire universe could be made visible to human sight, and human vision could encompass the universe in the same way that God can encompass the universe. Nicolaus Copernicus (1473–1543) presented the view that the sun was the center of the universe rather than the earth and fought persecution from the Church for this heretical belief.

Newton

Late in the Age of Enlightenment, another important European scientist, Sir Isaac Newton (1642–1727), developed the theory of the laws of gravity. In his treatise *Principia Mathematica,* Newton theorized that the universe could be explained completely through the use of mathematics. He also stated that the universe operated in a completely rational and predictable way and that one need not appeal to religion or theology to explain any aspect of the physical phenomena of the universe. Newton believed that all the planets and other objects in the universe moved according to a physical attraction between them called gravity. This scientific explanation did not deny the existence of God but rather posited that God did not involve Himself in the day-to-day workings of the universe but was the one who set it in motion.

Philosophy in the Industrial Revolution

Throughout the 19th century, the Industrial Revolution altered the perception of knowledge as new scientific understandings emerged. The sciences were divided into specialties rather than being considered a single entity. Chemistry, astronomy, physical science, and botany were created as areas of specialty within the realm of scientific study and knowledge. The microscope enabled scientists to hypothesize about the role of the cell and germs in health. Discoveries about energy and matter and the first theories about how the human mind and emotions were structured all created a fast-moving and exciting period in science. These advances led humans to believe that by taking things apart to their smallest particle, the unique aspects of each object could be understood.

Post–World War I Modernism

The next paradigm shift occurred after World War I, when the dominant philosophical movement in the English-speaking world was logical positivism. Logical positivism became popular in the mid-20th century and attempted to make philosophy more rigorous by creating criteria for evaluating the truth or falsity of certain philosophical statements. The main criterion for any statement is verifiability, which comes from two different sources: *empirical statements,* which come from science, and *analytical truth,* statements that are true or false by definition. Beginning in Vienna in the 1920s and 1930s, logical positivism heavily influenced philosophy of science, logic, and philosophy of language as well as other areas and remained influential until about the mid-1960s, by which time the movement had become less popular (another paradigm shift). Logical positivists had a high regard for natural sciences, mathematics, and logic. They tried to make philosophy more scientific.

Thomas Kuhn and Paradigms

In this scientific era, Thomas Kuhn (1922–1996) proposed the idea of paradigm and paradigm shift. He described normal scientific paradigms as the day-to-day activities in which scientists engage when their discipline is not undergoing revolutionary change. A paradigm consists of two main components:

- First is a set of fundamental theoretical assumptions that all members of a scientific community accept at a given time, and
- Second is a set of exemplars or particular scientific problems that have been solved by means of the theoretical assumptions and that appear in the textbooks of the discipline in question.

When scientists share a paradigm, they do not just agree on certain scientific propositions; they also agree on how future scientific research in their field should proceed, which problems are the pertinent ones to tackle, what are the appropriate methods for solving those problems, and what an acceptable solution to the problems would be. In short, a paradigm is an entire scientific outlook—a constellation of shared assumptions, beliefs, and values that unite a scientific community and allow normal science to take place.

According to Kuhn, science is primarily a matter of puzzle solving. No matter how successful a paradigm is, it will always encounter certain problems such as phenomena that cannot easily accommodate mismatches between the theory's predictions and the experimental facts. Kuhn suggested that the facts about the world are paradigm-relative and change when paradigms change. Truth then becomes relative to the paradigm.

Advancing Your Knowledge

Throughout history, we have seen that humans continue to strive for understanding and control over life and the environment in which they live. As more was learned about the workings of the universe and the human body, humans began to believe that they could understand and manipulate everything in creation and bend it to their will. In more recent times, theories concerning randomness and the inability to come to know a person fully outside of his or her experiences and beliefs have blossomed. As nursing strives to increase health and well-being among the population, theories for practice have evolved that require a larger view of human thought. Newman's theory of "health as expanding consciousness," Roger's theory of the "science of unitary human beings," and Parse's theory of "human becoming" all rely on a connection between subtle energies in the environment and the human mind as part of the health-care process.

1. Is it easier to create scientific thought that considers only what we can see and measure than to consider the science of what we cannot see or measure but what we sense or what is within the human soul or the universal consciousness?
2. Can you describe an experience in practice where you simply knew something to be true in patient care without being able to measure it or quantify a change? How did this experience or several experiences change your practice?

Modern Philosophical Theories From Outside Nursing

The previous discussion of the development of theoretical and scientific thought in the Western world highlighted different ideas about truth, realism, and the scientific process. In the modern world, paradigms in science shift more quickly as our ability to understand and explain phenomena expands exponentially, and we have come to understand that the more we know, the more we don't know. A brief discussion follows of theories from outside of nursing—but relevant to nursing—in the areas of science, human science, and social thought. These theories are summarized in Table 2-2.

Logical Positivism

New schools of philosophy today continue to theorize about and create meaning for science and society. However, the logical positivist paradigm continues to be popular as it theorizes that all things can be dissected into pieces and that

Table 2-2

Theories From Outside of Nursing That Are Integral to Nursing

Theory	Summary of Thought
Logical positivism	Form of empiricism that bases all knowledge on perceptual experience rather than using intuition or revelation
Existentialism	Meaning is derived from experience or the experience of existence; assumes that people are entirely free and responsible for what they make of themselves
Critical social theory	Theory that can provide the analytical and ethical foundation needed to uncover the structure of underlying social practices and reveal the possible distortion of social life embodied in them
Phenomenology	Theory based on the study of human experience in which considerations of objective reality are not taken into account

understanding each piece provides an understanding of the whole. This theory creates the idea that humans can understand and control the world through scientific thought and technology. Logical positivism is used to understand the workings of the human body, the structures of societies, and many other areas of human life. Although other theories posit that the whole is more than the sum of its parts, many scientists persist in using logical positivism to answer the questions of how the natural world works.

Existentialism

As paradigms expanded throughout the 20th century, another school of theoretical and scientific thought was emerging. First discussed in the early 1900s, existentialism hypothesized that individuals create the meaning and essence of their lives as opposed to it being created for them by deities or authorities or defined for them by philosophical or theological doctrines. Some of the most famous thinkers and philosophers of the existential movement were Swedish philosopher Søren Kierkegaard, Russian writer Fyodor Dostoyevsky, French writer Jean-Paul Sartre, and German philosophy professor Martin Heidegger.

Existentialist thinkers focused on the question of concrete human existence and the conditions of this existence rather than describing human essence, stressing that the human essence is determined through the choices one makes in life. For existentialists, humans exist in a state of distance from the world even though they are in the midst of it. A central proposition of existentialism is that existence and experience create the meaning of life. This means that the actual life of the individual is what constitutes what could be called his or her "essence," or the real meaning of life, instead of there being a predetermined essence that defines what it is to be a human. One goal of existential research is to "come to know" the experience of the other to begin to define the person's essence. Existential philosophers are interested in life experiences. Past experiences in a person's life are an important aspect of existential philosophy because past life experiences contribute to creating the person's essence in the present; however, to say that one is only one's past would be to ignore a large part of reality, which is the present and future. The core of existential learning is that a person must "find" himself or herself and live in accordance with that self.

Pierre Teilhard de Chardin (1881–1955) was a philosopher who took existential philosophy to a new level, defining the Earth as the core to human existence. De Chardin believed that all persons are connected through an evolutionary trend toward higher levels of consciousness. To express the idea of experience as the essence of humanity, de Chardin stated, "We are not human beings having a spiritual experience, we are spiritual beings having a human experience" (2003, p. 154). In de Chardin's philosophy, the heart and emotions were the most important aspects of humanity and a relationship to God. To this end, de Chardin said, "Someday, after mastering the winds, the waves, the tides, and gravity, we shall harness for God the energies of love, and then, for a second time in the history of the world, man will have discovered fire" (2003, p. 178). Although de Chardin's philosophical beliefs were not embraced by the church, he influenced many nursing theories, most notably Margaret Newman's nursing theory of health as expanding consciousness, which is discussed later in this chapter.

Advancing Your Knowledge

A nursing unit in a hospital is meeting to discuss the theoretical framework from which it practices. The clinical nurse specialist who works with these nurses and has completed her DNP is leading the discussion. There are many different ideas about practicing from a theoretical perspective. The group begins by discussing the difference between nursing science and theory and that of medicine. Many of the nurses believe that the paradigm of logical positivism, although incomplete, has significant meaning for nursing and patient care. Other nurses in the group believe that a more existential approach to nursing would better describe their practice and the way they view patient care.

1. How would you describe your nursing practice in terms of a theoretical focus on either logical positivism or existentialism? If both aspects are present, how can you describe both theoretical perspectives as working together in the practice setting?
2. How do you define the link between humans, environment, and health? What values and assumptions do these definitions hold, and how does your nursing practice reflect your ideas in this area?

Critical Social Theory

In the humanities and social sciences, critical theory is the examination and critique of the thoughts of society and literature that defines and presents societal realities. Originally presented as part of Marxist philosophy, the purpose of critical theory was to understand and overcome societal structures that dominated and oppressed society. More modern versions of critical theory attempt to draw from knowledge across social science and humanities disciplines to present a snapshot of what is happening in societies around the world at any given moment. Critical social theory is social theory oriented toward critiquing society as a whole; this contrasts with traditional theory, which is oriented only to understanding or explaining society. Modern critical theory explains "what is" without trying to explain "how it came to be." This has become one of the drawbacks of critical social theory because it criticizes and critiques societal norms, groups, and issues without offering alternatives that might improve society and increase social justice.

The first to define and use critical social theory was Max Horkheimer in 1937. Core concepts of critical social theory include the idea that the understanding of any society should consider the historical aspects of that society or how it came to be configured at a specific point in time. This theoretical approach held that critical social theory should improve our understanding of society by integrating all the major social sciences, including economics, sociology, history, political science, anthropology, and psychology. The theory remains prevalent today among social scientists and certain feminist theorists.

Phenomenology

Phenomenology is the study of *phenomena* (from Greek, meaning "that which appears") and how these phenomena appear to each human being from a first-person perspective. In modern times, it usually refers to the philosophy developed by Edmund Husserl, which is primarily concerned with consciousness and its structures or the ways in which phenomena appear to us. Phenomenology takes the intuitive sense of conscious experience and attempts to extract and describe fundamental essence. Because consciousness is supposed to be that which shows itself to everyone, phenomenology then becomes the study of consciousness.

An important element of phenomenology described by Husserl was the idea of intentionality (often described as "aboutness"), or the notion that consciousness always is consciousness *of* something. In other words, when a reference is made to a thing's *essence* or *idea,* or when one details the constitution of an identical coherent thing by describing what one "really" sees as being only these sides and aspects or these surfaces, it does not mean that the thing is only and exclusively what is described. For example, when we ask "what is a nurse," the answer depends on the person being asked. If the person is not a nurse, the answer might be very different than if a nurse were answering. To answer the question, "what is a nurse," we not only need to look at job descriptions, educational levels, and legal descriptions, but we also must ask both nurses and non-nurses "what is the experience of being a nurse or what is the experience of being cared for by a nurse," to understand fully what a nurse is. The ultimate goal of phenomenology is to understand *how* these different aspects are constituted into the actual thing as experienced by the person experiencing it.

Phenomenology has had a large theoretical impact on nursing. As part of the nature of nursing's paradigm of caring and defining each person as a unique individual, understanding the essence of experience explicates and illuminates the human condition. Through this understanding, nursing theorists and scientists are able to provide ideas about the human experience that lead to testable theoretical knowledge.

Critical Thinking Questions

Although the above-described theories are not "nursing" theories, they have a bearing on human science and the nursing paradigm of health, environment, person, and health.

1. How could each of these theories be used in nursing practice? How are these ideas from outside nursing practical in practice situations?
2. Evaluate the connection between philosophies through the ages and philosophies in nursing. Where has nursing come from, and how were its philosophical ideas developed?
3. When Florence Nightingale proposed that the role of nursing was to put patients in the right environment for nature to work on them for healing, what philosophical principles was she using?

Nursing Science, Theory, and Theory Testing: An Overview

To be designated a theory, a set of propositions and concepts must relate to a group of generalizations that provide a framework for ordering phenomena. For example, how do the concepts of early ambulation, deep breathing, and pain management lead to a theoretical framework for ways in which to care for postoperative patients? A theory needs to be complex enough to include multiple variables yet must be able to be understood and tested. An important aspect of nursing theory is that it must be useful in clinical nursing practice, and it must not be focused outside the discipline's paradigm. Finally, theory must be able to create order out of the complexity of concepts identified (Meleis, 2007).

How does nursing fit into a progression of philosophical thought and theory development? Nursing became a discipline with a body of knowledge later than many other professions, after Florence Nightingale (1820–1910) became interested in educating nurses and gathering data about nursing practice to develop a body of knowledge in the discipline. Nightingale was a pioneer in the development of theoretical ideas about nursing care. Nightingale was well read in the area of germ theories postulated by Louis Pasteur and Robert Koch in the 1860s, and her ideas stemmed largely from an understanding of the causes of disease (UNESCO, 1998). The idea of germs as the underlying cause of disease led to Nightingale's emphasis on hygiene for soldiers during the Crimean War

(1854–1856). She placed great importance on the nurse's role in management of the environment, including patient comfort, noise levels, water quality, fresh air, good nutrition, and sunlight. Consequently, she theorized that nurses, with their responsibility for maintaining hygiene, had a unique opportunity to discover the nature of God by learning his "laws of health" (Nightingale, 1969).

Nightingale was also interested in statistics and believed that using statistics to formulate outcomes was the best way to show the benefits of her ideas of creating healing environments. She used statistical information to develop and test theories that brought about fundamental changes in health care during and after the Crimean War. She statistically documented the devastation caused by poor sanitation in health-care facilities and the increased numbers of lives saved when changes were made. In 1859, through the Nightingale Fund, Nightingale began negotiations to establish a training school at St. Thomas' Hospital in London. The fact that she insisted on each probationer having her own private room in the Nightingale Home for study and reflection shows that she was not concerned merely with the practical side of nursing but also with each student nurse coming to understand the human condition.

Since Nightingale's time, there have been some shifts in the nursing paradigm. Meleis (2007) stated that nursing has moved away from an emphasis on natural science toward a paradigm and definition within the realm of human science. Meleis listed eight properties that define nursing as a human science, as follows:

- A human science focuses on humans as wholes and advocates understanding the particulars in terms of the whole (Mariano, 2001; Owen & Holmes, 1993).
- A human science has at its core an understanding of experiences as lived by its members.
- A human science does not separate the art and the science of nursing, which are the cornerstones of building nursing knowledge (Mitchell & Cody, 2002).
- A human science deals with meanings as seen and perceived by its members. Meanings attached to responses, symbols, events, and situations are included and guide practice of the science.
- To be able to understand meanings and experiences, a scientist needs to enter into meaningful dialogue with participants. Interactions are the prime source of meanings and perceptions of experiences, and participants in the activities of knowledge development are individuals who are developing and structuring knowledge and individuals about whom knowledge is developed. All participants have to verify the meanings of these experiences.
- "The scope for generalization for a human science is limited" (McWhinney, 1989, p. 298). A generalization has to be made within a context; generalization may be presented in terms of patterns.

- Responses and experiences form patterns. Patterns provide meaningful information about participants (Newman, 2002).
- Some conditions, situations, behaviors, and events are reducible for purposes of description (Meleis, 2007, p. 456).

Knowing is not static within any discipline, and patterns of knowing change as a reflection of the progress made. Nursing first used the received view of knowing, which comes from experience, embraces a positivistic view, and is resistant to change. Within a received view of knowing, there is thinking and doing that is steeped in tradition, and this view is still the most often used way of knowing identified by bedside nurses. The perceived view of knowing in nursing comes from the identification of trends and patterns. This way of knowing uses both phenomenological and philosophical methods of theory development. Coming to know in an intuitive way is an example of the perceived view of knowing.

The interpreted view of knowing is an extension of the perceived view, where the nurse is able to come to know the other through observing human behaviors and expressing an interpreted meaning that illuminates any given situation. Interpretive knowing provides full understanding of a situation and allows the nurse to respond in ways that are sensitive and appropriate. Nursing theories of all levels come from these ways of knowing. Newer nursing theorists talk about pattern recognition, using intuition and reflection to understand and come to know the patient. These theories look at the patient involvement in decision making as essential to demonstrate the effectiveness of the role. These theories look at all aspects of the human condition, such as gender, race, and culture, as essential to the uniqueness of each individual and essential as part of coming to know the other. This type of knowing challenges existing structures within the framework of theoretical knowledge to create new and limitless opportunities for nurses to change structures and organizations to meet the health and wellness needs of persons.

Fawcett (1984) proposed a metaparadigm, or an overarching paradigm, for nursing that consisted of four concepts: human, environment, health, and caring (caring and nursing are synonymous as a concept). This meta-paradigm has been widely accepted and formalized as the basis for the nursing profession. It allows nurses to understand the basic concepts of concern for the discipline and creates a framework for theory development and testing. Although nursing theory has developed and been used to build a distinct body of disciplinary knowledge, there remains a disconnection between nursing theory, theory testing or research, and nursing practice. Nursing theorists work in a philosophical realm, whereas nurses in practice focus on the "doing" of nursing. Many practice-focused nurses do not believe that theories are meaningful or helpful in everyday practice (Mars & Lowry, 2006).

The lack of connection between theory, theory testing, and practice has created a gap in nursing science (Meleis, 2007). Building bridges between knowing and doing enables the complexities of nursing to be discovered, tested, and understood better. In many health-care settings, the predominant link between professionals and patients is the medical model. This predominance of the medical model prevents nursing work from being recognized and valued because without theory, measurement is difficult, and without measurement, value is often disregarded. If Nightingale had been unable to present statistical data on the benefits of sanitation, it is unlikely that changes to the system would have been made. If nurses cannot demonstrate the value of caring through theory generation and testing, it is unlikely that changes in the level of autonomy and appreciation of nursing work will occur.

Because the primary mission of nursing is related to practice, it is important to understand how humans respond to health and illness to promote positive health behaviors and empower individuals to use the resources available to meet their needs in the areas of health and well-being. To accomplish this mission, nurses need to understand and use theoretical knowledge regarding issues such as pain, sorrow, comfort, confusion, and uncertainty (Mapanga & Mapanga, 2003). Instead of looking at nursing theory as a concept outside of routine practice, nurses must use theoretical knowledge to enhance practice and create interventions and help patients in ways that have been shown to be successful through theory testing. Using a theoretical framework for practice allows an advanced practice nurse to grasp the meaning of patient behaviors and connect with the patient in a meaningful way.

The use of middle range nursing theory is expanding quickly in an attempt to link practice and theory so that nursing knowledge can expand. Middle range theory is defined as abstract, with a limited scope and a limited number of variables. For example, Kolcaba's middle range theory of comfort (Kolcaba, 1994) deals with only that one construct and has a much smaller range of ideas than a grand theory. Middle range theories have a stronger relationship with research and practice because they are limited in scope to a definable construct or concept that has been well defined.

One of the fastest growing areas of middle range theory concerns the safety and welfare of patients. Middle range theories that can be tested and provide measurable outcomes to improve patient safety have already shown and will continue to demonstrate the value of nursing and nursing care (Meleis, 2007). Aiken, Clarke, Cheung, Sloane, and Silber (2003) tested a theory about the correlation between the level of education of bedside nurses and the safety and mortality of surgical patients. Testing of that theory confirmed that nurses educated at the baccalaureate level were able to identify better opportunities to rescue patients before the patients became critically ill or died than nurses educated at the associate degree level. The development and testing of this theory has led to many changes in nursing, including the American Nurses Credentialing Center Magnet Recognition Program requirement for an adequate percentage of all bedside nurses in a hospital to be prepared at the BSN level.

Theory development and testing is equally important in advanced practice nursing, which continues to be linked to the medical model rather than focusing on nursing knowledge. The term often used for an advanced practice nurse is *physician extender*, which seems to imply that nursing work has been abandoned by the advanced practice nurse, and the advanced practice nurse simply is an extension of the physician. This oversimplified and pejorative term is not used by people who understand the value of nursing care and nursing knowledge in the advanced practice arena. Nursing theorists and nurses in practice must value the contributions of one another and work together to enable nursing knowledge and the discipline of nursing to grow in a scientific and meaningful way to identify clearly the value of nursing in society.

Advancing Your Knowledge

T.T., a nurse practitioner, is working with a group of seven diabetic patients who seem unable to comply with their medical treatment plans. The physician in this practice has labeled these patients as "noncompliant" and has given up on them ever being successful in achieving and maintaining normal levels of blood sugar. In an attempt to discover the underlying problems faced by these patients, the nurse sets up a group treatment plan. T.T. uses the adaptation theory created by Sister Colista Roy to frame the plan. The underlying assumption in this theory is that patients' values and opinions are to be considered and respected and that a person's perceptions and experiences are the starting point of nursing (Whittemore & Roy, 2002). This theory proposes in part that people are adaptive systems and that within these adaptive systems are "cognator" subsystems, which provide meaning to behaviors.

T.T. uses the theoretical framework of adaptive systems to achieve the outcome as she attempts to help these patients overcome the stresses in their ability to cope with their disease process and maintain health and well-being. Adapting to the stress of disease may increase compliance with the treatment plan, and so T.T. designs interventions that include listening and creating trust between the patient, family, and nurse. She creates an atmosphere where no judgments are made on patient ideas, abilities, and thoughts. She finds common themes among the seven patients and develops interventions that promote adaptation to the notion of a chronic illness and the need for change in behaviors; she assists patients to compensate for behaviors that lead to compromised adaptation. Specifically, she discusses the psychological aspects of a disease that is long-term and chronic and allows patients to share feelings of hopelessness and discouragement that they will always have to take medications and watch their diet. She educates patients carefully on the outcomes of uncontrolled diabetes and helps them to understand the benefits of consistent monitoring, medication, and diet control to their long-term health. She allows for discussion with family members to determine the importance of keeping their loved one healthy and an active member within the family so that the family members support the patients in their treatment efforts. Finally, T.T. works with all seven

Continued on page 64

Advancing Your Knowledge *Continued from page 63*

patients to help them obtain the medications they need with cost assistance from the drug companies. Using the theoretical framework of Roy's adaptation model as a guide for practice, T.T. is able to have confidence in her interventions and is able to confirm the ability of the model to have an effect on patient outcomes as she works with the patients in her group.

1. How does theoretically based practice become real in the hectic and frenetic world of nursing care and health care today?
2. How could the link between theory and practice be strengthened?
3. How could theoretical testing be used by practicing nurses to create and improve practice models?

Nursing Theory for Advanced Practice

The objective of any theory is to explain observable phenomena, help the professional nurse "make sense" of what is happening, and provide a framework for how to care for patients in any situation. Theory can be explanatory (explain what is happening) or predictive (predict or anticipate what will happen). Theory testing provides the linkage between the theory and the real world of practice. As theory is tested, it provides evidence that guides practices and provides evidence for the most effective ways to care for patients, families, and society as a whole. Theory, through its clarification of relationships between evidence and practice, guides the nursing processes of assessment, diagnosis, and intervention. Nursing theorists have a different view of the work of nursing and have created nursing theories regarding the role of nursing and philosophical concepts of persons, caring, and the environment of care.

Theory can also be defined as a collection of concepts, including abstractions of observable phenomena expressed as quantifiable properties. Theory attempts to express relationships and aspects of the natural world and can be an organized system of accepted knowledge that applies in a variety of beliefs that are meant to guide behavior. Meleis (2007) stated that another use of nursing theory is to provide a common language to improve communication between nurses. For example, when nurses discuss a patient's use of *self-care* or *self-efficacy,* having an understanding of these concepts from a theoretical perspective makes communication more meaningful. Nursing theories are important to advanced practice nurses in creating visions of population-based care that produce effective responses to the complex challenges facing individuals, the health-care industry, and the world today.

Many nursing scholars have stated that nursing theory guides practice and provides a basic understanding about the role of nursing in society (Meleis, 2007). The gap between nursing theory, research, and practice exists because a gap exists in knowledge and leadership between nurses who develop theory and test it using research and nurses who are in practice. As experts in clinical practice with a higher level of knowledge regarding the value of nursing theory and using nursing theory in practice, the DNP is well positioned to act as a conduit through which theoretical ideas and research findings can be used to develop and implement evidence-based practice, clinical guidelines, and protocols for practice. Connecting theoretical ideas to practice situations is challenging in part because nurses steeped in practice are not as concerned with theory and theoretical propositions as they are with established guidelines for practice. In order for nursing to expand its body of knowledge and position itself as a profession in society, theory and theory testing are essential.

Because advanced practice nursing as a practice discipline is aimed at facilitating health promotion, disease prevention, and improved well-being for individuals, families, and communities, the opportunities for nurses to take on new levels of responsibility and gain value within society in practice situations are unprecedented. As the number of people who require health care and health knowledge increases and the idea of a finite health-care system that is unable to expand to meet societal needs completely is accepted, nurses will be asked to develop roles based on practice theory. Issues such as the aging population, ethnic diversity, health disparities, increased burden of chronic disease, genetic advances that have outstripped ethical consideration, and protection of the environment are challenges and opportunities for practicing nurses to respond and participate in change initiatives and the development of solutions. However, to avoid missteps and disappointing outcomes, these changes must be based on theory and the scientific testing of theory. Meleis (2007) stated that being a nursing scholar means having the ability to ask questions and make decisions based on disciplinary theoretical knowledge. Meleis also stated that after questions have been asked or decisions made, outcomes of these questions and decisions should be measured and communicated to others in the discipline to strengthen disciplinary knowledge and theory development. As nursing scholars, DNPs are the right professionals to use theoretical ideas and research findings to develop and implement evidence-based practice, clinical guidelines, and protocols for practice.

Advancing Your Knowledge

Five clinical nurse specialists from five cooperating hospitals meet regularly to discuss issues regarding patient care, nursing, and administrative policy. Each nurse has identified similar issues within the areas discussed, and the nurses hope to work together to facilitate improvements in patient care and outcomes and improvements in nursing job satisfaction, performance, and retention. After several meetings it is decided that the group should focus on a theoretical model that could be used to guide the changes group members suggest to meet their goals. The group members believe that by using a theoretical framework to identify and make changes to improve care and nursing satisfaction, the

Continued on page 66

Advancing Your Knowledge *Continued from page 65*

group will be better able to measure outcomes and create models for practice that will continue to grow.

1. Why do you think it would be useful for this group to decide on a theoretical framework as a fundamental foundation for their plans to improve care?
2. Can theory be used to change nursing behaviors and improve nursing satisfaction?
3. How would the theoretical concepts in the theories chosen lead to outcome measures and the creation of new models of practice and care in the hospitals where the clinical nurse specialists work?
4. Could the benefits from the work they are doing be used in other settings or hospitals? How could this be accomplished?

Theory in Nursing

Nursing theories assist in the understanding of phenomena and ultimately guide nursing practice (Ryan, 2009). DNPs can lead the way in using and testing theory and developing theory-guided practice as a standard for quality and professionalism. An essential characteristic of advanced practice nursing should be the use and testing of theory in practice (Falk-Rafael, 2005). As experts in clinical practice, the DNPs should focus on individual interventions and population-based and system changes to improve health and well-being. As leaders in health care practice, it is essential for DNP graduates with their advanced knowledge to use theoretical models with proven success as the initial and ongoing framework for designing interventions and to test the models for their effectiveness.

Basic knowledge of diagnosis, treatment, and pharmacology by advanced practice nurses has important implications for patients, and so does the development of theories of human health. Approaching care using a theoretical framework directed toward best-practice interventions to improve patient outcomes and create positive changes in health behaviors would enhance the management of complex clinical situations by providing holistic and comprehensive care. Without using theory as a guide for practice and intervention development, improvements in health behaviors and beliefs would be slow to develop, and many duplicate efforts to solve the same problems might slow the progress of nursing knowledge. This section provides an overview of the levels and types of conceptual and theoretical knowledge involved in nursing science. Table 2-3 summarizes levels of theory development.

Metatheory

At the highest level is the nursing metatheory, which is a conceptual definition of the phenomena of the discipline of nursing. Metatheoretical knowledge helps define the profession of nursing and nursing practice and provides fundamental perspectives for the discipline. Metatheories classify the values and beliefs of the

Table 2-3

Levels of Theory Development

Level of Theory Development	Definition
Metatheory	Metatheory is the highest level of theory. A nursing metatheory presents the most global perspective of the nursing discipline.
Conceptual models	Conceptual models represent how nursing thinks about a problem and define why complex concepts work the way they do. Models may draw on numerous theories to help understand a particular problem in a certain setting or context. A conceptual model "gives direction to the search for relevant questions about the phenomena of central interest to a discipline and suggests solutions to practical problems" (Fawcett, 2000).
Grand theory	Grand theory emphasizes a global viewpoint with a broad perspective of nursing. It is broad in scope and less abstract. Grand theory provides the foundation for middle range theory.
Middle range theory	Middle range theories include a set of related ideas that are focused on only one or two aspects of the nursing role (Smith & Liehr, 2008).
Microtheory	Microtheory uses specific nursing roles and tasks and provides direction on the best way in which to undertake these roles and tasks. Microtheory is specific and used primarily at the bedside.

profession and help describe what we know and how we know what we know in relation to concepts within the discipline. One example of a metatheory is the ways of knowing established by Carper (1978), who defined the basic structure of inquiry for nursing as "coming to know" in personal knowing, empirical knowing, esthetic knowing, and ethical knowing. The basic tenets of Carper's metatheory include the following:

- *Empirical knowing* comes from what can be felt, seen, and heard and is based on measurement of quantitative knowledge.
- *Ethical knowing* involves making judgments about what ought to be done, what is good, what is right, and what is responsible. Ethical knowing includes loyalty, advocacy, and social justice.
- *Personal knowing* concerns the inner experience of using personal experience to understand and help others. Awareness of self, being present in the moment, and being aware of the context of interaction create meaningful, shared human experience.
- *Esthetic knowing* involves understanding the meaning of a situation and the use of creative resources to transform experiences that might otherwise be impossible.

Because nursing metatheory creates a global model and perspective of the discipline, it is useful to understand these theories when one is attempting to define the profession of nursing in all of its aspects. In one application of the metatheory of Carper's ways of knowing, nurses found that knowledge within each of the four ways of knowing must be obtained and examined to avoid distortion in understanding and a narrow interpretation of data received (Lee, 2002). If knowing is used in isolation, inappropriate patterns of perception are formed, and the ability to know and understand the whole patient is lost. This metatheory establishes a fundamental philosophical perspective for nursing and clarifies the relationship between nursing science and nursing practice.

Metatheory is where nursing is defined as a discipline and the appropriate boundaries of disciplinary thought and ideas are expressed. Theory at this level is abstract and embraces possibilities and realities within nursing. At the practice level, metatheory tends to provide ways to view the profession as a whole and determine how to incorporate theoretical and scientific ideas in a general way. Metatheory provides definitions and dialogue regarding the underpinnings of nursing as a science and the progression of scientific thought in the discipline. Table 2-4 provides examples of meta-theory in nursing.

Advancing Your Knowledge

K.P. is a nurse practitioner who works with a physician in a family primary care practice. When providing care to elderly patients, K.P. asks them about their home environment. She includes questions about the physical environment (e.g., whether they have safety bars in the bathroom, stairs to climb), the social environment (e.g., is the patient engaged in social interactions; what does the patient enjoy doing; does the patient feel safe in his or her environment), and family environment (e.g., who do they call for help when they need it). K.P. is taking course work to obtain a DNP degree and wants to formalize some of these questions and determine how useful they are to patients not only in her practice but also in others. The physician with whom K.P. works tells her that he thinks this is not a good idea. Her questions are not medical; they are for a social worker to ask. He tells her that medicine and social work are separate and should not be mixed together in the office visit.

1. What metatheory could K.P. use to defend her idea for her capstone project?
2. How does the DNP "fit" into the metatheory or global understanding of nursing?
3. Why is it important for K.P. to address these issues during the primary care visit?

Conceptual Models

The second level of theory is a conceptual model, which creates ways to define nursing concepts and designs propositional statements that address the concepts. Propositional statements are made within the framework of the conceptual

Table 2-4

Examples of Metatheories in Nursing

Metatheory	Definition
Metaparadigm of nursing: A metaparadigm is a concept that is extremely general, one that serves to define an entire world of thought (Jacqueline Fawcett, 1984)	This metaparadigm or metatheory supports the idea that there are four aspects that come into consideration in the discipline of nursing: Person (this includes families and social groups; each person is unique and autonomous and should be treated as such) Health (a negotiable and contextual abstract concept in which each person defines his or her own health; in this way, a person with cancer could define himself or herself as in good health rather than as a person with a disease and in poor health) Environment (the environment in which a person lives, works, and interacts with others; understanding environment is crucial to understanding person and health) Nursing (the desire of nurses to ease suffering; in recent years, this fourth aspect has often been renamed "caring")
Humanistic nursing theory (Paterson & Zderad, 2008)	This metatheory was developed through the study of the existence and reality of nursing. Humanistic nursing theory is based on the idea that nursing is an intersubjective transactional relationship between a nurse and a patient who are human beings existing in the world
Integral philosophy and definition of nursing—metatheory of nursing (Olga Jarrin, 2007)	The central focus of the profession of nursing is using the art and science of caring to improve the health of human beings within their environments

model to confirm or deny the truth of a concept. For example, the statement that humans are open systems that interact with the environment is a propositional statement. Conceptual models do the following:

- Offer ways of thinking about a problem and ways of outlining and describing how complex things work the way they do
- Provide a mechanism by which different variables and different outcomes are interrelated and work together
- Use more than one theory to help develop an understanding of a problem within a particular context

Table 2-5 provides examples of conceptual models.

Table 2-5

Conceptual Model Examples

Conceptual Model	Ideas and Definitions
Family-centered care model (many different authors)	• Centered on meeting clients' needs within the context of the family • Emphasizes relationships and recognizes and builds on strengths and interconnectedness of family • Recognizes potentially harmful effects of caregiving on family members and that caregivers require the attention of health-care professionals
Science of unitary human beings (Rogers)	• Person and environment are energy fields that evolve negentropically (always moving forward/never moving backward) • Nursing was a basic scientific discipline • Nursing is using knowledge for human betterment • Unique focus of nursing is on the unitary or irreducible human being and the environment (both are energy fields) rather than health and illness
Model of human becoming (Parse)	• Indivisible beings and environment cocreate health • Theory of nursing derived from Rogers' conceptual model • Clients are open, mutual, and in constant interaction with environment • The nurse assists the client in interaction with the environment and in cocreating health
Health care systems model (Neuman)	• Reconstitution is a status of adaptation to stressors • Conceptual model with two theories—optimal patient stability and prevention as intervention • Neuman's model includes intrapersonal, interpersonal, and extrapersonal stressors • Nursing is concerned with the whole person • Nursing actions (primary, secondary, and tertiary levels of prevention) focus on variables affecting the client's response to stressors

Source: From Nursing Theories. Retrieved from http://currentnursing.com/nursing_theory/introduction.html

Advancing Your Knowledge

A group of DNP-prepared nursing leaders has been asked to make a presentation at a nursing conference to articulate the need for using nursing theory as a basis for practice. The group members are meeting to put together the presentation. In their discussion, they determine that starting with metatheory and definitions of nursing concepts that outline the profession and create boundaries for nursing would be beneficial. They discuss the concepts of person, caring, health, and environment as essential to their presentation. They also want to add the notion that human science is the focus of nursing rather than the physical sciences and discuss the idea of humans as open systems that are constantly evolving. Because they are presenting this information to nurses in advanced practice, they want to provide explanations and examples that reflect practice situations.

1. How would you define the concepts of person, caring, health, and environment in a way that relates to advanced practice nursing? Can you provide examples of the use of these concepts in your own practice experiences? How do you use the view of humans as open systems who are constantly evolving in the practice setting?
2. Could you assist advanced practice nurses to understand that the received view of nursing science may have a small place in the practice setting but that the perceived and interpreted view allows nursing to test theory and expand knowledge in the area of practice?

Grand Theories

Grand theories are the third level of theoretical and conceptual thinking; to frame the principles of nursing knowledge, these theories remain highly abstract. Although grand theories broadly review perspectives within nursing practice, they are not as global as meta-theory or as conceptual models. A grand theory is used to direct, explain, and predict nursing in particular situations. It is broad in scope and addresses the entire discipline of nursing rather than any one part. Grand theories of nursing have been developed to explicate the overall role and benefit of nursing in society and how nurses should approach the art and science of the discipline, rather than particular empirical knowledge of nursing practice. Tracing the evolution of the paradigms of nursing practice can be accomplished by following the time line of grand theories as they shift in emphasis and philosophy based on the evolution of nursing science and knowledge (Table 2-6).

Advancing Your Knowledge

In a large community primary care clinic run by nurse practitioners, a group of DNP-prepared advanced practice nurses wants to establish a theory base for practice. These nurse practitioners believe that using a theoretical model would allow them to complete application-based research and measuring outcomes from a theoretically driven perspective. Although they plan to use middle range theories for testing outcomes, they desire to have an overriding grand theory to guide practice.

The clinic has a large diverse client base and sees children from age 1 year to elderly adults older than 100 years. The clinic manages chronic diseases and diagnoses and treats acute problems. Many of the clients do not have insurance, and laboratory work, testing, and prescribing medications must be done

Continued on page 72

Advancing Your Knowledge *Continued from page 71*

with cost in mind. The patient base is equal parts white, Hispanic, African American, and Asian American.

1. What grand theory would you recommend for these nurse practitioners? Why? What types of outcome measures could they use that would be consistent with the theoretical perspective you have chosen?
2. How would using the theory you have chosen be beneficial to the practice? How could it be used to measure and improve practice patterns and patient care?

Table 2-6

Evolution of Nursing Science as Explained by Grand Theory

Grand Theory	Concepts
Self-care deficit theory in nursing (Dorothea E. Orem)	• Self-care creates and maintains wholeness • There are three general methods for providing nursing care: wholly compensatory (doing for the patient); partly compensatory (helping the patient do for himself); supportive-educative (helping the patient to learn self-care and emphasizing the importance of the nurse's role)
Adaptation model (Sister Callista Roy)	• Stimuli disrupt an adaptive system • The individual is a biopsychosocial adaptive system within an environment • Through two adaptive mechanisms, an individual demonstrates adaptive responses or ineffective responses requiring nursing interventions
Transcultural nursing, culture-care theory (Madeleine Leininger)	• Caring is universal and varies transculturally • Major concepts include care, caring, culture, cultural values, and cultural variations • Caring serves to ameliorate or improve human conditions and life base • Care is the essence and the dominant, distinctive, and unifying feature of nursing
Conservation model (Myra Estrin Levine)	Holism is maintained by conserving integrity Proposed that nurses use the principles of conservation of: • Client energy • Personal integrity • Structural integrity • Social integrity Conceptual model with three nursing theories: • Conservation • Redundancy • Therapeutic intention

Source: From Nursing Theories. Retrieved from http://currentnursing.com/nursing_theory/introduction.html

Middle Range Theory

In contrast to grand theories, which are abstract and apply to the entire discipline of nursing, middle range theory, the fourth level of theoretical and conceptual thought, applies to only one concept or a very narrow range of concepts. Middle range theories explicate the external substance and structure of nursing knowledge and create clarity for the empirical world of nursing. Middle range theories have fewer concepts and variables within their structure, are more easily tested, and more likely to pertain to specific issues in nursing practice (McKenna, 1997). Merton (1968) maintained that middle range theories were particularly important for practice disciplines because they concentrated on a few key variables, presented concrete propositions, and created opportunities for testing using clear hypotheses. Middle range theory is described as the next step in development of the nursing profession. These theories provide:

- A concrete link between grand theory and practice;
- A way to think about and measure actual practice concepts, such as uncertainty in illness;
- A theoretical framework for practice in specific areas of caregiving; and
- A benefit to the role of practicing nurses because they encompass the "what" of nursing knowledge, define the meaning of central concepts in nursing, and delineate the relationships among those concepts (Belgan & Tripp-Reimer, 1997).

Middle range theories are especially useful to advanced practice nurses because they are aimed at framing nursing practice. They focus on a narrow range of propositions that can be useful in specific practice situations. Middle range theories have a circular aspect because they often arise from themes, problems, and observations made in practice that are found to be generalizable to multiple practice settings and situations. Once theories have been developed that summarize and explain the observations made in practice, they can be used by practicing nurses to guide future practice.

Lenz (2007) stated that "middle-range theories are those that are sufficiently specific to guide research and practice, yet sufficiently general to cross multiple clinical populations and to encompass similar phenomenon" (p. 213). Lenz stated that middle range theory could assist the profession by explaining what happens in practice, designing effective interventions, and predicting and measuring outcomes related to theoretical propositions. The use of middle range theory to guide advanced nursing practice might be a step toward improving theory-driven practice and the overall adaptation of evidence-based nursing practice. One of the roles of the DNP is to be a leader in population-based health care. Middle range theories assist in developing models of care for populations based on their special circumstances and requirements.

Higgins and Moore (2009) stated that the "major role of middle-range theory is to define or refine the substantive content of nursing science and practice and it should be an important focus of both nurse scholars and practitioners" (p. 53).

Table 2-7

Middle Range Theories in Nursing

Middle Range Theories in Nursing
Maternal role attainment (Mercer, 1985)
Theory of comfort (Kolcaba, 1994)
Quality caring model (Duffy, 2005)
Health promotion (Pender, 1975)
Modeling and role modeling (Erickson, Tomlin, & Swain, 1983)
Theory of caring (Swanson, 1991)
Theory of transcendence (Reed, 1991)
Theory of resilience (Polk, 1997)
Theory of chronic sorrow (Eakes, Burke, & Hainsworth, 1998)
Theory of nursing transitions (Meleis, 2007)

To understand the applicability of middle range theory to nursing practice, we present four middle range theories with accompanying scenarios to describe ways in which each theory could be used to guide practice. Table 2-7 provides a partial list of middle range theories in nursing.

Middle Range Theory of Uncertainty in Illness

One of the most widely studied middle range theories is Mishel's theory of uncertainty in illness (UIT). This theory was initially developed to understand the uncertainty patients felt during the diagnostic and treatment phases of illness and was later expanded to include uncertainty during a chronic illness (Mishel, 1988, 1990). The development of this theory originated from observations that the uncertainty patients felt was detrimental to their health and well-being. *Uncertainty* is defined by Mishel as the inability to determine the meaning of illness-related events.

Three major themes of this theory are as follows:

- *Antecedents of uncertainty or what causes uncertainty to be felt.* Antecedents include familiarity with any event in diagnosis, treatment, or ongoing therapy and the understanding of congruence between these events and the disease that is present or potentially present. For example, teaching a person with diabetes about diagnostic tests such as fasting blood sugar, hemoglobin A_{1C}, or insulin levels reduces uncertainty. Learning how to take medications, signs and symptoms of the disease, and disease management through diet are ways that persons become familiar with the disease and understand the relationship between what they do and the outcomes of the chronic disease state of diabetes.
- *Ability of the person and provider to place value on the uncertain event or situation.* Value placed on the uncertainty of the disease process can be positive in the form of opportunity or adaptations.
- *Coping with uncertainty.* This involves understanding that there could be danger and possible harmful outcomes from the disease, but that there are

also opportunities and possibilities of positive outcomes. Adaptation and coping are the major activities in this theme.

The reconceptualized theory of the uncertainty of illness (RUIT) focuses on the uncertainty of how chronic illness will progress and what the final outcome will be. Among the themes in RUIT are the life changes experienced by individuals with chronic illness. Mishel posited that the parent theory for RUIT was chaos theory, which emphasized disorder, instability, diversity, and restructuring as part of the system of uncertainty. From the chaos of illness, uncertainty can extend into other areas of a person's life and feed on itself, generating further uncertainty and promoting instability.

How can advanced practice nurses use this theory in practice? Research reveals that providing information is a positive method of managing uncertainty because information provides a framework for patients to understand their disease or problem. Practitioners can recognize uncertainty and not only provide information but also make suggestions for adaptations, assist in planning for and mastering potential problems, and help patients and families cope with problems as they arise. Many studies confirm that RUIT is a theoretical framework for practicing nurses. In one study, Ritz et al. (2000) showed that follow-up from advanced practice nurses with women who had newly treated breast cancer reduced feelings of uncertainty in this group.

Advancing Your Knowledge

Mr. T. is a 50-year-old man who has been diagnosed with scleroderma, a widespread connective tissue disease that involves progressive changes in the skin, blood vessels, muscles, and internal organs. In most patients, the disease and accompanying disability slowly worsen, and death may result from gastrointestinal, heart, kidney, or lung involvement. For some patients, symptoms and problems develop quickly over the first few years and continue to worsen. Others get worse more slowly. The rheumatologist told Mr. T. that based on history and diagnostic findings, he may have only 5 years until the disease causes his death. Problems with the lungs are the most common cause of death in patients with scleroderma. The physician has asked Mr. T. to decide whether or not he wishes to be intubated and on life support when his condition worsens. The physician has also asked Mr. T. to consider a living will and a health-care surrogate.

Mr. T. is uncertain about the progression of the disease and what diagnostic tests indicate for the progression of the disease. He is uncertain about how his disability will affect his daily life, his family, and his ability to earn a living, and he is concerned about how much pain he will have to endure. All of these issues of uncertainty have led Mr. T. to experience profound depression. He has stopped leaving the house because he is uncertain of what might happen if he is out and gets overly fatigued. He tells the nurse practitioner that he spends most of his day in bed "trying to shut out the reality of his disease and where it is taking him."

Continued on page 76

Advancing Your Knowledge *Continued from page 75*

The DNP, Cary Thomas, who is Mr. T.'s primary health-care provider, realizes that uncertainty about his illness and about the progression of symptoms are affecting Mr. T.'s overall activities of daily living and his emotional and social health. Using the theory of RUIT, Cary understands that even though she may be unable to stop the progression of the disease, she can assist Mr. T. to cope and reduce his feelings of uncertainty. Cary has read studies about using RUIT to improve life perspective, creating new goals, redefining what is normal, and building new dreams through uncertainty (Bailey & Stewart, 2001). She develops a plan of care for Mr. T. and his family that includes the impact of uncertainty on his health and well-being.

When the family comes to the office, both Mr. T and his wife are concerned about the future and feel a high level of uncertainty about how to treat problems as they arise and how to cope with the disability and possible death as a result of the disease. Using the plan of care with the theoretical base of RUIT, Cary Thomas plans time during each visit to review what is known about Mr. T's disease, what diagnostic and therapeutic options are available, and services that Mr. and Mrs. T could access for assistance with daily care and other issues as they arise. Cary assures Mr. T that she will be available for questions as they arise and that he and his wife should feel free to call the office any time. She also informs Mr. T that if an emergency should arise when the office is closed, she will be alerted to his call via the answering service and will contact Mr. T. immediately. Additionally, she shares ideas about how Mr. T. can better manage his depression and feelings of fatigue. Mr. T. agrees to begin taking an antidepressant and to see a counselor to assist with his feelings of depression. Finally, Cary, Mr. T., and Mrs. T. sit together and discuss ways in which the family can enjoy the time they have left together, making plans for special time together, allowing Mr. T. to create a scrapbook of his life and experiences to leave for his grown children and grandchildren, and keeping in touch with recent and lifelong friends for support and love. Cary also discusses the idea of a living will, appointing a health-care surrogate, and initiating hospice care at the appropriate time. Mr. T. was very confused regarding the meaning of these documents and how to make his end-of-life wishes known. After a few visits, Mr. T. and his wife both signed living wills and appointed one of their children as their health-care surrogate.

The ability of Cary Thomas to meet the needs of this family, which was struggling with a difficult diagnosis and continuing deterioration of a loved one, was very satisfying for her and her patients. The use of theory and theory verification through research findings helped Cary to provide appropriate care and ease the uncertainty of Mr. T. and his family. In addition, Mr. T. had fewer office visits to his rheumatologist, reducing health-care costs, because his questions and concerns were being addressed.

1. List other chronic disease situations where this middle range theory might be beneficial.

2. What outcome measures could be put into place to determine the effectiveness of this theory and whether it was beneficial to patients?
3. Can you recall a patient or group of patients who might benefit from the middle range theory on "uncertainty"?
4. How could an interpretive view of knowing be used to create better practice models using the theory of uncertainty in illness?

Middle Range Theory of Unpleasant Symptoms

The middle range theory of unpleasant symptoms was created by Lenz, Suppe, Gift, Pugh, and Milligan (1995). Because symptoms are perceived differently by different individuals, this theory is applicable at the level of individual patients and in groups of patients with similar symptoms. The purpose of this theory is to design interventions to prevent or lessen the effect of unpleasant symptoms. The desire to decrease the effect of unpleasant symptoms is the focus of this theory, and developing interventions for individual or populations of patients is the overall goal. The authors suggest that symptoms can be physiological, psychological, or situational and observable or not observable. These factors may act alone or together to create the unpleasant symptoms. Another theoretical assumption is that unpleasant symptoms may impede recovery. For example, the pain associated with early breastfeeding may impede a mother's desire to continue with breastfeeding. The theory of unpleasant symptoms also proposes that identifying the factors that may increase unpleasant symptoms and attempting multiple interventions might increase symptom relief.

To practicing nurses, the concepts and propositions in this theory may seem like common sense rather than theoretical knowledge. Nevertheless, although symptom management is one of the most important aspects of clinical nursing practice and nurses have a great deal of autonomy in creating solutions, unpleasant symptoms remain problematic in health-care settings and are often inadequately addressed. The theory of unpleasant symptoms suggests that nurses should determine the possibility and existence of multiple symptoms and multivariate causes of unpleasant symptoms and consider experiences, situations, and emotions as well as biophysical issues to be influencing factors. Main points in this middle range theory include the following:

- Unpleasant symptoms are detrimental to patient care and recovery.
- Four variables that can be measured in unpleasant symptoms are intensity, timing, distress level, and quality of symptoms.
- Other factors affecting symptoms include physiological factors, psychological factors, and situational factors.
- All factors and variables must be considered to address unpleasant symptoms in patient care.

Advancing Your Knowledge

Mrs. S. is an 82-year-old woman who was admitted to the hospital for hip replacement surgery after a fall at home. Mrs. S. lives with her husband, who was diagnosed with Alzheimer's disease 5 years ago. The couple has two children who live in another state and who both have families with small children and cannot come to help Mr. S. at this time. Mr. and Mrs. S. have a neighbor who looks in on Mr. S. and brings him supper each night. Mrs. S. feels as though her life is spinning out of control. She has always been a strong and self-sufficient person who cared not only for herself but for her husband as well. As Mr. S. becomes more cognitively impaired, it has been necessary for Mrs. S. to be physically active in her husband's care; she helps him into and out of the shower and up and down the stairs to the front door of their house. Mrs. S. is active in community groups as well. She attends church and is a member of the altar guild, in which her role is to decorate the church with flowers. She is an avid gardener, and the flowers she uses in church often come from her garden.

Dr. John Stiers (DNP) is a clinical nurse specialist on the orthopedic floor at the hospital where Mrs. S. is a patient after surgery. John is aware of the theory of unpleasant symptoms and is attempting to address Mrs. S.'s unrelieved pain during postoperative day 2. The physician ordered pain medication every 4 hours as needed after the pain pump was removed on day 2. Mrs. S. has asked for pain medication several times and complains of breakthrough pain between doses. John obtains a complete history from Mrs. S. and realizes that there may be multiple causes of her pain, some related to the surgery and some unrelated to the surgery, and that multivariate issues may be causing her pain to be unrelieved with narcotic analgesics. Some of the nurses on the unit believe that Mrs. S. is addicted to the narcotics and asks for them even when she does not need them for pain.

John outlines the issues related to Mrs. S.'s pain. One issue is that the pain medication is ordered as needed rather than on a regular schedule. This means that Mrs. S. asks for medication when the pain becomes intolerable because she believes that she is strong enough to "bear" some pain. By the time Mrs. S. actually receives her dose of pain medication, however, the pain is severe, and the medication cannot "catch up" with her level of pain. To decrease the negative effect of as-needed pain medication on the unpleasant symptom of pain for Mrs. S., John encourages the nursing staff to offer pain medication every 4 hours instead of waiting for Mrs. S. to request it. He educates the nurses concerning the benefits of adequate pain management in Mrs. S. and reassures them that she is not addicted to the pain medication.

The second assessment of unpleasant symptoms that John makes is Mrs. S.'s emotional state after the surgery. Mrs. S. is concerned for her husband who is alone at home. She is also concerned that she will be unable to take care of him when she is released from the hospital and recovered from her surgery. Mrs. S. is also concerned that her life may be curtailed and that she may be unable to garden or take part in the social groups she enjoys. This worry and emotional stress adds to her unpleasant symptom of pain. In an attempt to help Mrs. S. with this aspect of her pain symptoms, John consults the social worker to determine whether Mr. S. is eligible for home health care for the few days his wife is in the hospital and while she recovers in a rehabilitation hospital. The social worker sends a nurse to evaluate Mr. S. and finds that he is eligible for home health care for dressing, bathing, and giving his medications. John calls the home health agency and asks them to prioritize the initiation of visits to Mr. S. because of his cognitive condition. This intervention significantly reduces Mrs. S.'s emotional stress and allows her to rest more comfortably.

John invites the rehabilitation hospital intake coordinator to visit Mrs. S. to discuss her rehabilitation and what she can expect after she is released from the rehabilitation hospital. The coordinator assures Mrs. S. that based on her present level of health and the fact that she would like to resume her former level of activity, there is no reason she cannot eventually go back to gardening and being socially active. The coordinator provides Mrs. S. with information about the expected levels of activity for most patients who receive rehabilitation and follow the recommendations of the physical therapists and other health-care providers. Mrs. S. is smiling for the first time since admission, and she tells John that she is encouraged by what she has heard.

Finally, John prepares an in-service for the nursing staff on the orthopedic unit to review pain assessment and management. He includes the theory of unpleasant symptoms as a framework for beginning the class. The nurses discuss the prevalence of unmanaged pain on the unit and create assessment sheets that include an investigation of multiple causes for pain, including physical, emotional, spiritual, and psychological. Part of the educational session also deals with appropriate ideas about acute pain management, particularly in the area of postoperative pain medications. As a result of this work, the general patient satisfaction on the unit is improved, and the management of pain is greatly improved.

Using the theory of unpleasant symptoms allowed John to uncover a common problem on the orthopedic unit and devise appropriate methods for reducing the problem from a multivariate perspective.

1. How did the middle range theory of unpleasant symptoms guide John in his care of Mrs. S.?
2. How could John measure the effect this theoretical framework has had on the care of Mrs. S.?
3. Do you see ways in which you could use this middle range theory in your practice?

Middle Range Theory of Interpersonal Relationships

Peplau's middle range theory of interpersonal relationships was published in 1992. In this theory, Peplau (1992) defined communication as an essential nursing skill that is needed to understand the wishes, needs, and desires of patients and fellow nurses. She identified interpersonal relationships as core to nursing practice to understand and interact with others in a healing manner. According to this theory, one of the essential duties of nursing is to identify patterns that promote or undermine personality development among patients and work with those patterns to strengthen interconnectedness and decrease anxiety (Peterson, 2009). The two guiding assumptions within the theory of interpersonal relationships are that the nurse's own growth and development are important and that growth and development among nurses are the only ways to improve interpersonal relationships with patients.

Peplau identified the following functions that are important in the theory of interpersonal relationships:

- *Phase of orientation:* Nurse is a resource, counselor, and surrogate
- *Phase of identity:* Identify goals; patient, family, and nurse work together; trust is developed

Tasks the nurse and patient take on together include the following:

- Ability to count on others
- Ability to identify strengths and weaknesses
- Ability to participate with others

This theory answers the following question: What aspects of a relationship are able to be improved by strengthening the relationship and building trust?

Advancing Your Knowledge

Dr. Sally Hill (DNP) is the chief nursing officer of Great Valley Hospital, a 334-bed tertiary care center in a suburban community. The board of directors of Great Valley is interested in obtaining magnet status for the hospital and has met with Sally several times to determine what can be done to facilitate this. Sally has worked hard to create a good relationship with middle managers and nursing staff at the hospital; however, the staff members are unsure they want to put effort into obtaining magnet status for the hospital. During staff meetings, many nurses have asked Sally "what is in it for us?" when discussing magnet status.

Sally uses Peplau's theory of interpersonal relationships to determine how to help the nurses understand the benefits for them, for patient care, and for the hospital in obtaining magnet status. She first assesses her own growth and development in the position of chief nursing officer, which she has held for 5 years. She determines that her strength in interpersonal development is that she has always listened to the nurses before determining the best course of action and that she believes all staff members are interested in making Great Valley an excellent hospital that provides quality nursing care. Sally prepares a fact sheet for the nurses listing all of the benefits of magnet hospitals and how nurse retention at these facilities is higher than at nonmagnet hospitals. She prepares a list of what must be done to move Great Valley toward magnet status and outlines the benefits that would be provided as the work is completed. For example, to encourage nurses to obtain higher levels of education, Sally has deemed that they can receive time off from work to attend class, classes will be paid for by the hospital, and pay raises will accrue as educational levels are completed.

Sally invites nurses to discussions about the magnet journey. Consistent with the theory of interpersonal relationships, Sally acts as a resource and counselor to the nurses as she answers their questions and participates in discussions. She assists the nurses not only in agreeing to participate in the magnet journey but also in embracing the changes that will take place as beneficial to themselves and their patients. Through this process of interpersonal relationship building, both the nursing staff and Sally are made stronger, trust each other more, and create better working conditions for everyone at Great Valley Hospital.

1. How would you use the middle range theory of interpersonal relationships in your workplace?
2. How could you measure the effects of this theory in the practice setting?
3. How could this middle range theory be used to improve communication and collaboration skills among all types of health-care professionals in practice?

Middle Range Theory of Behavior Change

One of the most important aspects of health care today is encouraging and assisting patients to change their health behaviors. Numerous diseases are the result of unhealthy behaviors, including smoking, obesity, sedentary lifestyle, and alcohol and drug consumption. Researchers suggest that poor health behaviors account for more than 50% of illness (Ryan, 2009).

The theory of health behavior change is important as a theoretical basis for improving health outcomes. Behavior change is an essential component of health promotion and disease prevention and the underpinning of advanced nursing practice. The creators of this middle range theory found that socio-demographic status can have a positive or negative impact on behavior change. In addition, simply providing information, no matter how thorough or creative, is insufficient to sustain long-term behavior change. The integrated theory of health behavior change is aimed at maintaining behavior change to prevent a relapse into poor health behaviors, which occurs often early in the change process.

The components used to sustain health behavior change in this middle range theory are fostering knowledge and beliefs, creating and strengthening self-regulation abilities, and enhancing social facilitation (Ryan, 2009). Establishing a philosophy of self-management in daily habits is the goal of behavior change in this model.

- The first goal of this theory is to increase confidence in the patient's ability to change behaviors successfully in both normal and stressful situations.

- The second goal is to create self-regulation so that the health behavior becomes incorporated into the daily routine.
- The third goal is to develop social support for the behavior change.

All of these goals lead patients to establish a sense of self-management for the behavior change, ultimately helping them to sustain the change over a lifetime.

Advancing Your Knowledge

Dr. Linda Kramer (DNP) is the director of a community health center in an inner-city area. Funds for the center come from the city and federal government by way of grant funding. The center offers primary care, dental care, women's health care, pediatric care, mental health counseling, and educational services for both individuals and groups for a community of approximately 20,000 that has no other access to care. Of the patients at the center, 50% are Hispanic, 32% are African American, 10% are white, and 8% are Asian American. Patients primarily receive Medicaid or other federal health insurance. This community center is a model for others that have been developed in inner-city areas around the United States, and Linda and her staff of nurse practitioners, nurses, medical assistants, billing personnel, psychologists, and pharmacists are proud of their accomplishments. A new program aimed at improving diabetic blood sugar levels is being developed at the center. The clinic currently has 2800 diabetic patients, of whom less than 20% have their blood sugar under control. In a discussion with staff, it was determined that several health behavior changes would assist these diabetic patients to maintain better blood glucose control. First, the patients would do better if they understood the nature of diabetes; second, taking medication correctly would have a positive impact on blood sugar; and third, learning about and using good nutrition would help the patients to reduce diabetes.

The health-care provider group chose the middle range theory of behavior change as the theoretical framework for the development of guidelines to assist diabetic patients with regulating their blood sugar levels. A team was formed to review literature on the theory and on effective ways to reduce blood sugar among populations similar to those served by the clinic. It was decided early in team meetings that to foster self-management, some of the diabetic patients who came to the clinic should be included on the team. To meet the theory's first goal of increasing confidence in the diabetic's ability to change behaviors to improve blood sugar levels in both normal and stressful situations, the group developed a self-monitoring program for diabetics in which each diabetic patient was asked to keep a chart at the clinic of his or her hemoglobin A_{1C} levels.

A class was scheduled for anyone with diabetes and their family members to review carefully the diabetic diet, medications, and a rewards program. The rewards program was developed so that patients who were able to reduce their hemoglobin A_{1C} levels by 10% in any given 3-month period received a free ticket to the local movie theater, a coupon for a free massage at the center, and an invitation to a celebration party held at the clinic. Any diabetic patient who had a normal hemoglobin A_{1C} level was also invited to the celebration, given a coupon for a free massage and a free movie ticket, and was given a pin stating that they were an "A_{1C} Player." Similar rewards were offered to patients who lost weight over a 3-month period. Movie tickets were provided by a local theater as a gift to the clinic, and the local massage therapy school sent students to perform the free massages. The party featured healthy snacks, games that helped review good dietary habits and diabetic facts, and music and dancing for exercise. The cost to the clinic was almost nothing, and the program was a success with the diabetic patients.

To meet the second goal of the theory of behavior change, which was to create self-regulation so that the health behavior becomes incorporated into the daily routine, participants were asked to keep a diet and blood sugar diary. At group meetings, members were asked to discuss the challenges they overcame and successes they had achieved during that week. In this way, each person was responsible for self-regulation and had the ability to share his or her experience with a group to get feedback and support.

To assist with the third goal of the theory of behavior change, which is to develop social support for assistance with health-care behavior change, the group decided to create a mentorship program. All patients with newly diagnosed diabetes were provided with a mentor who was a regular member of the diabetic program and whose blood sugar was under control. The mentoring role assisted both the mentor and the mentee to establish self-regulation and self-responsibility for meaningful and lasting behavior change.

1. Choose a different scenario where this middle range theory could be applied.
2. How would you measure the success of this theory in practice settings?
3. How could the advanced practice nurse help other groups see the need for using middle range theory in practice settings?

Microrange Theory

The final level of theory is microrange theory. This is the least formal and most restrictive type of nursing theory. At this level, theory is developed to describe outcomes of practice interventions. Also called *practice theory*, each microrange theory is related to a distinct aspect of practice. Microrange theories are often used to create policies and procedures in health-care settings and are based on common scientific principles. Microrange theories are only now beginning to emerge in nursing as an attempt is made to link practice and theory more closely. The use of evidence-based practice principles is expected to increase greatly the number of microrange theories available to nurses in the practice setting. Possible areas in which microrange theory could be useful include:

- Skin and wound care,
- Pain medication administration,

- Patient falls,
- Nursing injury prevention, and
- Patient risk assessment for deep vein thrombosis or pulmonary embolism on admission to the hospital.

Advancing Your Knowledge

A group of nurses, nursing assistants, and nursing administrators in a nursing home noted that the nursing home began to experience an increase in decubitus ulcers. To address the problem, a multidisciplinary team of nurses, nursing assistants, nutritionists, and administrators developed a risk assessment tool to identify residents at risk for skin breakdown and created a team to monitor and intervene to decrease the risk for skin breakdown. If a decubitus ulcer occurred, the team would be proactive in addressing the problem before it became more serious. From this work, the team developed a microtheory regarding skin care in elderly adults that identified a need for a multidisciplinary team approach to both risk assessment and treatment. They drafted a manuscript outlining their microtheory and subsequently had it published in a geriatric nursing journal. Other nursing homes requested permission to use their risk assessment and intervention guide, and the system is currently being used in many nursing homes across the United States.

1. How could the development of microtheory assist DNP-prepared nurses to care better for populations of patients in a practical way?
2. What other microtheories could be useful in advanced practice? How could DNP-prepared nurses be instrumental in creating and disseminating these types of theories?

Critical Thinking Questions

Can you develop a theoretical base for the practice you are working in currently? If you are not currently working, use a practice with which you are familiar. As you think about theory-guided practice (either grand theory or middle range theory), use the following as a template to develop the base for practice.

1. What concepts within the theory are relevant to the practice setting?
2. How will the concepts be operationalized in the practice setting?
3. What rationale is there for using this particular theory?
4. Has anyone else used this theory as a basis for practice? You can usually find articles regarding the use of a theoretical basis for practice in a database search.
5. What would be the benefits of using this theory in a practice setting? How would it benefit nurses, patients, families, and administrators?

Ethical considerations and concepts are an essential part of theory development and testing and decision making. As a profession gains more independence in practice, ethical decision making becomes even more important.

Ethical Decision Making in Advanced Practice Nursing

Ethics is an important aspect of the scientific underpinnings of nursing and of the value of nursing in society. Ethics is especially important within advanced practice nursing. Respect for human dignity is the foundational principle of health-care ethics and an essential component of advanced practice nursing. Advanced practice nurses may not realize that the decisions they make on a daily basis have an ethical component, but ethical decisions are at the forefront of all health-care practice whether they are made consciously or unconsciously. Emphasis on high-technology interventions, financial limitations, and measuring performance based on cost-effectiveness remains the predominant focus of employers and payers of health care and often overshadow ethics in health-care decision making. This section discusses:

- Ethical decision making;
- The need to respect human dignity;
- The ideals of autonomy, beneficence, nonmalfeasance, and justice;
- The American Nurses Association Code of Ethics;
- Privacy and confidentiality;
- The ethics of impaired practice; and
- Accountability, responsibility, and respect.

The ideal of respect for human dignity underlies ethical decision making. Respect for human dignity encompasses respect for self and for others. Doane, Pauly, Brown, and McPherson (2004) examined the ideal of human dignity in practice. In their study, advanced practice nurses described having a sense of "self as moral agent" and felt that trusting colleagues and having a background of ethical understanding were integral to resolving ethical issues in practice. Advanced practice nurses obtain ethical knowledge and ideas from diverse spheres, including medicine, philosophy, religion, and bioethics, as well as from nursing itself.

When contemplating and beginning doctoral study focused on clinical practice and clinical excellence, it is essential that ethics has an important role in educational discussion and practice decision making. Creating a full understanding of ethical principles and testing those principles in practice settings promote effective ethical practice among advanced practice nurses who are prepared to serve individuals, families, and communities with respect for human dignity. See Table 2-8 for definitions of major terms involved in ethics discussions.

At all levels of practice, ethical considerations are influenced by work-related policies and authority within the health-care setting. Supplying ethical knowledge is not enough to strengthen respect for human dignity as the cornerstone of nursing practice; rather, ethical knowledge must be reviewed, investigated, and discussed in the context of actual health-care settings and situations. In the practice setting, enormously diverse ethical issues are experienced, and each issue has slightly different characteristics that make it unique to the individual,

Table 2-8

Definitions of Ethical Terms

Ethical Term	Meaning
Autonomy	Principle that recognizes the rights of individuals to self-determination. This is rooted in society's respect for ability of individuals to make informed decisions about personal matters.
Beneficence	Refers to actions that promote the well-being of others. In the medical/nursing context, this means taking actions that serve the best interests of patients.
Nonmaleficence	Concept that is embodied by the phrase, "first, do no harm"; it is more important not to harm a patient than to do the patient good.
Justice	A principle of fair and equal treatment for all, treating people in a nonprejudicial manner.
Truth telling/ informed consent	Truth telling requires the provider to tell the patient what is happening and what to expect about health, health-care testing, and treatment. Obtaining consent for testing and treatment requires the provider to inform the patient about the procedure, the risks and benefits from the test or procedure, and the possible outcomes of the test or procedure. After being informed, the patient can provide consent in writing to undergo the test or procedure.
Conflict of interest	Occurs when an individual or organization is involved in multiple interests, one of which could *possibly* corrupt the motivation for an act in the other. In health care, a conflict of interest can occur when providers receive money for ordering a certain drug or test and therefore may order it more often or in lieu of other medications or tests. Physicians should not allow a conflict of interest to influence medical judgment.
Futility	Concept that has been an important topic in discussions of medical ethics. What should be done if there is no chance that a patient will survive, but the family members insist on advanced care?

the setting, and the creation of an equitable outcome. Although ethics is not a situational proposition, ethical decision making can have situational aspects. The nurse must use the ideas of caring, coming to know the patient and family, and authentic presence and positive communication to be able to treat patients ethically and advocate for fairness and compassion.

In a review of the literature regarding nurses' ethical decision making in practice, Goethels, Gastmans, and de Casterle (2010) found that ethical decision making among nurses is a complex process that involves reasoning, decision making based on reasoning, and implementation of the decision made in the practice setting. The process of ethical decision making is more than a cognitive one; it is influenced by personal knowledge and experience in any given situation, evidence-based knowledge, and understanding of the situation in which the decision is being made. In addition to these processes, nurses encounter ethical dilemmas linked to rules, regulations, and underlying factors in the work environment. For example, if hospital policy states no visitors, but a patient is dying and the family wants to be at the bedside, the ethical dilemma is whether the nurse's responsibility is to the patient or to the hospital for which the nurse works. An example for advanced practice nurses could be that the insurance company wants detailed information about a patient that the patient does not wish to share. Is the nurse's responsibility to the insurance company, who pays the nurse for the care provided, or to the patient?

Ethical Principles and DNP Education

The idea for the DNP and the need to educate advanced practice nurses at this level was created in response to a need for increased social responsibility among nurses in advanced practice (Silva & Ludwick, 2006). The following four ethical principles are strongly tied to the essentials of DNP education and practice:

1. Social responsibility, or the ability to assist all persons to obtain what they need to be healthy;
2. Respect for persons, which includes cultural competence and effective communication skills;
3. Do no harm when in the clinical area by being competent and knowledgeable in practice; and
4. Fairness, so that everyone is treated equally, regardless of their ability to pay, their attitude toward the nurse, or any other problems they have.

With DNP programs still in their infancy, insufficient data exist to determine whether DNP-prepared advanced practice nurses make an ethical difference and have an improved notion of respect for human dignity. With appropriate preparation and dialogue regarding ethical decision making, the DNP presents an opportunity for nurses to ground practice in an ethical framework and to lead the health care field in respect for human dignity and social justice.

Advancing Your Knowledge

M.O. is an advanced practice nurse who works in a large urban clinic. As part of his professional practice, M.O. strives to be fair to all patients no matter their ethnicity or financial situation. M.O. is often challenged to treat people who he knows are destroying their bodies and the bodies of others by taking or selling drugs. He finds it difficult to be respectful to women who come to the clinic with multiple pregnancies by different men, all of whom do not want to care for the children or their mothers. Sometimes he tells his wife that he is just tired of trying to help people that don't seem to want or appreciate his help. He knows that he makes a difference in the lives of some of the patients, but overall he is unsure and feels defeated in his attempt to make a difference.

Continued on page 88

Advancing Your Knowledge *Continued from page 87*

M.O. sits with the clinic director, an advanced practice nurse who has a DNP. She tells him that even though he may not always see the difference he makes in the lives of the people in the clinic, there are things that he does do that make a difference in their lives. She relates a story of a patient who was an alcoholic and drug addict and lived on the street who came into the clinic for an infected tooth. His face was swollen and he was feverish and the tooth had to come out. M.O. gave him antibiotics and made an appointment for him at a free dental clinic. As the patient was leaving, he spoke to the director and said that although he had made a mess of his life, when M.O. treated him with respect and cared about him it helped him to realize that he was still a human being and a child of God. As he said this, a tear rolled down his cheek. The director gave M.O. several other examples of how his caring for patients with respect and dignity and always being honest and fair with them had made a difference.

1. Take each of the four ethical principles listed earlier and provide an example of how they could be used in practice.
2. In the larger picture of health-care policy and access to care, how can ethical principles be applied and needed services be fairly provided?
3. What are some of the most difficult ethical issues you have had to deal with? How can the aforementioned principles be applied to those situations?
4. When patients, families, or coworkers seem unreasonable in their demands or create difficulties in the practice setting, how can ethical principles be used?
5. Does treating someone ethically mean giving them everything they want or even need?
6. What is the difference between being ethical and protecting yourself legally?

American Nurses Association Code of Ethics

To highlight and define ethical responsibilities and actions and to provide a framework for ethical decision making in nursing, the American Nurses Association (ANA) published a code of ethics for nursing (2005). This code creates a standard for practice that the ANA affirms is "non-negotiable" and is "an expression of nursing's own understanding of its commitment to society" (ANA, 2005, p. 2). The code of ethics lists the fundamental ethical and moral values of professional nurses and the duties and responsibilities of nurses toward their patients. Box 2-1 lists the nine provisions of this document.

Highlighted in the ANA code of ethics is the worth and dignity of all humans regardless of health status, health beliefs, or practices. The goal of nursing is to promote physical, social, emotional, and spiritual well-being to all patients regardless of any factor such as race, culture, ethnicity, gender, religion, or belief. Professional nurses must respect human dignity and the autonomous right of

Box 2-1

Nine Provisions in the Nurses Code of Ethics

Provision 1: The nurse, in all professional relationships, practices with respect and compassion for the inherent dignity, worth, and uniqueness of every individual, unrestricted by consideration of social or economic status, personal attributes, or the nature of health problems.

Provision 2: The nurse's primary commitment is to the patient, whether an individual, family, group, or community.

Provision 3: The nurse promotes, advocates for, and strives to protect the health, safety, and rights of patients.

Provision 4: The nurse is responsible and accountable for individual nursing practice and determines the appropriate delegation of tasks consistent with the nurse's obligation to provide optimum patient care.

Provision 5: The nurse owes the same duties to self as to others, including the responsibility to preserve integrity and safety, to maintain competence, and to continue personal and professional growth.

Provision 6: The nurse participates in establishing, maintaining, and improving health-care environments and conditions of employment conducive to the provision of quality health care and consistent with the values of the profession through individual and collective action.

Provision 7: The nurse participates in the advancement of the profession through contributions to practice, education, administration, and knowledge development.

Provision 8: The nurse collaborates with other health professionals and the public in promoting community, national, and international efforts to meet health needs.

Provision 9: The profession of nursing, as represented by associations and their members, is responsible for articulating nursing values, for maintaining the integrity of the profession and its practice, and for shaping social policy.

each individual to make his or her own health-care decisions and choices. In the area of self-determination, although nurses teach, counsel, listen, and create learning opportunities, patients must be able to make their own decisions without fear of recrimination or reprisal.

Patient as First Priority

In certain situations, nurses must choose between the rights of an individual and the rights of a community. Patients with tuberculosis who choose not to take medication that reduces the communicable nature of the disease are sometimes incarcerated to protect the community from contracting the disease. When this type of situation arises, nurses must be aware of the violation of self-determination and consider carefully how to move forward with patient care while protecting the larger community. The self-determination of the patient must be acknowledged even if the patient's wishes cannot be honored. If a patient wishes to die because he is in pain or because he has become a burden to his family, the ANA code would ask the nurse or advanced practice nurse to acknowledge the patient's wishes, provide a sympathetic understanding response to the wishes that include the inability of the nurse or health-care provider to assist the patient in this way and an honest attempt by the provider to make the patient more comfortable, ease the care burden on the family, and provide the patient with an improved quality of life where possible.

Because of the foundational tenet of the nursing profession to recognize the uniqueness of every human being and to honor the right of all humans to self-determination, the preeminent commitment of the nurse is to the individual receiving care. When conflicts arise between the patient or person receiving care and others in the health-care setting, including family members, other health-care providers, and payers, the first responsibility of the nurse is to the patient. The ANA code of ethics points out that advanced practice nurses and nurse administrators are at particular risk for conflicts of interest in this area and must be ever vigilant in putting the patient's interests first and maintaining integrity. Nurse practitioners and clinical nurse specialists must be aware that financial interests, cost concerns, and benefit to the health-care organization are secondary to the well-being of the patient. However, this awareness does not mean that cost is not considered; it means that the nurse should be knowledgeable regarding the best course of action for the lowest cost. Likewise, nurse administrators must be cognizant of the ethics related to decisions they make that affect the welfare of patients. Patient welfare should be the most important consideration, with the welfare of the health-care institution a close second.

Collaboration as an Ethical Imperative

Collaboration is mentioned in the ANA code of ethics as an ethical imperative. Nurses must work through interdisciplinary and multidisciplinary collaboration to ensure the best outcomes for patients. Discussing the best course of action and ensuring everyone on the health-care team is informed about the condition and needs of the patient improve patient outcomes and reduce costs and waste in the health-care system. It is incumbent on the advanced practice nurse to ensure that her concerns about the patient are addressed and that the patient's well-being is maintained, even when working with others who are unwilling to listen.

Effective and efficient communication in general is an important aspect of collaboration. Effective communication improves relationships between individuals working toward the common goal of respect for human dignity and optimal patient care, creates a smooth transmission of ideas, and builds trust among colleagues. Dixon, Larison, and Zabari (2006) described professional communication as a complex process and identified components of skilled communication as education, teamwork, commitment, evaluation, and ongoing vigilance. Each of these qualities is essential when caring for patients. For collaboration to occur, excellent communication is needed to provide a smooth, effortless flow of work and support between caregivers. Sound nurse-physician communication is a cornerstone of safe, efficient, and effective patient care. Good communication is assertive rather than aggressive, calm rather than frenetic, flows logically, provides all necessary information, and does not assess blame but rather makes the situation known so that it can be rectified. In this sense, using good communication skills and effectively communicating areas of concern to fellow health-care providers are ethical and uphold the provisions of the ANA standards of ethics for nurses.

Privacy and Confidentiality

The ethics code addresses the need for privacy and confidentiality that can affect primary care provided by advanced practice nurses. Honoring the patient's wishes for disclosure or nondisclosure of information about his or her health can be a difficult ethical decision for advanced practice nurses but must always be made with the patient's wishes at the forefront. Although laws such as the Health Insurance Portability and Accountability Act (HIPAA) protect patients' privacy and confidentiality, nurses are held to an even higher standard for the protection of privacy by the code of ethics (ANA, 2005). HIPAA makes privacy a legal standard. This standard addresses the use and disclosure of individuals' health information by organizations. It also addresses individuals' rights to understand and control how their health information is used. A major goal of the Privacy Rule is to ensure that individuals' health information is properly protected, while allowing the flow of health information needed to provide and promote high-quality health care and to protect the public's health and well-being.

Nurses not only must protect the patient's privacy but also must maintain confidential information in an appropriate way. Nurses often obtain confidential patient information based on a relationship of trust; patients assume that health information will not be divulged except in ways that have been previously agreed on (e.g., for treatment, for payment of services, or for use in monitoring the quality of care that is being delivered). This relationship of trust is especially important in the area of advanced practice nursing because the patient often develops a long-term relationship with the health-care provider and may disclose confidential information because of the privileged respect and trust the patient has for the provider. This information must be kept confidential unless that confidentiality could physically harm the patient or others.

Impaired Practice

The ANA code of ethics addresses the need for nurses to act in situations where there is questionable and impaired practice. In a study entitled "Silence Kills," the researchers found that less than 10% of health-care professionals confront their colleagues about safety and practice concerns (Maxfield, Grenny, McMillan, Patterson, & Switzler, 2005). These researchers also found that only 10% of the 1700 health-care workers interviewed were confident in their ability to raise concerns and questions about patient care. Although 10% is a small number, the health-care workers who were confident enough to raise concerns and questions believed that they worked harder, were more satisfied with their jobs, stayed in their jobs longer, and were able to demonstrate better patient outcomes than the health-care workers who were less able or willing to raise concerns about practice. The ANA code of ethics requires ethical nurses to raise concerns, to speak up, and to bring to light questionable practices.

Consider the case in Texas where two nurses were charged with "misuse of official information," a third-degree felony that carries a large fine and jail term, for filing a complaint against a physician for poor practice and a pattern of improper prescribing and surgical procedures. These nurses were supported by the ANA and finally exonerated of the charges pressed against them by the local authorities. The media portrayed this as a win for patients as well as nurses because it highlighted the need for and support of nurses and other health-care providers to speak out against bad practice. Speaking out takes courage but has proven in the long-run to improve job satisfaction and patient outcomes.

Accountability, Responsibility, and Self-Respect

The ANA code of ethics calls for nurses to accept accountability and responsibility for the care they provide; this is especially important for nurse practitioners and clinical nurse specialists because they have increased autonomy and responsibility for patient care. Nurse practitioners, clinical nurse specialists, and nurse administrators should remain up-to-date and competent regarding guidelines for patient care and safety and take the initiative to institute the best possible standards of care for patients.

Nurses demonstrate personal ethics when they have self-respect, continue to grow professionally, and maintain competence. Caring for self improves the nurse's ability to care for others. Having respect for the dignity and uniqueness of self allows the nurse to encourage dignity for others. Although this seems to be an easy concept, research shows that nurses often neglect their own well-being and disregard self-care to the detriment of their own health and their ability to care for others.

Nurses have an ethical obligation to become involved in health-care policy to advocate for patients and their families. Nurses are better qualified to act as advocates by maintaining standards in education, competence, and clinical practice. Social reform is an ethical role in nursing as nurses advocate for the community, family, and individual persons. Higher levels of educational attainment allow DNPs to position themselves to speak for nursing and for individuals who need care in the community but do not have a voice. Becoming involved in legislative and policy issues is appropriate for the DNP because these nurses have an advanced understanding of population-based health-care needs, the policies affecting health care, and the ethical responsibility of nurses to put the needs of the patient first.

As mentioned earlier, no studies have evaluated improvements in respect for human dignity with the advent of the DNP degree. As greater numbers of DNPs are graduated and become involved in practice and as the entry into advanced practice becomes the DNP degree, studies will determine the ethical impact of the DNP on health care. Promoting leadership as part of the educational experience may provide DNP graduates with the courage and will to increase respect for human dignity within health care and promote ethical actions among all health-care professionals.

Critical Thinking Questions

Consider the following ethical dilemmas that could occur in the practice setting:

1. Mr. R.T. is a patient who comes to the office and reeks of alcohol. It is obvious he has not bathed in several days, and he appears not to have a place of residence. The nurses in the office grumble about caring for this man because he is smelly and dirty. He asks if he can have a cup of coffee from the pot in the corner of the office. The nurse asks him, "Who do you think you are; get and pay for your own coffee." The nurse is asked by the advanced practice nurse to get R.T. some samples of vitamins and an antibiotic for his skin infection from the sample closet. The nurse says, "Why should we give him stuff? He is a bum and probably will only sell them on the street for alcohol." What is the ethical dilemma here? What should the advanced practice nurse do? How should this whole situation be handled?
2. L.G. is starting her own independent practice, which is based on home visits for patients with end-stage chronic obstructive pulmonary disease. She has met all the local, state, and federal requirements for opening a practice, including hiring a collaborating physician and developing a large group of patients who want her services. She has been approved to be on several insurance panels for reimbursement. Dr. R.M. writes a letter to the local hospital and states that L.G. should not be allowed to admit patients to the hospital because she is practicing illegally and will get the hospital in trouble. What ethical principles are at risk in this scenario? How should L.G. handle this problem?
3. A wound care advanced practice nurse who goes to nursing homes all over his state is asked by the agency he works for to increase revenue for the agency by increasing the number of visits to patients even when they do not currently have a wound and to use a higher billing code for the work he does than is necessary. The agency says that "up coding" his visits will not be noticed by insurance companies or Medicare, and if he can increase revenue, the agency might be able to give him a raise. What is the ethical dilemma here? How should the advanced practice nurse handle this problem?
4. M.T., an advanced practice nurse, has a patient who has been referred to a cardiologist. The patient returns to the office and tells M.T. that he went to the cardiologist and had some tests but does not know what the tests showed or if there should be any change in his treatment for coronary

Continued on page 94

Critical Thinking Questions *Continued from page 93*

artery disease. He is still having angina pain weekly and is worried that things might be getting worse. M.T. calls the cardiologist and is told that he will not speak to her because she is not a medical doctor and that she should not be seeing patients. The nurses in the office also tell M.T. that they have been instructed by the cardiologist not to provide M.T. with results or treatment plans. What is the ethical dilemma here? How should the advanced practice nurse handle this problem?

5. S.T. is a clinical nurse specialist (CNS) at a hospital. Several of the nurses on the unit where she works tell her that there is a physician who does not see his hospitalized patients for several days at a time and then writes inappropriate orders for their care. They are concerned for his patients and ask the CNS what they should do.

What other examples of ethical dilemmas have you experienced in practice?

Using the metaparadigm of nursing articulated by Fawcett (1984), which proposes that nursing is interested in person, environment, health, and nursing, social justice is an essential element within practice. Because advanced practice nurses are working with patients in primary care settings, they are well aware of many of the injustices of society and should be advocates for patients to reduce injustice.

Issues of Social Justice in Advanced Practice Nursing

Social justice is defined as the fair distribution of resources and responsibilities among members of a population. Although the many layers of issues and concepts within social justice are not fully covered here, it is important that advanced practice nurses—especially nurses educated at the doctoral level—be aware of the basic tenets of social justice. Social justice seeks to resolve health disparities among the population, including access to care, food, security, adequate housing, acceptable working conditions, employment, access to education, social acceptance, and the presence of a social safety net (World Health Organization, 2008). Using the ideals of social justice to improve aspects of society that have a negative impact on health and well-being of the poorest and most underserved individuals in a society may create positive outcomes that improve the health and well-being of society as a whole.

Social justice has been at the core of nursing philosophy since the days of nursing activists Lillian Ward and Lavinia Dock, who held a vision of health as a social concern (Bekemeier & Butterworth, 2005). Fahrenwald et al. (2005) theorized that the five essential core values in professional nursing are human dignity, integrity, altruism, autonomy, and social justice. Linking social justice to professional nursing is crucial because research indicates that if societal relationships are more equal, population health indicators between diverse groups become more stable nationally and globally (Boutain, 2005).

In a publication prepared by the Canadian Nurses Association (2006) regarding social justice, many questions were proposed to allow advanced practice nurses to evaluate the social justice aspects of their personal practice:

- "Do I routinely associate patient 'noncompliance' with the possibility that the patient has no money for transportation or prescribed treatments?"
- "Is lack of action on my part a form of discrimination?"
- "Does my practice setting consider methods to decrease inequities in access to care and emphasize the social determinants of health with all patients equally?"
- "Does my workplace implement policies that explicitly address social justice? Are these policies reviewed regularly to determine if the policies are implemented?"
- "How does my political party perform on social justice issues such as child poverty and homelessness at the national, state, and local levels?"
- "How do I personally contribute to improve social justice in my community and state?"
- "As an advanced practice nurse, how do I focus on social justice, and how do I help others understand the impact of inequality of the health and well-being of my community and nation?"

In the areas of economics and human effort, health-care rationing is a necessity and requires careful analysis regarding the level of care provided and the equal distribution of care. In the United States, there has long been a debate over whether access to health care is a right or a privilege. That debate remains at the forefront of the social agenda of Americans. Although many other countries of the world take a societal view of the right of all individuals to a minimum level of health care, the United States takes a more individualistic view that people who are able to afford care should be able to purchase it, whereas people who cannot afford to pay for health care either through insurance or privately may be unable to receive what they need. DNPs will be challenged with the duty to overcome the moral hazards of the "fee for services" health-care system now in place and replace it with a system that is socially just, provides care at a level that is cost-effective, and combines the advances of science and technology with the determinants of health and well-being among all people.

Advancing Your Knowledge

A group of advanced practice nurses has decided to open a free clinic for underserved people. Each nurse will volunteer his or her time for a set number of hours per week. The group has a collaborating physician who will also donate hours to the clinic. They have worked with the local medical association and

Continued on page 96

Advancing Your Knowledge *Continued from page 95*

the Health Department to arrange for specialty care and referrals. Several civic leaders are lobbying to keep the clinic from opening because they say it will attract undesirable people to the area. They have asked for a meeting between the nurse practitioners, physicians, and the town council to discuss the issue.

1. How can this be presented as a social justice issue?
2. Some Americans are concerned that too much help makes people less likely to help themselves, that too much governmental intervention creates a "welfare" state. How can these concepts be reconciled with social justice?
3. Take each of the determinants of health provided in the discussion on social justice, and describe how advanced practice nurses could create improvements in these areas for the populations you serve in practice. Remember, populations can include older adults, nursing staff, or ethnic or cultural groups.
4. *Social Work Today*, a journal for social workers, has outlined the top four issues in social justice in the United States:
   - Celebrating diversity
   - Health-care reform
   - Child welfare and protection (20% [1 in 5] of American children live in poverty)
   - Poverty and economic injustice

What is your feeling about each of these issues? How can nurses affect and help to resolve some of these social inequities? Should nurses even get involved? What are the barriers to providing social justice in the United States? How does social justice link with democratic values and legislative issues in the United States today?

Nurses work within organizations, whether they are hospitals, community organizations, government organizations, or large health-care organizations outside of the hospital environment. It is essential for DNP-prepared nurses, as leaders in health care, to work within organizations to advocate for patients, commit to social justice, and improve patient outcomes. To be as effective as possible in large organizations, the DNP-prepared advanced practice nurse should be familiar with organizational science and systems theory.

Organizational Science: Systems Theory

The study of organizations from multiple viewpoints and levels of analysis is termed *organizational science*. Understanding how organizations work, the cultures within organizations, and the idea of organizations as communities is the work of organizational science. Components of organizational structure include decision making; organizational design; and understanding the effect of personality, stress, and motivation within organizations. Using a systems framework to analyze and create opportunities for improvement in organizations is a positive way to improve personal health within communities and health-care organizations.

Organizations—whether families, communities, or health-care organizations—are systems, and systems thinking should be used to assess, evaluate, and change behaviors within each system. Systems thinking views any organization as a whole and focuses on interrelationships and patterns to understand the dynamics of the organization. Systems thinking is a holistic approach to the understanding and pattern recognition within organizations. Refuting the claims of Descartes that a system could be broken into its smallest parts and analyzed independently to understand the entire entity, Ludwig von Bertalanffy (1901–1972) theorized that systems can be comprehended only by understanding the interaction between components and the nonlinear aspects of these interactions (von Bertalanffy, 1950).

Systems theory is an interdisciplinary field of science that studies complex systems in nature, society, and science. More specifically, it is a framework by which one can analyze or describe any group of objects that work together to produce some result. The DNP-prepared nurse may be responsible not only for patient care but also for the management of a group of interdisciplinary health-care providers and workers and must understand the complex nature of any group.

General systems theory was first outlined by von Bertalanffy in 1928. He believed that logical positivism was wrong in its assumption that studying the various components of a system in a linear fashion would create a description of the whole system. According to von Bertalanffy, systems can be studied in three ways: (1) A *holist* approach examines the system as a complete functioning unit. (2) A *reductionist* approach looks downward and examines the subsystems within the system. (3) The *functionalist* approach looks upward from the system to examine the role it plays in the larger system. All three approaches recognize the existence of subsystems operating within a larger system.

In a closed system, interactions occur only among the system components and not with the environment. In an open system, input is received from the environment, and outputs from the system are released into the environment. The basic characteristic of an open system is the dynamic interaction of its components. Medical practices are open systems, where the workers interact with patients, families, and other social groups. In this way, the medical practice receives input from insurers and the developer of guidelines for health promotion. The outputs of this group are patient assessments, testing, treatments, and management of chronic diseases. The identification of how these inputs and outputs are managed in any practice or medical care setting is essential for the practice to be successful financially, in the area of patient outcomes, and in meeting legal and legislative requirements.

A system is composed of regularly interacting or interrelating groups of activities. Organizations are complex social systems; reducing the parts from the whole reduces the overall effectiveness of organizations. Conventional models center on individuals, structures, departments, and units as separate from the whole instead of recognizing the interdependence between groups of individuals, structures, and processes that enables an organization to function. Kuhn (1974) referred to the detector, selector, and effector functions of a system:

- The *detector* is concerned with the communication of information between systems, such as between health-care systems and patients.
- The *selector* is defined by the rules that the system uses to make decisions, such as who receives care and at what level.
- The *effector* is the means by which transactions are made between systems, such as the health-care organization and the community.

Communication and transaction are the only intersystem interactions, and they determine what happens within any given system. Communication is the exchange of information, whereas transaction involves the exchange of matter-energy. All organizational and social interactions involve communication or transaction or both. Communication and transaction provide the methods for a system to achieve equilibrium. Culture within an organization is the learned patterns of behavior communicated throughout all levels of the system. When society is viewed as a system, culture is seen as a pattern in the system.

Using the principles of systems theory, Janecka (2009) reviewed the U.S. health-care system for effectiveness and efficiency. Findings from his research determined that the U.S. health-care system is incomplete and is threatened because it is chaotic in function. Recommendations from this research include a statement that the health-care system in the United States would dramatically improve its value to society and increase its long-term sustainability by taking several concrete steps. These include prioritizing health over care by promoting health and supporting changes in health behaviors rather than simply caring for the sick and introducing health and life insurance for all. Janecka (2009) stated that the guideposts are easily visible, but the future of health care in the United States is up to the citizenry.

Critical Thinking Questions

- You are the administrator for a large health-care company that operates 35 primary care offices in three states. This company hires physicians, nurse practitioners, and office staff and has a billing company that provides services. You are asked to analyze why three of these offices seem to be less able to attract patients than the others. Each of the practices is in similarly populated areas with similar demographics. How would you use systems thinking to determine the issues for these three clinics? If you found the reasons, what would be the next step?
- You are the director of a federal qualified health clinic in a predominantly Hispanic community. Your clinic services 11,000 people. Diabetes is a common disease that you treat. Epidemiologic data from the clinic show that less than 50% of the diabetics in the clinic are at goal for blood sugar, weight, and blood pressure. How would you use a systems approach to determine how to fix this problem and help these patients?

- You are a clinical nurse specialist in a hospital, and you notice a problem with patients who have chest tubes. These patients seem to do poorly compared with patients with chest tubes in other hospitals, especially in the area of infection and the time it takes for the lung to reinflate and the chest tube to be removed. The nurses complain about the current chest tube being used, and they tell you that they often have to wait for new tubing or supplies to care for these patients. The hospital has recently had a high turnover of nursing staff, and about 25% of the nursing staff has less than 2 years of experience. How would you approach these problems using a systems theory method? How would you make things better?
- Describe the organization in which you work. Use organizational science to create a picture of the workings of this organization. If you wanted to make changes in organizational thinking, structure, or culture, how would you do this using systems thinking?
- How could the values, theories, and ideas in systems and organizational science assist the United States to create a less fragmented and more efficient health-care delivery system?
- How could you use systems and organizational thinking in your own practice to improve health promotion and disease prevention among your patients? If you are an administrator, how could you use systems and organizational thinking to improve the job satisfaction and performance of staff?

Conclusion

This chapter reviewed the progression of scientific thought and the development of theory throughout the Western world, starting with the Greek philosophers. Nursing as a profession has developed amid all of these philosophical ideas. Because professions are created to meet the needs of society, theory development and testing are used to determine and identify the boundaries of nursing as a profession and the ability of nurses to meet societal needs. Because nursing is a practice discipline, theories must be linked to practice, and practicing nurses must use theory to create a framework for everyday practice. Theories have different levels of abstraction and use. For nursing, metatheory frames the entire discipline and provides an overarching idea of the ways in which the profession should frame the work that is done in practice. Nursing models are the second level of theory and provide ideas about ways of being with others. Grand theory provides a broad idea of the role of nursing practice and defines the concepts involved in practice. Middle range theories are discussed in detail in this chapter because they are among the most useful for advanced practice nurses. Middle range theories have a limited number of variables, are more specific, and can be tested in practice. Microrange theory is very specific to a task or functions within nursing and is valuable as a tool for understanding the best way to complete a task, such as caring for a decubitus ulcer. DNPs are important to theory testing and the advancement of nursing as a discipline and profession.

This chapter discussed the ethical issues relevant to advanced practice nursing. The ANA code of ethics for nursing outlines ethical responsibilities for the profession. Ethics is a central concept in caring theory, and it is the way nurses envision themselves as a profession. Respect for human dignity is an important priority in practice, and nurses are required to put the patient first in their ethical and moral practice. Acting in an ethical manner requires nurses to use effective communication skills and have a willingness to act in concert with others in the health-care professions. The concept of social justice was also discussed as an adjunct to ethics. Social justice is an issue that focuses on resolving health disparities and providing humans with the tools to remain healthy, such as good food, clean water, a clean environment, safety, and acceptable working conditions.

Finally, this chapter discussed organizational science. Organizational science enables advanced practice nurses to understand the idea of organizations as communities and the cultures and work habits of organizations. Organizational science uses systems theory to understand the complexities and workings of organizations. Further readings on topics from this chapter are listed in Table 2-9.

Table 2-9

Further Readings on Topics From This Chapter

Social Justice

Barry, B. (2005). *Why social justice matters*. Cambridge, UK: Polity Press

Kenny, M., Horne, A. M., Orpinas, P., & Reese, L. (Eds.) (2009). *Realizing social justice: The challenge of preventive interventions*. Washington, D.C.: American Psychological Association

Raaman, R., & Steinler, B. (2008). *The moral foundation of public health and health policy: Issues in bio ethics*. Oxford, UK: Oxford Press

Systems Theory

Lazlo, E. (2001). *The system view of the world: A holistic vision of our time. Advances in systems theory, complexity and human science*. Cresswell, NJ: Hampton Press

von Bertalanffy, L. (1969). *General systems theory: Foundation, development*. New York: Brazilla Inc

Philosophy of Science

Godfrey-Smith, P. (2003). *Theory and reality and introduction to the philosophy of science*. Chicago, IL: University of Chicago Press

Ladyman, J. (2002). *Understanding the philosophy of science*. New York: Rutledge Press

Samir, O. (2002). *Philosophy of science: A very short introduction*. Oxford, UK: Oxford University Press

Ethics

Benjamin, M., & Curtis, J. (1992). *Ethics in nursing*. Oxford, UK: Oxford University Press

Butts, J., & Rich, K. (2005). *Nursing ethics across the curriculum and into practice*. Ontario, Canada: Jones & Bartlett

References

Aiken, L. H., Clarke, S., Cheung, R., Sloane, D. M., & Silber, J. (2003). Educational levels of hospital nurse and surgical patient mortality. *Journal of the American Medical Association, 290*(12), 1617–1623.

American Association of Colleges of Nursing. (2006). Essentials of doctoral education for advanced nursing practice. Retrieved from http://www.aacn.nche.edu/publications/position/DNPEssentials.pdf

American Nurses Association. (2005). Code of ethics for nursing with interpretive statements. Retrieved from http://www.nursingworld.org/MainMenuCategories/EthicsStandards/CodeofEthicsforNurses.aspx

Bailey, D. E., & Stewart, J. L. (2001). Mishel's theory of uncertainty in illness. In A. M. Mariner-Tomey & M. R. Alligood (Eds.), *Nursing theorists and their work* (5th ed.) (pp. 257–273). St. Louis, MO: Mosby.

Bekemeier, B., & Butterworth, P. (2005). Unreconciled inconsistencies: A critical view of the concept of social justice in 3 national nursing documents. *Advances in Nursing Science, 28*(2), 152–162.

Belgan, M. A., & Tripp-Reimer, T. (1997). Implications for nursing taxonomies for middle range theory development. *Advances in Nursing Science, 19*(3), 37–49.

Boutain, D. M. (2005). Social justice as a framework for professional nursing. *Journal of Nursing Education, 44*(9), 404–408.

Canadian Nurses Association. (2006). Social justice: A means to an end; an end in itself. Retrieved from https://www.ethicshare.org/node/716955

Carper, B. (1978). Fundamental patterns of knowing in nursing. *Advances in Nursing Science, 1*(1), 13–23.

de Chardin, P. T. (2003). *The human phenomenon*. East Sussex, UK: Sussex Academic Press.

Dixon, J., Larison, K., & Zabari, M., (2006). Skilled communication: Making it real. *Advances in Critical Care, 17*(4), 376–382.

Doane, G., Pauly, B., Brown, H., & McPherson, G. (2004). Exploring the heart of ethical nursing practice. Implications for ethics education. *Nursing Ethics, 11*(3), 240–253.

Duffy, J. (2005). Implementing the quality care model in acute care. *Journal of Nursing Administration, 35*(1), 4–6.

Eakes, G. G., Burke, M. L., & Hainsworth, M. A. (1998). Middle range theory of chronic sorrow. *Journal of Nursing Scholarship, 30*(2), 1547–1569.

Erickson, H. C., Tomlin, E. M., & Swain, M. A. (2005). *Modeling and role-modeling: A theory and paradigm for nursing* (8th printing). Cedar Park, EST Company. (Original printing by Prentice Hall, 1983).

Fahrenwald, N. L., Bassett, S. D., Tschetter, L., Carson, P. P., White, L., & Winterboer, V. J. (2005). Teaching core nursing values. *Journal of Professional Nursing, 21*(1), 46–51.

Falk-Rafael, A. (2005). Advancing nursing theory through theory-guided practice: The emergence of a critical caring perspective. *Advances in Nursing Science, 28*(1), 38–49.

Fawcett, J. (1984). Analysis and evaluation of conceptual models of nursing. *Research and Nursing in Health, 7*(4), 334–335.

Fawcett, J. (2000). *Analysis and evaluation of contemporary nursing knowledge: Nursing models and theories.* Philadelphia, PA: F.A. Davis.

Goethels, S., Gastmans, C., & de Casterle, B. D. (2010). Nurses' ethical reasoning and behavior: A literature review. *International Journal of Nursing Studies, 47,* 635–650.

Higgins, P., & Moore, S. (2009). Levels of theoretical thinking in nursing. In P. Reed & N. B. Shearer (Eds.), *Perspectives on nursing theory* (5th ed.). Philadelphia, PA: Lippincott Williams & Wilkins.

Janecka, I. P. (2009). Is the U.S. health care an appropriate system? A strategic perspective from science. Healthcare Research International, 7:1.1 doi:10.1186/1478-4505-7-1

Jarrin, O. F. (2007). An integral philosophy and definition of nursing. *School of Nursing Scholarly Works.* Retrieved from http://digitalcommons.uconn.edu/son_articles/47/

Kolcaba, K. Y. (1994). A theory of holistic comfort for nursing. *Journal of Advanced Nursing, 19*(6), 1178–1184.

Kuhn, A. (1974). *The logic of social systems: A unified deductive system based approach to social science.* San Francisco, CA: Jossey-Bass.

Lampert, L. (2010). *How philosophy became Socratic.* Chicago, IL: University of Chicago Press.

Lee, P. (2002). Applying Carper's patterns of knowing to children's nursing today. *Contemporary Nurse, 23*(2), 217–223.

Lenz, E. (2007). Mid-range theory: Impact of knowledge development and use in practice. In C. Roy & D. Jones (Eds.). *Nursing knowledge development and clinical practice.* New York, NY: Springer Publishing Company.

Lenz, E., Suppe, F., Gift, A. G., Pugh, L. C., & Milligan, R. A. (1995). Collaborative development of middle-range theories: Toward a theory of unpleasant symptoms. *Advances in Nursing Science, 17*(3), 1–13.

Mapanga, K. G., & Mapanga, M. B. (2003). A community health nursing perspective of home health care management and practice within the Zimbabwean health care system. *Home Health Care Management and Practice, 15*(5), 429–435.

Mariano, C. (2001). Holistic ethics. *American Journal of Nursing, 10*(1), 24a–24c.

Mars, J. A., & Lowry, L. W. (2006). Nursing theory and practice: Connecting the dots. In P. Reed & N. B. Shearer (Eds.). *Perspectives on Nursing Theory* (5th ed., pp. 18–39). New York, NY: Lippincott Williams & Wilkins.

Maxfield, D., Grenny, G., McMillan, R., Patterson, K., & Switzler, A. (2005). Silence Kills: The seven crucial conversations in healthcare. Report from VitalSmarts. Retrieved from http://www.silencekills.com/UPDL/SilenceKillsExecSummary.pdf

McKenna, H. P. (1997). *Nursing models and theories.* London, UK: Routledge.

McWhinney, I. R. (1989). An acquaintance with particulars. *Family Medicine, 21*(4), 296–298.

Meleis, A. F. (2007). *Theoretical nursing development and progress* (4th ed.). Philadelphia, PA: Lippincott Williams & Wilkins.

Mercer, R. (1985). The process of maternal role attainment over the first year. *Nursing Research,* 34(4), 198–203.

Merton, R. K. (1968). *Social theory and social structure*. New York, NY: The Free Press.
Mishel, M. H. (1988). Uncertainty in illness. *Image: Journal of Nursing Scholarship, 20,* 225–231.
Mishel, M. H. (1990). Reconceptualization of the uncertainty of illness theory. *Image: Journal of Nursing Scholarship, 22,* 256–262.
Mitchell, G. J., & Cody, W. K. (2002). Ambiguous opportunity: Tolling for truth of nursing art and science. *Nursing Science Quarterly, 15*(1), 71–79.
Newman, M. A. (2002). The pattern that connects. *Advances in Nursing Science, 24*(3), 1–7.
Nightingale, F. (1969). *Notes on nursing: What it is and what it is not.* New York, NY: Dover Publications.
Owen, M. J., & Holmes, C. A. (1993). "Holism" in the discourse of nursing. *Journal of Advanced Nursing, 18*(11), 1688–1695.
Patterson, J., & Zderad, L. (2008). Humanistic Nursing. Being and Becoming. Retrieved from http://www.gutenberg.org/files/25020/25020-8.txt
Pender, N. (1975). A conceptual model for preventive health behavior. *Nursing Outlook, 23*(6), 385–390.
Peplau, H. E. (1992). Interpersonal relations: a theoretical framework for application in nursing practice. *Nursing Science Quarterly, 5*(1), 13–18.
Peterson, S. (2009). Interpersonal relations. In S. Peterson & T. Bedrow (Eds.), *Middle range theory: Application to nursing research* (2nd ed.). New York, NY: Lippincott Williams & Wilkins.
Polk, L. V. (1997). Middle range theory of resilience. *Advances in Nursing Science,* 19(3), 14–27.
Reed, P. (1991). Toward a theory of self-transcendence. *Advances in Nursing Science,* 13(4), 1–84.
Ritz, L., Nissen, M. L., Swenson, K., et al. (2000). Effects of advanced nursing care on quality of life and cost outcomes of women diagnosed with breast cancer. *Oncology Nursing Forum, 27,* 923–932.
Ryan, P. (2009). Integrated theory of health behavior change: Background and intervention development. *Clinical Nurse Specialist, 23*(3), 161–170.
Silva, M., & Ludwick R. (2006). Ethics: Is the doctor of nursing practice ethical? *The Online Journal of Issues in Nursing*. Retrieved from http://www.medscape.com/viewarticle/536482
Smith, M. J., & Liehr, P. R. (2008). *Middle range theory for nursing*. New York, NY: Springer Publishing Company.
Swanson, K. (1991). Empirical development of a middle range theory of caring. *Nursing Research, 40*(3), 132–191.
UNESCO: International Bureau of Education. (1998). Florence Nightingale. *Prospects: The Quarterly Review of Comparative Education, 28*(1), 153–156.
von Bertalanffy, L. (1950). An outline of the general systems theory. *British Sociology, Philosophy and Science, I*(2), 134–165.
Whittmore, R., & Roy C. (2002). Adapting to diabetes mellitus: A theory synthesis. *Nursing Science Quarterly, 15*(4) 311–317.
World Health Organization. (2008). *Health equity through action on the social determinants of health*. Geneva: Author.

CHAPTER

3

CLINICAL SCHOLARSHIP AND ANALYTICAL METHODS FOR EVIDENCE-BASED PRACTICE

Translating Research into Practice

Objectives:

By the end of the chapter, students should be able to:

1. Define and describe clinical scholarship and the role of the doctor of nursing practice (DNP) as a clinical scholar by:
   - Identifying the ways of knowing in nursing, analyzing the need for creating inquiry in nursing practice areas, and relating the ways of knowing to clinical inquiry.
   - Assessing barriers and challenges in crossing the research-to-practice gap in nursing.
2. Define and evaluate research by:
   - Discussing innovative ways in which to improve nursing through research and evidence-based practice.
   - Analyzing the differences between and appropriate uses of research studies and quality improvement projects.
   - Evaluating and critiquing quantitative and qualitative research for rigor, appropriateness, validity, reliability, and generalizability.
   - Defining evidence-based research, mixed methods research, and participatory action research and how these types of research can be beneficial to evidence-based practice.

3. Analyze the need for multidisciplinary research teams, and describe the role of the DNP in these teams.
4. Describe examples of evidence in practice, examples of DNP capstone projects, and the ability of these projects to be translated into practice.
5. Review methods for development of practice and clinical guidelines.

Scholarship is a method of uncovering, testing, and accepting knowledge. Nursing scholars concentrate on uncovering knowledge through research and exploration and then applying that knowledge in practice. Inquiry aimed at uncovering knowledge is used by scholars within a discipline to make claims about the world, validate discipline-specific theory, and create new knowledge. Scholars are responsible for uncovering facts and truths in a defined area and making these facts and truths known to the public. To accomplish this type of scholarship, researchers use investigation, theory testing, and dissemination of the new knowledge. Scholars take research findings and test and retest them in practice for the purpose of creating standards of care that are foundational to a profession.

Applying research findings in a practice area and changing practice habits with any regularity can be challenging. The Agency for Healthcare Research and Quality (2007) reported that there can be a 10- to 20-year gap between the uncovering and dissemination of research findings and the implementation of these findings into standard health-care practice. The gap between research and practice continues to be a stumbling block for health-care professionals. This chapter describes and defines clinical scholarship as it relates to the doctor of nursing practice (DNP) and delineates methods for translating research into practice. The chapter also defines and evaluates research methods, discusses the need for multidisciplinary teams of researchers, and reviews examples of DNP-specific research.

Clinical Scholarship

Clinical scholars use new knowledge developed from research evidence to change and improve practice. Clinical scholarship is critical to the DNP. The DNP performs literature reviews, uses practice-based intervention design based on findings from reviews, and tests the interventions developed in practice. The arena of clinical scholarship includes the following:

1. The scholarship of discovery and application entails clinical scholars testing research findings in practice areas and creating standardized protocols and treatment guidelines based on the success of application.
2. The scholarship of integration allows for connections to be made across disciplines to coordinate care and provide solutions to common health-care problems that are not discipline-specific. It incorporates the ideas and solutions of groups of health-care professions.

3. Scholarship can also be recognized in the application of solutions beyond the phase of discovery where interventions are proven to be successful in specific situations. This type of scholarship directs evidence toward larger groups of communities, patients, and families.

In "The Essentials of Doctoral Education for Advanced Practice Nurses," the American Association of Colleges of Nursing (2006) listed the following objectives as important for the preparation of DNP students in the area of clinical scholarship:

- Use analytical methods to appraise existing literature and other evidence critically to determine and implement the best evidence for practice.
- Design and implement processes to evaluate outcomes of practice, practice patterns, and systems of care within a practice setting, health-care organization, or community against national benchmarks to determine variances in practice outcomes and population trends.
- Design, direct, and evaluate quality improvement methodologies to promote safe, timely, effective, efficient, equitable, and patient-centered care.
- Apply relevant findings to develop practice guidelines and improve practice and the practice environment.
- Use information technology and research methods appropriately to:
  - Collect appropriate and accurate data to generate evidence for nursing practice,
  - Inform and guide the design of databases that generate meaningful evidence for nursing practice,
  - Analyze data from practice,
  - Design evidence-based interventions, and
  - Predict and analyze outcomes.
- Function as a practice specialist or consultant in collaborative knowledge-generating research.
- Disseminate findings from evidence-based practice and research to improve health-care outcomes.

For practice-based inquiry to be successful in health-care settings, advanced practice nurses should champion research initiatives. The role of these advanced practice nursing leaders is to use their expanded knowledge and skill in research, research evaluation, and clinical nursing to move the discipline forward and advance the value of nursing in society.

Creating Inquiry Within Practice

In terms of the research skills expected of DNPs, nursing leadership groups such as the American Association of Colleges of Nursing focus on clinical inquiry within practice settings and evaluating research findings for application to practice. Clinical inquiry informs practice through the use of research findings and experiential learning (Hardin & Kaplow, 2005). Clinical inquiry requires evidence from research findings and evidence from the nurse's experience to determine and define best practice. As a leader in the nursing profession, the DNP should be involved in inquiry, should motivate other nurses at the practice level to increase the use of evidence-based practice, and should direct evidence-based change in the practice setting (Kleinpell, 2008).

Clinical inquiry creates positive outcomes for patients, improves nurses' sense of autonomy, and allows for the expansion of nursing knowledge (Gross & Fogg, 2001). A sense of awareness of the importance of research to clinical practice, identification of best practice initiatives, the development of research projects that target quality indicators, and emphasis on research in areas of special interest increase positive attitudes of nurses toward clinical inquiry.

It is important that nurses come to examine nursing and nursing interventions in light of current knowledge and nursing experiences to determine methods to improve work and patient outcomes. Applying findings from nursing research studies is one method of stimulating interest in clinical inquiry. For example, if creating a clinical support group for women with osteoporosis is found to be beneficial based on research studies, replicating this type of group in a particular practice setting would create a sense of engagement with the research findings, extend research findings to a larger group, and create a method to develop programs that are specific to the population receiving care.

Another strategy for increasing interest in clinical inquiry is to work with nurses to highlight research studies pertinent to their practice area. There are many ways to highlight or present research findings, including poster presentations, journal clubs, and staff meetings. Suppose a hospital is initiating a rapid response team to assist in early recognition and response to clinical problems in individual patients. The hospital could use posters and other presentations of research evidence that illustrates that these teams improve both patient outcomes and the nursing work environment. When this type of strategy is employed, nurses are more likely to accept and welcome innovation because it is supported by research evidence (Mikos-Schild, Endara, & Calvario, 2010).

Advancing Your Knowledge

Because of government regulations and patient safety issues, the nurses at a small hospital have been assigned to devise a method for assessing the risk for deep vein thrombosis (DVT) and pulmonary embolism (PE) in patients admitted to the hospital. The nurses are charged with proposing a method for increasing the use of appropriate prophylaxis measures in patients who have significant risk levels. The team includes a nurse from each unit and is led by a nurse practitioner with a DNP. The group began by gathering all of the information they could find about the risk factors, incidence, and prevalence of hospital-acquired DVT and PE and appropriate levels of prophylaxis for prevention of these problems. Based on the findings of the literature review, the nurses developed a risk assessment tool, which they used to evaluate the risk of all persons who had experienced DVT or PE in the hospital for the prior year. They matched the mean scores on the assessment tool of persons who had DVT or PE against persons who did not and found that the individuals who had DVT or PE had a higher mean score than the individuals who did not have hospital-acquired DVT or PE. Because the nurses were able to validate the risk assessment tool, the rest of the nursing staff members were willing to test it out in the hospital. Nurses were very pleased with the outcomes of their work and were especially pleased when a manuscript describing what they had done was published in a peer-reviewed nursing journal. The DNP leader of this group was pleased with the ability of the nurses to embrace research findings, combine them with their own experience, develop the tool, and test it for validity.

1. Choose a problem that you have experienced in providing care to patients or in an administrative role. Complete a literature search, identify five to seven research-based articles about this issue, and compile an evidence-based opinion of how this problem might be resolved.
2. The components of evidence-based practice include research evidence, experience, and patient preference. Why are these three components necessary to make a difference in patient care?

History of Nursing Clinical Inquiry

Discipline-specific clinical inquiry is necessary to increase the understanding of clinical practice issues and best practices. Clinical scholars must be empowered to participate in multidisciplinary research teams to bring nursing values, principles, and standards into the research plan. Similarly, clinical scholars must be able to coordinate research dissemination, integration, and application with nurses of other backgrounds to promote continuous quality improvement and to close the gap between research and practice. The creation of a group of clinical scholars in nursing that is distinct from researchers with an orientation in traditional basic knowledge and theory development would increase the visibility of nursing work. The DNP with expert clinical knowledge and an understanding of research would be able to create an atmosphere in practice where use of research is the norm.

The idea of basing practice on the findings of evidence was introduced by Florence Nightingale as she compiled statistical evidence to demonstrate the positive effects of cleanliness in the operating room and during recovery from surgery (Nightingale, 1869). Nightingale combined the knowledge gained in practice with the statistical evidence from research studies to create guidelines for physicians, nurses, and health-care institutions regarding cleanliness and healing environments. These guidelines are credited with saving lives and propelled Nightingale into the forefront of health care in England for that period. Following her return from the Crimea in 1860, Nightingale established schools of nursing that used scientific methods and evidence-based practice to educate nurses.

As scientific and technological advancements emerged and the male-dominated profession of medicine gained authority and power over health-care practice, the profession of nursing became more focused on tasks. Usual practice or habit replaced evidence as the primary method for educating nurses. In the United States, nurses were trained in hospital settings where they performed nursing tasks as part of their training and learned from others with more experience. Because many hospitals were attached to religious orders, teachers came from religious backgrounds rather than educational backgrounds. These "diploma" nurses were well trained in tasks and processes but were not well informed in methods of gathering and using data to provide evidence for best practice in patient care. Leaders in health care at the time were opposed to advanced education for nurses because they considered it unnecessary and costly (Rogers, 2009).

However, as the complexity of health care increased, the role of the nurse became more complicated, and the need for nurses to be educated using an evidence basis for practice became essential. Nurses were charged with higher-level assessment and intervention skills, and their ability to use these skills became increasingly important. As nurses assumed more responsibility for patient safety, patient outcomes, and cost, the ability of nurses to use evidence as the basis for practice became more necessary.

Kim (2000) reviewed the emergence and history of evidence-based practice in modern nursing. In the 1970s, the emphasis was on quality improvement and cost-effectiveness. In the 1980s, nursing leaders centered their efforts on doing the right thing, at the right time, but these decisions were not based on nursing scholarship. Rather, they were based on what may have been best for the health-care institution. At the present time, the emphasis in nursing is on using the evidence of research, drawn from the various ways of knowing, to design nursing interventions that improve patient outcomes and increase satisfaction.

Ways of Knowing

Enhancing clinical inquiry requires various methods to create and evaluate new knowledge and translate that new knowledge into standard nursing practice. Both academic and clinical nurses acknowledge the significance of multiple *ways of knowing* in nursing that influence the questions asked in clinical inquiry and how answers are framed. Nursing is a multidimensional discipline within itself. It is shaped not only by the empirical sciences but also by shared experiences; relationships with patients; and ethical, esthetic, sociopolitical, and personal ways of knowing.

Carper (1978) wrote a seminal article that outlined, identified, and explored four different ways and patterns of knowing in nursing: personal knowing, esthetic knowing, empirical knowing, and ethical knowing. These patterns of knowing provide the discipline with perspective and significance, and they link theory and research to practice by providing a foundation from which nursing work can be conceived and understood. Using the ways of knowing in practice provides nurses with an increased awareness of the complexity and diversity of the discipline.

Personal patterns of knowing are created through attitudes and knowledge from personal understanding or self-understanding. When a nurse puts himself or herself in the patient's position and tries to empathize with what the patient is experiencing, the knowledge gained comes through personal knowing. *Esthetic knowing* encompasses the awareness of the immediate moment and being authentically present in that moment to understand a patient's circumstance as uniquely individual. Perceiving persons as whole and complete in the moment and coming to know them as whole and complete are aspects of esthetic knowing.

Empirical knowing is factual and scientific in the truest sense. Measurements of vital signs and laboratory results are empirical. Knowing that a patient can walk because the patient has demonstrated that he or she can do so is also empirical knowing. *Ethical knowing* takes into account the moral choices that are made regarding a patient or attitudes toward patients and families. An example is identifying patterns of abhorrent objectionable behavior by a patient and then being able to care for the patient despite the behavior.

Since the first description of the ways of knowing, several other patterns have been added, such as sociopolitical knowing (Barker, 2009). *Sociopolitical knowing* takes into account how we come to see and know patterns that are socially or politically developed. Nurses who work with undocumented persons often see patterns of fear and distrust in all aspects of communication. Reflective knowing is another later addition to the ways of knowing and identifying patterns. *Reflective knowing* comes from the reflection of the nurse as situations arise and the ability to recognize patterns and know persons based on those reflections (John, 2008). A final way of knowing has been proposed called *unknowing* (Holtzlander, 2008). Unknowing is achieved by allowing all of the other ways of knowing and pattern recognition to fall away in order to be in the moment and, without any preconceived ideas, hear the patient's call for nursing care at that specific moment.

Science tries to control and predict the occurrence of phenomena; however, when working with human beings, control and prediction are not always possible because of multiple confounding variables and situations. Although nursing science has different professional aims than traditional science, it is no less important that nurses use evidence gathered through the multiple ways of knowing to promote positive patient outcomes, increase patient safety while undergoing health-care procedures, and increase the satisfaction of patients receiving nursing care. All of these ways of acquiring, processing, reflecting, and evaluating nursing knowledge are important in developing a comprehensive clinical perspective.

Using Reflection, Intuition, and Introspection to Uncover Evidence

Using an evidence-based approach to nursing interventions and being able to understand the findings of research are important aspects of advanced practice nursing. The development of evidence-based plans of care to ensure patient health, well-being, and safety should be central to advanced practice nursing. Using reflection, intuition, and introspection as tools to uncover clinically applicable evidence is common in nursing. Reflective practice is a conscious process that enables the advanced practice nurse to evaluate practice as he or she draws from work experiences or situations (Manthey, 2004). Using reflection in practice implies a conscious focus and an individual evaluation of the outcomes of practice. In reflective practice, nurses engage in an analysis of any situation by questioning the meaning of the situation itself and reflecting on the best method for approaching the situation. Atkins and Murphy (1993) provided the phases through which a reflective practitioner moves when faced with a complex patient situation. The first phase is a thought or feeling that the current knowledge is insufficient to explain what is happening. In the second phase, the nurse critically assesses the situation to be unique and to require new knowledge. The final phase is the development of a new perspective for the treatment of this unique situation that meets the needs of all involved.

Cirocco (2007) found that when nurses used reflective practice—including journaling and discussion with other nurses—it enhanced their critical thinking and problem-solving ability. Maloney and Hahessy (2005) stated that the ability to reflect is a critical component for the development of competency and is vital to professional growth. These authors proposed that using reflection in practice makes knowledge explicit and tangible and creates a sense of ownership of the knowledge imbedded in practice.

Intuition is knowledge based on a deep grasp of a subject, even without being able to articulate how the understanding was reached (Silva, 2011). Introspection can be described as a looking inward—specifically, the act or process of self-examination, or inspection of one's own thoughts and feelings; the cognition that the mind has of its own acts and states; self-consciousness. Contemplating and examining thoughts and observing personal feelings that come from patient and family interactions and determining the meaning of those interactions and personal feelings are uses of introspection that reveal evidence.

The discipline of nursing requires interaction with patients in ways that are therapeutic. Reflection, intuition, and introspection are essential elements in the development of evidence for clinical excellence and scholarship in nursing practice. Reflection on past events and interactions with patients and the outcomes of these interactions can be used as evidence. For example, when caring for a "difficult" patient, you may reflect on interactions during the patient's last visit and, through introspection, examine your feelings to uncover evidence that may lead you to be more successful in caring for this patient even though he or she is difficult.

Advancing Your Knowledge

Many women's health practices in the United States require women to have a yearly pap smear to obtain a prescription for contraceptive medications or receive a contraceptive injection. There is no relationship between pap smear findings and the safety of contraceptive medication use. Health-care providers create this requirement to increase the numbers of women who get pap smears yearly as a preventive measure. The evidence and nursing experience point to a flaw in this plan. Women without health insurance or the ability to pay for a pap smear or who find the experience distasteful do not have a pap smear and so are unable to get contraceptive medications. Unwanted pregnancies result. One nationally known gynecologist has stated that if we really followed evidence-based practice, oral contraceptives would be over-the-counter (because they have very well-defined contraindications that can be understood by patients), and patients would need a prescription to obtain cigarettes (Grimes, 1995).

1. How do you feel about this issue? Do you agree with the current policy about pap smears and oral contraceptives?
2. In what circumstances would you override this policy?
3. How does evidence-based practice in this instance use research evidence, nursing experience, and patient preferences?

Advancing Your Knowledge

B.W. is a patient in a primary health-care practice and generally sees the advanced practice nurse for her care. B.W. works as a physical therapist and is knowledgeable about her health and well-being. Blood work revealed that B.W. is anemic. As part of the evaluation of the anemia, B.W. was referred to a gastroenterologist where she underwent an upper and lower endoscopy. The upper endoscopy revealed a tumor in the stomach, which on biopsy was found to be adenocarcinoma of the stomach. The gastroenterologist sent B.W. to a surgeon who told her they would schedule surgery to remove most of her stomach within the next 2 weeks. B.W. told the surgeon that she wanted to explore alternative options and wanted to speak with an herbal specialist she had seen in the past. The surgeon became angry and said he would not see her again. B.W. came back to the primary care office to see the nurse practitioner. As expected, she was devastated by and afraid of her diagnosis. She told the nurse practitioner that she was afraid of having her stomach removed because she would never be able to eat again. The nurse practitioner comforted B.W. and told her to make her appointment with the herbal specialist and come back to see her in 2 or 3 days.

During that time, the nurse practitioner reflected on the situation. She realized that surgery was the best and almost only option for B.W., but she also realized that if B.W. resisted or was uncomfortable with this procedure, she might not do well. Over the course of the next 2 weeks, B.W. came to see the nurse practitioner four times. Between each visit, the nurse practitioner reflected on what the patient said, how her situation was unique, and what could be done to assist her in this time of crisis. Each time the nurse practitioner and

Continued on page 114

Advancing Your Knowledge *Continued from page 113*

B.W. met, they discussed what the herbalist had said, and the nurse practitioner gently guided B.W. by sharing with her information about adenocarcinoma of the stomach and treatment options. Over these weeks, the nurse practitioner and B.W. agreed that the patient required surgery and that she could continue with the recommended herbs and other supplements that might strengthen her for this procedure. B.W. and the nurse practitioner also discussed the fact that B.W. was the best judge of what was right for her body. B.W. and the nurse practitioner cried together and discussed what would happen after surgery. They talked about B.W.'s life, what she hoped for as she aged, and her ideas about how to cope. After 2 weeks, B.W. flew to the city where her sister lived, consulted a surgeon, had the surgery, and recovered at her sister's home. The nurse practitioner realized that her reflection on this patient's problems allowed her to reason that the patient needed to be able to see her herbalist and needed some time to adjust to the idea of surgery. B.W. still sees the nurse practitioner for checkups and frequently expresses her gratitude for the nurse practitioner's patience and care. The nurse practitioner was able to see that this situation was unique and analyze the situation critically to develop a plan that allowed the patient to remain in control and make a decision in her own time.

1. Can you think of a situation in which you used reflective practice to create new ideas about care?
2. How does reflective practice create opportunities for advanced practice nurses to use clinical scholarship in practice?
3. How is this type of practice scientific?

Ways of Knowing as Clinical Inquiry to Develop Evidence

Both academic and clinical nurses acknowledge the significance of multiple ways of knowing in nursing practice. These ways of knowing direct clinical inquiry and create evidence that can be used to direct patient care. In her metatheory on the ways of knowing in nursing, Carper (1978) proposed that nurses have multiple ways of "coming to know" and assist patients in ways that are not based on traditional scientific methods but that are effective and essential to providing care. Nursing is a multidimensional, holistic discipline shaped not only by the empirical sciences but also by shared experiences; relationships with patients; and ethical, esthetic, sociopolitical, and personal ways of knowing.

In an effort to expand the definition of evidence-based practice in nursing, McKenna, Cutliffe, and McKenna (1999) discussed the myths that surround what constitutes evidence and the need to use multiple ways of knowing to provide effective nursing interventions. They began their exploration by describing the methods nurses use to establish evidence of the effectiveness of an intervention, including findings of traditional research investigation, testing interventions supported by the opinion of experts in the field and continuous quality improvement activities, and the use of traditions that have been proved successful over the years and handed down from one generation of nurses to another. These authors posited that Carper's ways of knowing can be equated with the types of evidence used in nursing practice. Empirical knowing can be created through traditional scientific research; esthetic knowing is the art or intuition of nursing; ethical knowing is the ability to use expert opinion and tradition about what is just, fair, and right as well as using the nurse's own perceptions of justice and fairness; and personal knowing is the ability of the nurse to use personal experience and experience that has been handed down from other nurses to develop solid evidence-based practice interventions.

Advanced practice nurses are charged with caring for patients in many different areas of health care with complex physical, psychosocial, cultural, emotional, and geopolitical issues. It is essential that practitioners perceive all types of knowing as valuable and that they use all of the methods for gathering evidence to promote the most effective interventions and provide the best in patient outcomes, safety, and satisfaction. Although the remainder of this chapter focuses on research evidence (because it is the most foreign concept to most advanced practice nursing students), that focus should not be viewed as discounting the importance of all of the other types of evidence when developing practice patterns and guidelines. Advanced practice nurses are charged with using the multiple ways of knowing—and their accompanying evidence-gathering modes—to create more appropriate care methods, to assist patients to make life changes to improve health behaviors, and to provide comprehensive and compassionate care to all patients. Translating knowing and the ways of knowing into the practice setting creates interventions and behaviors that are evidence-based and cross the research to practice divide.

Barriers to Crossing the Research to Practice Divide: Obstacles to and the Imperative of Evidence-Based Practice

Crossing the research to practice divide is a focus of many nursing leaders who are searching for innovative methods to develop evidence-based practices that improve quality, effectiveness, and safety in the health-care setting (Rogers, 2009). Nevertheless, significant barriers remain to introducing research evidence into practice. Change must be gradual, and too many changes in too short a time frame can cause confusion and make it difficult to evaluate what works and what does not in a particular nursing area. Sustaining change is also challenging. Nurses who are challenged to change must be supported and encouraged to sustain the level of commitment to the change. The effect and outcomes of the change must be evaluated routinely to determine the effect on patient outcomes, nursing workload, and acceptability of the new intervention.

Obstacles to creating evidence-based practice in health-care settings remain and continue to impede the progress of nurses toward using research and experiential evidence as the foundation for practice. These obstacles include the following:

1. Favoring usual practice rather than embracing change and creating new practice patterns based on evidence.
2. Inability of nurses at the bedside and in practice to find, obtain, and understand research.
3. Inability to translate research findings into practice interventions.
4. Inability of nurses to use translation research to measure the success of new practice interventions based on research findings.

To overcome the barrier of "favoring usual practice," nurses must decrease their dependence on "usual practice patterns" and embrace change, creating new practice patterns that improve patient outcomes. Developing a willingness to change requires champions who (1) understand and welcome research and evidence-based practice and (2) possess the skill to identify, evaluate, and translate evidence into the practice setting. To become such a champion, the DNP must overcome the second barrier (ability to obtain and understand research) and develop an advanced level of knowledge about research and research evaluation. One educational experience that compels DNP students to take on the idea of developing change based on the findings of research is the completion of the capstone project, which is discussed later in this chapter. After becoming comfortable with finding and evaluating research, the DNP-prepared nurse should teach other nurses to find and use research in their practice. This teaching can be accomplished through journal clubs and research committee work and can employ the assistance of the hospital librarian. As a leader in nursing, the DNP-prepared nurse should make scientific evidence available in a readable and usable form and should design evidence-based practice interventions that meet the needs of the organization, the patients, and the health-care providers. In this way, the DNP can assist in making research or evidence-based practice a reality.

To overcome the fourth barrier, DNP-prepared advanced practice nurses should be able to translate research findings of all types into practice standards and guidelines, test them for relevance in the setting in which they work, and educate others in the use and benefits of these interventions. One of the most important tools needed to translate research into general application is the ability to evaluate the quality of the research and research findings; this is also discussed later in the chapter. Although research is a cornerstone of clinical scholarship, not all research findings are applicable to all settings and practice areas.

The ability of nurses to translate research findings into applicable nursing interventions is critical. Although opportunities to improve practice through the use of research findings are apparent, challenges have been noted when attempting to translate evidence into real-world practice settings. Some experienced researchers have noted that using an intervention in practice may require a redesign of the intervention to improve its acceptability in different settings. In other words, instead of the nurse or care setting adapting to the new intervention, the new intervention should be adapted to the nurse or care setting (Duan, Braslow, Weisz, & Wells, 2001). It is important to evaluate the current practice environment and the prevailing culture of the organization before the implementation of the new intervention, even when the new intervention has proven to be successful in other areas.

Creating Champions for Change

One of the important aspects of creating change in nursing care is identifying and mentoring champions for change. For example, consider a new insulin protocol for postoperative patients. Although these types of protocols have shown a positive patient outcome in general, the initiation of the protocol would be unsuccessful without taking into account the staffing and work flow that exist on the specific unit where it is being tried. The nursing leader advocating the change should meet with staff members who are champions of the new intervention and should build support for the change by providing evidence of the benefits of the new intervention. Meeting with staff members who are resistant is also important to establish a level of confidence that the change can occur without greatly disrupting staff or patients.

Kitson (2007) created a three-step framework for successful implementation of new evidence-based interventions. This framework is entitled Promoting Action on Research Implementation in Health Service (PARIHS). The three main steps in this framework involve context, evidence, and facilitation. *Context* refers to an evaluation of the situation into which the evidence would be implemented. Is the evidence best used in an outpatient, hospital, or clinic setting? *Evidence* refers to an evaluation of the research evidence to ensure that the research being used is robust and scientifically sound. Examiners must be able to determine the rigor of the methodology, the threats to validity and reliability, and the strength and generalizability of the findings. The final step in this process is to formulate a method to *facilitate* the introduction of the intervention or practice, taking into account service delivery and organizational and unit characteristics. This step is very important because the organization as a whole must be willing to make changes in process and care delivery to create this change in practice. There are many ways that nursing leaders can develop support for new evidence-based interventions.

Starting a journal club is one way to increase nursing knowledge and interest in evidence-based practice. A journal club is a group of individuals who meet to evaluate critically recent research-based articles from the literature. Nursing journal clubs are often led by advanced practice nurses who are able to conduct a literature search, critique an article, and pick topics of interest. Journal clubs have been used within medicine since the late 1800s and are still used in medical schools today. Journal clubs have proven to be effective in creating excitement about research, furthering an understanding of research findings, and establishing a willingness to implement research findings into practice. Rogers (2009) analyzed the ability of a journal club to cross the research to practice divide.

Results revealed that nurses who participated in journal clubs were better able to read and understand research publications. These nurses were also better at critiquing research and implementing research findings into practice and were more confident about using evidence in care delivery.

Another common way to improve the understanding of research and the need to translate research findings into practice interventions is the research committee. There are many different structures for research committees; however, they are often composed of at least one member from each nursing unit in the health-care setting. The nurses on the research committee often discuss common issues and choose topics for exploration. This group may review and critique research articles and present them on the nursing units, hold discussions to support and guide nurses in setting up research studies, and sponsor research nursing grand rounds during which interesting cases and important nursing interventions are discussed.

No matter what type of organization, support for using research is an essential aspect of translating research into practice-based interventions. Before beginning any change in practice based on research findings, a competent facilitator is necessary to create and sustain the change in practice (Tucker et al., 2006). Stetler (2001) noted that at whatever level the translation of research into practice takes place, there is usually an individual clinician pushing for the change. Until more recently, these champions were physicians or administrators.

As DNP nurses become more prominent in clinical situations, they will be facilitators and champions for the translation of research evidence into practice. When nurses are not present in deciding on and implementing new interventions, it makes the change that much harder to sustain. In some instances, nurses educated as DNPs have assumed responsibilities as the director of nursing translational research within health-care settings (Barnsteiner, Reeder, Palma, Preston, & Walton, 2010). Placing strong leaders in the area of translational research would provide nursing with the ability to include a nursing framework when new interventions are considered.

Another important aspect of creating support for new research-based practice interventions is the provision of adequate education regarding the change. Nurses who are being asked to adopt new ways of practice should understand the theory, principles, and skills associated with this new way of practice. Nurses who are involved in the planned change should have input into the process of change and the implementation of the intervention itself to uncover areas where the process could be improved. This process engenders support from all individuals involved to increase the chance of successful and sustained change.

Several other factors that increase success of translation of research into practice include strong leadership, organizational support, collaboration, teamwork (discussed in Chapter 8), and shared goals among staff members. All members of the team are important in the effort and must be made to feel as though their contributions are valued for them to sustain changes that are implemented.

Advancing Your Knowledge

A group of advanced practice nurses who work in a large community clinic are attempting to create a method for smoother transitional care for patients who move from hospital to home or extended care. This project is in response to several problems the clinic has encountered lately where patients were transferred without important orders for medications and laboratory work. Most recently, a 32-year-old patient with a pelvic fracture was transferred from a hospital setting to extended care, and orders for a blood thinner to prevent clots did not follow the patient. After 2 days in the extended care facility, the patient developed a pulmonary embolism and died. Several of the physicians and nurse practitioners in the practice had seen this patient in the extended care facility, and no one noticed the missed medication order. In their effort to improve patient care overall, the nurse practitioners reviewed the literature on best practices for transition care and developed a proposal for the practice to adopt.

1. What barriers might these nurse practitioners face in changing practice?
2. How could they work to implement a culture of change within the practice in this specific area?
3. How could the measurement of outcomes from this new proposal be used to facilitate the needed changes?
4. How should these nurse practitioners disseminate the findings for the measurements of change so that others can benefit?

Identify a research-based scientific advancement in health care. How can this scientific finding from the laboratory be translated into practice? How could the DNP assist in the application of this knowledge in the practice area? Include the concepts of Promoting Action on Research Implementation in Health Services (PARIHS) (context, evidence, and facilitation) in your discussion.

Nursing Research

Nursing research is the systematic study of a problem pertaining to nursing and is essential for the continued development of the profession (Burns & Grove, 2008). Nursing research is designed to improve patient care, develop nursing skills and abilities, and identify meanings within situations so that the nurse can better understand and empathize with patients. Through nursing research, nurses are able to ask questions about "why they do what they do." The nurse asks the question, "Is this the best intervention for this patient situation?" or, "Could there be a better course of action?" The knowledge gained from research guides practice and improves the outcomes of nursing care at all levels. This section distinguishes quality improvement from research; it offers an overview on how to evaluate, translate, and critique research; and it covers several different types of research.

Quality Improvement Versus Research

Before delving deeper into nursing research, it is important first to clarify the distinction between research and quality improvement. Many clinical nurses who are already familiar with and engaged in quality improvement projects are not engaged in or familiar with nursing research. Differentiating between what is true research and what is quality improvement is important to nurses and health-care settings.

Generally, quality improvement is a method that is used to improve care, create positive patient outcomes, and create efficient systems and processes within a specific health-care setting. Quality improvement is usually not generalizable because it is so specific to the setting in which it is performed, whereas the findings of research can be generalized outside the immediate example to other settings. Quality improvement begins with a plan for solving a problem; research activities usually begin by studying what the problem is and what is already known about the problem through literature review. Research provides new data on a subject or problem, whereas quality improvement measures change from implementing interventions to solve a problem. Both quality improvement and research are important aspects of nursing care; nurses should understand the difference in approach to each. Table 3-1 presents an overview of the differences between quality improvement and research.

Although quality improvement is an intrinsic part of providing good clinical care, it is distinct and different from research. Research either creates new knowledge or builds on knowledge from other research to develop and create a better understanding of the human experience and better methods of caring for patients.

Table 3-1

Differences Between Quality Improvement and Research

Feature	Quality Improvement	Research
Purpose	Improve local care process and outcomes	Create generalizable knowledge
Who asks the questions	Clinicians, leaders, local clinical setting	Researchers, funders, public
Measures and sample size	Few, simple, small	Many, more complex
Confounders and analysis	Confounders not usually considered, analysis simple	Measures of control Complex analysis of data obtained for full understanding
Resources and time line	Few, usually local health care setting provides resources Time line usually short	Can use funding from local or national sources Time line usually longer to study the issue fully

Source: Solberg, et al.(1995). Assessing the impact of continuous quality improvement. *Joint Commission Journal of Quality Improvement, 23,* 136.

The science of research manipulates one aspect of a process to determine the effect of that process on outcomes being measured. Research is a systematic investigation that uses prescribed methods to answer questions or solve problems. Research designs are meant to control for as many variables as possible to establish a secure link between the intervention being studied and the outcome measures. Research is designed to produce new knowledge in an area. This new knowledge can be generalized to other situations and in similar circumstances in other health-care environments.

Quality improvement encourages participants to use previous experience and insight to identify ways to implement and study changes in systems and processes to improve patient care. The process of improvement considers many variables that influence outcomes and influence the quality of care.

One of the most frequently used frameworks for quality improvement projects is *plan-do-study-act* (Alexander & Herald, 2010). This process occurs during the quality assurance cycle to:

1. *Plan* (develop new ways of delivering care)—call patients after discharge to make sure they have been able to obtain needed medication and home health assistance and reduce readmission.
2. *Do* (carry out the new ways developed)—implement the plan and have three nursing staff members who make these calls, log responses, and report patient problems with medications or home assistance.
3. *Study* (observe and learn lessons from the outcomes)—observe the numbers of patients who are sent home without prescriptions for needed medications and are unable to obtain them.
4. *Act* (determine if further changes are required or if the new plan can be implemented)—create a mechanism for nurses to intervene and ensure that patients have prescriptions for needed medication before they are discharged.

Quality improvement is narrower in scope and is not generally useful outside of the institution in which it is undertaken. Usually quality improvement (sometimes called *quality assurance*) is undertaken by a group of individuals within a workplace to improve systems and processes that can improve care. Quality improvement work is generally not based on theory, does not measure other variables that might affect results, and often lacks the ability to make causal inferences from the data collected. An example of a quality improvement project is as follows. A group of managers in a hospital review the processes for obtaining medications from the pharmacy only to find that nurses must go to the pharmacy themselves, leaving the unit three or more times before actually retrieving the medication. The managers reviewed the process and established a new system for prioritizing medication needs on the nursing units. The hospital ultimately purchased a robot that could be dispatched to the unit from the pharmacy with the medication after it was prepared. This process improved care by speeding up the time it took to obtain urgent medications from the pharmacy and allowing o stay on the unit caring for patients rather than making trips to t... ...cy. This work improved patient care and allowed nurses to stay with patients, ...owever, it did not develop new knowledge, and it cannot be used outside of the studied institution. Also, this outcome is not based on any theoretical knowledge, and all of the variables that could have caused the outcome are not accounted for.

Benchmarking is another term that is used in conjunction with quality improvement. Benchmarking is a process whereby a facility measures and compares functions, systems, and practices against others in the community or region. When a group or organization is unable to meet the benchmark that is met by others in the community, programmatic changes are often made to catch up and meet benchmarks. For example, if a hospital has a shortage of nurses, it might undertake to benchmark salary levels compared with other hospitals in the community. If the hospital is lower than the benchmark average salary, it may decide to raise salary levels to be competitive. Benchmarking is a way to make improvements based on measuring how one institution "stacks up" against another.

Although evidence-based research and quality improvement are different, they both derive evidence that can be used to create and change practice. Research provides a higher level of evidence, whereas quality improvement provides real-life experiences and descriptions of processes and organizational issues that need attention.

Critical Thinking Questions

1. Choose a topic that might be explored to improve patient care. Create two programs—the first a research program and the second a quality improvement program. How are they different?
2. In what areas might research be needed, and in what areas might quality improvement undertakings work better?
3. Discuss the concepts of the research of application and integration as ways that DNP graduates are well suited to do research.

Evaluating and Translating Research for Application in Practice Settings

A critical step in translating research evidence to practice settings is determining what research evidence applies to a given situation, finding that evidence, and evaluating the evidence for quality and rigor. Appraisal of all types of research evidence to determine the usefulness and applicability in a given clinical situation is an important role for the DNP and is foundational to clinical scholarship. A straightforward definition of research describes it as systematic inquiry that uses disciplined methods to answer questions or solve problems. From that definition, many questions arise for the advanced practice nurse—Was the research method sound? Is there a theoretical basis in nursing for the study? Is the sample adequate?—before the research is ready to be used in general practice.

Generally, four methods of critical thinking must be used when evaluating research studies in nursing, as follows (http://nursingplanet.com/Nursing_Research/critiquing_nursing_research2.html)

- *Comprehension:* Understanding the terms and concepts in the report; identifying the elements or steps in the research process, theoretical framework, and design
- *Comparison:* Examining the extent to which the researcher followed the rules of an ideal study
- *Analysis:* Evaluating the links that connect each element within the study to the rest of the study
- *Evaluation:* Uncovering meaning and significance of the study and the ability to generalize findings to other similar situations

Evaluating research is an important aspect of evidence-based practice. Using a consistent approach to evaluating research reports allows the DNP to weigh the evidence in a structured manner that removes bias and allows for the development of treatment guidelines that are evidence-based. The steps to research evaluation are as follows:

- Choose a research manuscript to review.
- Identify the research questions, aims, problem statement, or hypothesis.
- Identify the purpose and objectives of the research.
- Identify the conceptual framework for the study and whether the framework fits with the research purpose and objectives. How does this particular research expand nursing theoretical knowledge?
- Identify the dependent and independent variables within the research study. Are these variables appropriate for the research purpose? Are there confounding variables that have not been identified?
- Is the review of literature current, complete, and relevant to the purpose of the research? Does it identify gaps in the research that would be filled by the proposed study?
- Are ethical considerations addressed adequately?
- Is the research design appropriate to the purpose, objectives, and aims of the study?
- Is the population that is being studied identified? Are key aspects of the sample described, such as age, gender, ethnicity, or educational level? Is the sample used similar to the population being studied? How was the sample group recruited? If the sample is divided into groups, how was this done? Were the groups similar before any intervention?
- Identify the measurement tools or instruments used in the study. Does the author present studies on the reliability and validity of these instruments? Are these instruments appropriate for the population being studied (e.g., if the study population is children, the geriatric depression scale would be inappropriate)? If interviews are used, are the interview questions listed? How are the interviews conducted, where are they conducted, and by whom?

- Is a quantitative or qualitative method used? Is the method appropriate for the type of data gathered? Are data gathered that do not appear to have been analyzed in the research report? Is the sample large enough to use parametric statistical tests? Are there controls in place for analysis of confounding variable influence on data? Does the research identify any personal bias in data analysis of qualitative data?
- In the discussion section, what is the researcher's interpretation of the study findings? Are study limitations clearly presented? Are the findings consistent with the results and population studied? Are recommendations for future studies made?
- How much confidence can be placed in the study findings?

Finding articles that present research studies from journals and other publications is the first step in reviewing and evaluating research findings on a topic of interest. Research articles from peer review journals are considered more credible. *Peer review,* as discussed in Chapter 8, is a process whereby a profession maintains standards and regulates the quality of materials that appear in print or during presentations. Articles submitted to peer review journals for publication are read by a person or several persons of equal standing in the profession who are experts in the area being discussed. Peer review is used to determine the quality and acceptability and rate the clinical value of the article. Peer review is done anonymously so that the reviews can be completed in an impartial manner without bias. Although peer review is not a perfect method for evaluation, the process does allow for screening to maintain standards of clarity and writing quality, determine whether the research methodology and data analysis are adequate, and create a method to measure the importance of the work for nursing. Peer review journals describe themselves as such and are easy to identify when undertaking to review literature on a specific topic. The ability to perform a *data-based search* for pertinent research articles is an essential part of the development of clinical databases. Table 3-2 outlines steps used in a systematic data-based search for research information.

When research articles have been collected, each article must be assessed for quality and appropriateness in providing evidence for the topic under investigation. The research article must fit specifically with the topic in your evidence search; for example, it would be inappropriate to include "geriatric depression" in your search for evidence about the appropriate treatment of depression in teenagers. Generally, research articles should be current or within the last 5 years to be useful in providing evidence. Older research may have become outdated or surpassed by new research and not be as useful. However, some research studies may be considered seminal to the area you are exploring. Seminal research can be defined as providing the seed or beginning knowledge in an area from which all other knowledge grows. These types of research articles can be included in your evidence search because they provide background and beginning information about the research being evaluated. After a representative group of articles has been compiled that provides a full picture of the research available on the

Table 3-2

Steps in Performing a Database Search

1. Choose a database that is appropriate for the study.
2. Describe the search topic: Think of a question, a phrase, or a sentence that includes all the important aspects (or concepts) of your topic.
3. Break up the sentence developed above into key terms or phrases that can be used to search for articles.
   You can usually link two key words with "and" to make the search more specific (e.g., music and pain).
   You can usually use "or" between two words to make your search more extensive (e.g., HIV or AIDS).
4. Be prepared to modify the search to find all of the available articles on a topic.
5. Look for articles that are "full text" within a database, or make note of "full text" articles that might be found in other areas.
6. Make sure the articles you find are peer reviewed so that they provide the quality of evidence required.
7. Look at the words used in the full text articles available to determine if other key words might prove useful in a database search.
8. Look at the reference lists for articles that are full text on a database to determine if there are useful articles there that could be found online or in hard copy.
9. Keep refining search terms and methods of searching until enough quality research material is found to make a good literature review of available knowledge on a subject.
10. Review database information frequently to determine if new information on a topic has emerged.

topic of interest, the next step is to critique and accumulate evidence regarding the topic of interest.

Qualitative Versus Quantitative Research

The first question that should be asked when reviewing research evidence is whether the correct approach was used to obtain research results. Table 3-3 presents the differences between quantitative research and qualitative research. When attempting to identify a problem and come to understand the components of a problem, the preferred method is qualitative research. When the goal of research is to predict outcomes and control for variables that could affect outcomes, quantitative research is the method of choice.

Assessing and Evaluating Quantitative Research

The quantitative research method is used to gather empirical or measurable evidence to test a hypothesis, theory, or research question. Quantitative research is based on traditional scientific methods, which generate numerical data, seek to establish causal relationships between two or more variables, and use statistical methods to test the strength and significance of the relationships. This type of research follows a strict design structure to ensure that evidence gathering is

Table 3-3

Differences Between Quantitative and Qualitative Research

Purpose	Types of Questions in Quantitative Research	Types of Questions in Qualitative Research
Identification	This is not a proper question in quantitative research	What is this phenomenon? What is its name?
Description	How prevalent is the phenomenon? How often does the phenomenon occur? What are the characteristics of the phenomenon?	What are the dimensions of the phenomenon? What variations exist? What is important about the phenomenon?
Exploration	What factors are related to the phenomenon? What are the antecedents of the phenomenon?	What is the full nature of the phenomenon? What is really going on here? What is the process by which the phenomenon evolves or is experienced?
Explanation	What are the measurable associations between phenomena? What factors cause the phenomenon? Does the theory explain the phenomenon?	How does the phenomenon work? Why does the phenomenon exist? What is the meaning of the phenomenon? How did the phenomenon occur?
Prediction and control	What would happen if we alter a phenomenon or introduce an intervention? How can we make the phenomenon happen or alter its nature or prevalence? Can the occurrence of the phenomenon be controlled?	Prediction and control are not used in qualitative research because the point of this type of research is to come to know what is without prior prediction or control

standardized, regardless of the type of evidence gathered. When critiquing a research study that uses a quantitative methodology, guidelines for determining the quality of the research are based on the guidelines set by the research to measure the consequence of an intervention or the outcome of the independent variable on the dependent variable being studied. For example, in a study to determine the effect of a low-carbohydrate diet on diabetic blood glucose control, the independent variable would be the low-carbohydrate diet. Some study participants would be placed on this type of diet and others would not so that the effect could be compared. The dependent variable would be blood glucose because it would vary depending on whether or not the participant was on the low-carbohydrate diet.

The process of critiquing research articles requires the advanced practice nurse to read the entire study carefully and examine the organization and presentation of information. The nurse needs to make note of each step in the research process, beginning with what is being studied, the study population, method and outcome measures, method used to analyze the data, results, and finally implications and conclusions drawn from the study findings. The nurse needs to determine what the authors list as limitations, and note limitations that have not been listed. Examples of limitations include small sample size, inability to generalize findings, inability to adjust for confounding variables that may have influenced findings, and problems with the research design and implementation.

Overall, when critiquing quantitative study results, the reviewer should be able to answer the following questions: (1) Were the aims of the research met? (2) Could the research questions be answered? (3) Was the hypothesis accepted or rejected? (4) Were there limitations in this study, and were they defined by the researcher? (5) Did the results of this study agree with research findings of similar studies in the background and significance portion of the research paper? (6) Were there unexpected findings? If so, were they explained and evaluated by the researcher? (7) Did the outcomes of the research have implications for nursing practice, nursing education, or public policy? (8) Did the findings of the study add to nursing theory or theoretical knowledge?

Based on all of this information, readers can determine the validity and value of the research article. One can then decide whether or not to include the research presented as part of the response to the research question. Table 3-4 summarizes the steps in critiquing quantitative research studies.

Table 3-4

Steps in Critiquing Quantitative Research

1. In what journal is the study published? Is it peer reviewed? Is it a reputable journal in the field?
2. What was the general purpose of the study?
   - What is the research question?
   - What are the aims of the research?
   - What is the research hypothesis?
3. What quantitative design is used? Is the design appropriate for the question being asked?
   - Quasiexperimental
   - Experimental
   - Descriptive
   - Survey
4. How does answering the research question(s) add something new to what is already known?
5. Who or what was studied?
   - How was the sample obtained?
   - Were participants randomly assigned to groups?
   - Are the samples homogeneous?
   - Is the sample representative of the population being studied?

Continued on page 128

Continued from page 127 Table 3-4

Steps in Critiquing Quantitative Research

6. What data were recorded and used for analysis?
7. What kind(s) of data analysis was used? Is the analysis appropriate for the study?
8. What were the results? What conclusions are drawn from the results?
   - Do the conclusions fit with the data and analysis?
9. What are important reservations?
   - What limitations did the author list?
   - What limitations were not listed but were obvious in the study?
10. What particularly interesting or valuable things did you learn from reading the report?
11. Is the study important for nursing practice? Do the outcomes of the study warrant implementing the intervention in practice?
    - How useful is this study to everyday practice?
    - Would implementing the findings of this study in practice be beneficial for patients?
    - What is the cost-benefit ratio for implementing this intervention in practice?

The value of quantitative research is often defined and evaluated within a hierarchy of the strength of the method used. The traditional hierarchy of quantitative scientific research is presented in Table 3-5. The hierarchy in Table 3-5 does not evaluate the strength of specific research designs but rather ranks the types of quantitative research methods used, according to their reliability.

Table 3-5

Hierarchy of Scientific Research: Highest Level to Lowest Level

Type of Research—From Highest to Lowest Level	Definition of Research
Meta-analysis	Reviews and examines multiple studies on a specific topic. Combines and analyzes statistical results as though they were one large study. Includes critical appraisal of each study and of the studies as a whole. *For example:* Taking all of the literature regarding the effect of music listening on blood pressure, reanalyze the statistics and combine the analysis to form an overall picture of the effect.
Systematic reviews	Focuses on one clinical topic and answers a specific question. An extensive literature search is conducted to identify all studies with sound methodology on a specific topic. The studies are reviewed and assessed, and the results are summarized according to the predetermined criteria of the review question. *The Cochrane Collaboration* has done a lot of work in the area of systematic reviews (Cochrane Reviews, 2010). *For example:* Review all studies regarding treatments for childhood obesity and analyze the results. From this analysis, a guideline for the most successful interventions for childhood obesity could be developed.

Continued from page 128 Table 3-5

Hierarchy of Scientific Research: Highest Level to Lowest Level

Type of Research—From Highest to Lowest Level	Definition of Research
Randomized controlled clinical trials	Carefully planned research studies that determine the effect of a therapy on real patients. They include methodologies that allow for comparison between the interventional group and a control group not receiving the intervention. These types of studies attempt to reduce the potential for bias by randomly assigning participants to either the intervention or the control group, creating homogeneity between the two groups and blinding researchers who collect the data as to which participants are in which group. *For example:* Recruit a group of participants and divide them into two groups. The division is done by having them choose a sealed envelope inside of which is a slip of paper. Participants who have a "C" on their paper are in one group (the control group), and participants with an "E" on their paper are in another group (the experimental group). An intervention is provided for the experimental group but not for the control group. Both groups are measured for whatever the research is measuring (e.g., blood pressure, weight, stress, anxiety) and compared. Because the groups were randomly assigned, and therefore equal at baseline, the results of the measurement comparison can be assumed to be caused exclusively by the intervention.
Cohort studies	Studies that follow patients who have a specific condition or receive a particular treatment over time and compare them with another group that has not been affected by the condition or treatment being studied. Cohort studies are observational and not as reliable as randomized controlled studies because the two groups may differ in ways other than in the variable under study. *For example:* Observing the weight of a group of children who are allowed to run and play at recess and after school and comparing them with a group of children who must remain inside the school during recess and after school.
Case control studies	Are similar to cohort studies except they compare subjects with a certain condition with subjects who do not have the condition in more general terms. *For example:* Observe the health status of older adults who have diabetes compared with older adults who do not.
Case series and case reports	Consist of collections of reports on the treatment of individual patients or a report on a single patient. Because they are reports of cases and use no control groups with which to compare outcomes, they have no statistical validity. *For example:* Report on three women with Marfan's syndrome in terms of length of life, ability to work, and ability to care for their children.

Critical Thinking Question

Choose a quantitative research article and use the steps in Table 3-4 to evaluate the study. How does your expertise and experience in the clinical setting help you to evaluate this research study? How could you plan a change in practice based on this study?

Validity and Reliability in Quantitative Studies

A study is valid if the finding of the study is true. Bias can destroy validity. Bias is the result of any unknown or unacknowledged error in research where the findings deviate from the truth. Bias and threats to validity can occur in any study design, but they are most often found in quasiexperimental studies. Threats can occur to internal validity (e.g., Is the intervention being studied responsible for the changes that occurred?) and external validity (e.g., Are results generalizable to similar groups?). Table 3-6 provides a list and explanation of common threats to the validity of the findings in quantitative research.

Table 3-6

Threats to Study Validity

Threat to Validity	Explanation of Threat
Mortality	The loss of a significant number of participants could decrease the validity of the findings of a study. It is always important for the researcher to state how many participants dropped out of the study and why.
Selection bias	Bias can come from methods used to select the population and the method used to place participants into intervention and control groups for study.
History	Events that occur between the first and second data collection points that could affect the outcome.
Maturation	The natural changes in the population being studied over a long period. If you were studying the effect of pollution on health in a group and the study lasted 10 years, the aging of the population being studied may cause health problems unrelated to pollution and reduce the validity of the study results.
Repeat testing	If participants take the same test several times, there is the risk that they will become better at answering the questions as time goes on
Instrument change	Changes in the measurement instrument during the study or having different people obtain information in different ways, creating a threat to the validity of findings.
John Henry effect	This happens when subjects know you are studying their reactions to an intervention. They often are more positive about the intervention or work harder to create better outcomes to help the study.

When critiquing a research article, the reader should look for acknowledged and unacknowledged threats to the validity of the research findings. Within the article, the research should state how the threat was minimized to the extent possible. If the person critiquing the research is able to identify a threat that has not been addressed, he or she should perform an assessment of the influence of the threat on the validity of the study.

Assessing and Evaluating Qualitative Research

Qualitative research is undertaken to create an understanding of human experience, perceptions, motivations, intentions, and behaviors based on description and observation. It uses a naturalistic interpretative approach to a person that includes the contextual setting. The goal of qualitative research is to understand and describe a phenomenon or a human experience or to examine the quality of an experience or happening in a population or group. Qualitative research methods were first used in social work and anthropology, but nurses began to use qualitative methodologies as a natural consequence of the desire to come to know human beings and their experiences. Qualitative research methodologies allow nurses to understand human experience in the context of the individual, the family, and the community (Burns & Grove, 2008). Although many practice-based nurses find the quality of qualitative evidence to be weak because it deviates from the traditional scientific method, qualitative research provides unique insights into the perception of patients and their view of the world. For example, understanding the experience of having a child with autism may assist nurses to develop interventions that are helpful to the child and the family in coping with this condition. Table 3-7 lists the assumptions used in qualitative research.

Table 3-7

Assumptions in Qualitative Research

1. Qualitative researchers are concerned primarily with process, rather than outcomes or products.
2. Qualitative researchers are interested in how people make sense of their lives, experiences, and their structures of the world.
3. The qualitative researcher is the primary instrument for data collection and analysis. Data are mediated through this human instrument, rather than through inventories, questionnaires, or machines.
4. Qualitative research involves fieldwork. The researcher physically goes to the people, setting, site, or institution to observe or record behavior in its natural setting.
5. Qualitative research is descriptive in that the researcher is interested in process, meaning, and understanding gained through words or pictures.
6. The process of qualitative research is *inductive* in that the researcher builds abstractions, concepts, hypotheses, and theories from details.

Source: Creswell, J.W. (1994). *Research design: Qualitative and quantitative approaches.* Thousand Oaks, CA: Sage Publications.

Findings from qualitative studies can create insight into problems and promote empathy among nurses. Stimulating empathy and knowledge of "what it is like" may allow nurses to develop the ability to pay attention to subtle cues from patients in situations where interventions may improve health and well-being. Miller (2010) stated that the findings of qualitative research are valuable for planning anticipatory guidance and coaching and help the nurse to understand patients' decision-making processes in a given situation. Many nursing researchers believe that the findings from qualitative research provide valuable evidence for practice in nursing because nurses focus on the individual person as whole and unique. Several categories of qualitative research methodologies and approaches exist, and each has a different way of explaining and expanding nursing knowledge.

Polit and Beck (2008) listed six characteristics of qualitative research, as follows:

1. Blending of data collection strategies.
2. Flexibility—capable of adjusting to what is being learned.
3. Strives to understand the whole.
4. Requires researcher involvement in different ways.
5. Researcher becomes an instrument of the research.
6. Requires ongoing analysis of the data to determine and uncover meaning, themes, and essences within the research.

When critiquing a qualitative study, the first step is to determine if the questions asked by the researchers fit with the type of qualitative study used. Does the research identify the experience being examined? Are the conclusions drawn from the study data consistent with the experience being examined? Participants for the sample in qualitative studies are drawn from people who are the best sources of information about a phenomenon, and sample size is generally small. Each participant is observed or interviewed several times until no new information is being received and all new material has been obtained, which is considered to be the point of saturation.

One of the most difficult aspects of critiquing a qualitative study is determining the validity and reliability of the findings. The terms *validity* and *reliability* are not often associated with qualitative research; rather, the term *trustworthiness* is used to describe the ability of the qualitative process to produce true understanding of a situation. This term is used because findings are not based on measureable data but rather on understanding the meaning of individual dialogue or observation and extracting thematic material from these data. In a seminal work, Lincoln and Gupta (1985) coined the term *trustworthiness* to describe the findings of qualitative study and developed a foundation for understanding the quality of a qualitative research study. These authors established four measures of trustworthiness: credibility, transferability, confirmability, and dependability.

A study is considered to be *credible* if the researcher has used the exact words spoken or observations made to provide conclusions from the evidence. This measure can be tricky because researchers can be tempted to put meaning into evidence that is not really exhibited in the narratives or observations collected. For qualitative research to be credible, the findings must be able to be directly linked to the narratives or observations made.

Transferability refers to the degree to which the results of qualitative research can be generalized or transferred to other contexts or settings. The qualitative researcher can enhance transferability by describing the research context and the assumptions in detail. The person critiquing the transferability of the research results to a different group can make the judgment of how closely themes from one research group can be transferred to a similar group in other contexts or settings.

The *confirmability* criterion involves establishing that the results of qualitative research are credible or believable from the perspective of each participant in the study. Do the findings accurately and adequately describe what the participant meant in interviews and observational data? Because the purpose of qualitative research is to describe or understand the phenomena of interest from the participant's eyes, the participants are the only ones who can legitimately confirm the results. Many qualitative researchers share the findings of their research with participants to determine whether the findings accurately reflect the information provided by the participants. The opinion of participants regarding the accuracy of these findings should be contained in the research report.

Dependability as a criterion for qualitative research is met when researchers determine that the same results would be obtained if researchers repeated the study with a group of similar participants. The idea of dependability emphasizes the need for the researcher to account for the ever-changing context within which research occurs. The research is responsible for describing the changes that occur in the setting and how these changes affected the way the researcher approached the study.

Each of these measures of trustworthiness should be evaluated when critiquing qualitative research. Does the research use exact words from the participants to develop themes and essences of study findings? Can a link be made by readers between the material gathered for the study and the findings? Does the researcher describe the context and assumptions in the study in sufficient detail so that readers can put themselves within the context of the study and understand the experience the research is trying to capture? Did the researcher share findings from the research with participants to confirm that the themes extracted were those intended? Finally, could this study be re-created using a similar group of participants, or if the context is so unique, is it fully explained by the researchers?

Critical Thinking Questions

Choose a qualitative research article and critique it using the steps described. How did the authors demonstrate trustworthiness in their findings? How can qualitative research studies be useful in clinical practice? What would be the benefit of replicating qualitative studies or of taking qualitative data and designing a quantitative study to provide further evidence for the research findings?

One Frequent Type of Nursing Clinical Inquiry: Evidence-Based Research

If we define evidence as proof supporting a theory and research as the investigation, collection, and interpretation of facts, we can say that evidence-based research is a research methodology used when the researcher is already aware of evidence from previous research but wishes to explore this evidence further in a particular situation. Because evidence-based research is focused on specific evidence and how to use or apply that evidence in the practice setting, it is the basis for translating evidence of research into practice. Evidence-based research is not focused only on empirical evidence but also on the evidence of nursing experience, intuition, and reflection. Evidence-based research enables practicing nurses to make decisions about best practices and appropriate guidelines. If a group of studies shows a positive correlation between moderate exercise and weight loss in women older than 55 years of age, designing a study in a specific practice setting that treats a large number of female Haitian immigrants older than 55 years old would be an example of evidence-based research. Taking information that has already been established and expanding the knowledge to examine a specific group provides a way to improve guidelines for care.

Evidence-based practice has become a buzzword for many other health professions, including medicine. Evidence-based medicine differs from evidence-based nursing in several ways. In evidence-based medicine, research findings are the primary method used for decision making to determine what is best for the patient because medicine concentrates on the sciences of biology, physiology, and chemistry, where control and manipulation are used to inform scientific understanding. In nursing, which uses both science and art as a foundation for practice, a combined concentration on physical, psychosocial, cultural, and emotional factors is important. All of these aspects of care are used equally as the basis for evidence-based practice and decision making. Evidence is combined with nursing intuition, reflection, knowledge, and patient preference to create the fundamentals of evidence-based practice.

Advancing Your Knowledge

The nursing administration team at a hospital has completed a literature review on research regarding self-governance models. They would like to explore the possibility of implementing a model at the hospital to determine the success of the model in increasing nursing job satisfaction and retention and improvements in patient outcomes. The team gathers a group of nurses from each unit in the hospital and reviews with them what is known about self-governance and the research that shows the benefits of such a program. The team devises a complete plan for education and implementation of self-governance throughout the hospital. The team also uses the research literature to help determine how to measure the outcomes of this project.

1. How would you classify this project in terms of type of research or level of research?
2. If the outcomes of this new program are similar to the outcomes of other research studies in the literature, is this important?
3. How can these nurses share the knowledge they have gained through this process with others to create and solidify nursing knowledge about shared governance as a process?

Translational Research

Many types of research methodologies are needed to advance nursing knowledge, and some methods are more suited to the DNP-prepared nurse as opposed to the PhD-prepared nurse. Translational research has been discussed as an appropriate avenue for DNPs with advanced education in clinical research and a firm knowledge of and experience in practice. Translational research is one of the priorities for the National Institutes of Health to help bridge the research to practice gap that currently exists. Translational research refers to taking the results of scientific experiments completed in a laboratory (often called *bench science*) and translating the findings of that research into the practice arena to determine its overall effectiveness in real-life situations.

Lauer & Skarlatos (2010) defined three types of translational research (T1, T2, and T3). T1 is the challenge to use the findings of bench research to create new understandings of disease mechanisms and develop these into new methods for diagnosis, therapy, and prevention of disease in humans. Although the T1 components are often beyond the scope of nursing practice research, advanced practice nurses can be instrumental in gathering and classifying data in this area. T2 is the challenge to translate and test the results from research studies into everyday clinical practice and health-care decision making. This translational challenge is relevant to advanced practice nursing. Implementing new research findings in practice and continuing to evaluate the effectiveness of research-based results in practice are part of advanced nursing practice, especially for nurses with a DNP degree. T3 is the challenge to disseminate the findings of both T1 and T2 research. Lauer & Skarlatos (2010) stated that too often T1 research is funded over T2 research, but that the time has come for a major effort to support T2 research.

In nursing, translational science (the broader area of study within which translation research is completed) has been defined specifically as the ability to translate clinical knowledge into evidence-based practices for the improvement of patient care outcomes. At the center of translational science is a commitment to quality care, using evidence to improve quality of care and patient safety and intraprofessional and interprofessional communication about research findings and implementation.

The DNP is uniquely situated to identify, evaluate, translate, apply, and evaluate research findings in practice. Nurse scientists and practice specialists must re-examine the gap that exists between theory, research, and practice to determine how research findings fit within and contribute not only to the development of new knowledge but also to the translation of that knowledge to the care of diverse communities and populations.

Advancing Your Knowledge

F.L. is a nurse practitioner in a primary care setting. She notes that many of the children in her practice are overweight. F.L. has read that childhood obesity leads to poor health outcomes and is the primary risk factor for adult obesity. F.L. reads about a research project in a large urban setting where overweight children and their families participated in a program that included education regarding diet and healthy eating and a fun program in which the children earned points for walking and other forms of exercise and points for reducing hours of television watching and video games. The points were redeemable for prizes, including movie tickets and tickets to a local water park. F.L. gets funding and other assistance for a similar program for the children in her practice from local gyms, movie theaters, the local zoo, and miniature golf course. She advertises the program to families in her practice and gets a positive response. Other families join the practice as the word spreads of this innovative program for overweight children.

1. How should F.L. measure the success of her program?
2. Think of a scenario in your own practice experience where research has been used. Were you part of the group that implemented the research findings? Did you implement the findings on your own within your own practice? What were the barriers and opportunities that developed from this work for you and for your practice?
3. Can the findings of this research be used in other practices? How can F.L. apprise others of her research and findings?

Mixed Methods Research

Multimethodology, or mixed methods research, is an approach that combines the collection and analysis of quantitative and qualitative data. Flemming (2007) asserted that mixing methodologies in a single study improves the design and effectiveness of the study to provide evidence for practice. Flemming listed four main ways to design mixed methods research:

- Triangulation,
- Using the results of qualitative studies to create quantitative research,
- Using the findings of quantitative research to create qualitative questions, and
- Completing a qualitative and a quantitative study to determine different aspects of a phenomenon.

The first way is triangulation, in which both types of data are procured independently and compared to provide study results that consider both the qualitative and the quantitative aspects of the study. The second way is to use qualitative research to facilitate quantitative studies. In other words, researchers complete a qualitative study to determine the meaning and understand the phenomenon, followed by a study through control and manipulation using a quantitative design. The third way is to use quantitative research to facilitate qualitative research in which a phenomenon is controlled and manipulated using quantitative methods and then explained better by undertaking a qualitative study. The final way to design mixed methods research is to complete two separate studies on a phenomenon, one qualitative and one quantitative, to investigate two different aspects of the phenomenon.

Mixed methods research is useful in bridging the transfer gap between research and practice because of the multiple types of data and broader scope of results this type of research produces. Creating research findings that both come to understand a phenomenon and measure the outcomes of manipulation and control on the phenomenon provides an enhanced basis for using evidence in practice. Mixed methods research may reflect the complex and diverse nature of the nursing profession better because it approaches a phenomenon or question from different perspectives—the quantitative or data driven and the qualitative or that of coming to know. This type of research allows for the many areas of knowledge within the discipline to be uncovered and translated into practice. When evaluating mixed methods research, criteria for both qualitative and quantitative methods should apply. There should be a summary of how the results of both the qualitative and the quantitative perspectives provide unique and blended findings.

Participatory Action Research

Another type of research that is uniquely suited to the DNP is participatory action research, also called *collaborative inquiry, emancipatory research, action learning,* and *contextual action research*. Action research has focused much on health within communities. Participatory action research involves learning by doing, where a group of people identify a problem, develop a plan to resolve the problem, implement the plan, evaluate the success of their effort, make adjustments if needed, and implement a new plan to start the process again. Although these steps form the essence of the approach, other key attributes of action research differentiate it from common problem-solving activities. Participatory action research includes cooperative community members that work with the researcher in a colearning process to develop systems in local environments. This type of research is empowering for the participants in part because it increases control over their lives by involving them in problem solving and nurturing community strengths. One group defines participatory action research as follows:

> "Research that aims to contribute to the practical concerns of people in an immediate problematic situation, and to further the goals of society simultaneously. Thus,

there is a dual commitment in action research to study a system and concurrently to collaborate with members of the system in changing it in what is together regarded as a desirable direction. Accomplishing this twin goal requires the active collaboration of researcher and client, and thus it stresses the importance of co-learning as a primary aspect of the research process." *(ABL Group, 1997, p. 25).*

Minkler (2000) found that participatory action research helps to create healthy communities by employing:

- Information and problem solving from the grass roots rather than from a top-down approach,
- Democratic participatory processes and social learning,
- An emphasis on strengths of people and communities in the problem-solving process, and
- Ideas driven by community priorities

Table 3-8 describes one way of undertaking a participatory action research project. Participatory action research represents an attractive research method for advanced practice nurses primarily because it allows them to participate in a collegial collaborative environment, it is population based, and it emphasizes

Table 3-8

Steps in Participatory Action Research

Steps	Focus	Actions
One	**1.** Reflection	The group and thematic concerns are identified through discourse between researchers, nurses, and the community.
	2. Plan	The plan is developed to determine concerns and the social situation in which these concerns occur. *All* stakeholders are identified and brought together to decide how to proceed and collaborate.
	3. Action **4.** Observation	The plan is put into action, and the group collects its observations.
Two	**1.** Reflection	The group reflects on its findings to define more accurately its thematic concern. This reflection would also include self-reflection by the participants.
	2. Plan	The group can plan a change in practice to improve health. Potential problems need to be resolved, and approval from ethics committees needs to be obtained.
	3. Action	A change in practice is effected, and the research commences.
	4. Observation	The group observes the consequences of the change in practice and uses the research method outlined in the plan to examine the results.
Three	**1.** Reflection	The possibility of the project not reaching an end is realistic. This does not mean the original problem remains the same or that the group never finds any change to its situation or social justice in its community or setting.

naturalistic and humanistic scientific methods. Advanced practice nurses often are closely connected to and trusted by the communities they serve. DNPs, with skills in clinical practice, population-based health, and leadership, are perfectly positioned to participate in this type of research.

Advancing Your Knowledge

R.M. is a nurse practitioner who has a primary care practice in a rural setting where there are a large number of new immigrant families who come to work on farms. These families often bring older adults with them as they move from their homeland. Some of the older adults become very isolated in their homes because they are not assimilated into the community through work or school. This isolation leads to cognitive and physical impairments in the older adults, and R.M. seeks ways to overcome this isolation. Most of the immigrant families attend one of two churches in the town, and R.M. meets with the leaders of these churches to discuss ways to integrate the older adults into their new community. A county senior center has a day program for older adults where they can socialize, play games, learn new skills, and receive lunch each day. Schoolchildren often come to sing or to put on plays for the seniors, and students in health-related fields come to do blood pressure screenings and other health-related projects. R.M. visited the senior center and noticed that none of the new immigrant older adults were in attendance. When she asked the director why this might be so, he told R.M. that the immigrant older adults did not attend because most of them did not speak English and some of the seniors already in attendance did not like the group of new immigrant older adults. The pastors of the two churches indicated that the immigrant older adults did not feel comfortable at the senior center because no one spoke to them. The pastors also indicated that transportation to and from the center could be a problem for these older adults.

R.M. obtained funding from a local charity group interested in assisting underserved populations and was able to create a program at the senior center specifically designed to integrate the immigrant older adults into the center. The first step was to go to the two churches and the senior center and discuss the idea and how the integration would benefit both groups. Second, she found a translator who would go with the older adults each day to the center, act as a translator, and begin to teach the immigrant older adults English words and phrases. She found that the county-owned transportation system had free bus passes for older adults, but that to obtain these passes individuals had to go to the bus center 45 miles from this area and had to speak English. R.M. arranged for the transportation authority to come to the community and help the immigrant older adults apply for and get the free bus passes that allowed them to come to the center. By the end of the program, more than 50 immigrant older adults attended the senior center regularly. Even though

Continued on page 140

Advancing Your Knowledge *Continued from page 139*

language remained a problem, these older adults were able to play dominoes and other games with the other seniors and establish a sense of community and belonging in their new home.

1. What outcomes could be measured (quantitative or qualitative) in this research?
2. Why is this important work in communities? How can community keep people healthy?
3. How could you use participatory action research in your work? Would this type of research benefit your practice? How? Why should clinical scholar nurses be involved in community participatory action research?
4. How could a multidisciplinary approach be used to foster this type of research?

Compiling Evidence From Research

After collecting and critiquing the research, evidence emerges that can be used to make decisions about changes to practice. One way to compile the evidence findings is through evidence tables. Table 3-9 is an example of an evidence table that can be used to compile the findings of multiple research studies and guide the development of changes in practice patterns and habits. After the evidence has been combined and decisions made about the strength of the evidence for changes or new innovations in practice, translational research can be undertaken.

Table 3-9

Sample Evidence Table

Article Name and Author	Number of Participants and Sampling Method	Research Question or Aim or Hypothesis	Research Design	Method of Analysis	Findings	Limitations

Multidisciplinary Research Teams

DNP-prepared nurses are uniquely positioned to become members of a multidisciplinary research team and work in patient care areas where research protocols are initiated. As members of multidisciplinary teams, DNPs are able to use clinical knowledge to integrate research findings from diverse sources and use data from other disciplines to improve the health and well-being of populations.

As health-care practice becomes more complex and requires a broader knowledge base to promote health, prevent disease, and care for patients with chronic and acute diseases, no one member of the health-care team can do all that is necessary. Health-care agencies at the national, state, and local levels strongly endorse a multidisciplinary approach to health care, obtaining ideas and creating solutions at many levels of care and practice. The same is true for uncovering or establishing the evidence for effective practice (National Academy of Sciences, 2004). No one group has all of the answers, but groups working together may be able to establish multilevel, creative, and lasting solutions to health-care issues. There are powerful drivers for multidisciplinary research with major research funding agencies urging professionals to include a multidisciplinary approach in research proposals.

True interdisciplinary research moves beyond simple collaboration and teaming to integrate data, methodologies, perspectives, and concepts from multiple disciplines to advance fundamental understanding or to solve real-world problems. Interdisciplinary research requires either that an individual researcher gain a depth of understanding in another discipline and be fluent in the languages and methodologies or, more frequently, that multidisciplinary teams assemble and create a common language and framework for discovery and innovation.

Evanoff, Potter, Wolf, Dunagen, and Boxerman (2006) found that nursing and medicine had different priorities when caring for patients and that this was an impediment to multidisciplinary work between the two professions. It is essential for teams of professionals to develop an understanding of the disciplinary priorities and framework for practice of the other to work together effectively to develop useful evidence. In many medical research studies, a drug or treatment is shown to be beneficial, but no mention is made in the research study as to how to motivate patients to spend money to purchase the medication, to take a medication even though they have no obvious symptoms, or to take the medication despite side effects. Using a multidisciplinary approach to research could involve finding answers to the previous questions and creating evidence that the medication is effective.

Creating well-functioning multidisciplinary teams requires special abilities, including leadership abilities. The DNP may be involved in the creation of this type of team or may be a member of the team. Establishing roles and responsibilities between multidisciplinary partners is one of the first challenges that should be negotiated between group members. Understanding the interests of each member of the team in relation to the research topic and goals provides a better understanding of the priorities from each discipline involved.

Examples of Evidence in Practice

Many hospitals have developed evidence-based research and practice committees. These groups often begin by establishing a journal club. These groups ask members to read, evaluate, and present research articles pertinent to a clinical topic. Discussions about research presented allow committee members and others who are interested to reflect on their own practice and propose new nursing interventions and policies to improve patient care. Finally, the ideas and changes recommended by the committee are discussed at the bedside during grand rounds. Grand rounds involves short presentations and discussions that take place at regularly scheduled intervals on all hospital shifts to allow questions to be raised and further discussion on any topic.

Following is an example of the process and outcomes from an attempt of one hospital to institute an evidence-based practice protocol. The evidence-based practice committee, which consisted of one nurse from each unit in the hospital, discussed the need for nursing practice improvements. The topic chosen was assessment of patients for risks of venous thromboembolism (VTE) after admission. VTE, including DVT and PE, was found to be the most preventable cause of hospital mortality. A study of research literature addressing this problem revealed that more than 300,000 Americans die each year of hospital-acquired VTE and that assessment of each patient's risk for VTE on admission and after any change in clinical status plus the early initiation of prophylactic protocols could prevent VTE and save lives. The literature review also listed the diagnoses, treatments, and hospital issues that are the most frequent causes of hospital-acquired VTE. The nurses were surprised to find that evidence showed that 80% of hospital-acquired VTE occurred on medical units as opposed to surgical units. Finally, the research literature outlined the most effective treatment options. After reading and evaluating the data collected, the nurses created a VTE assessment tool. The tool consisted of a numerical rating of all risk factors possessed by each patient on admission and on change of status during the hospital stay. There were three levels of final risk: high, medium, and low.

To test the accuracy of the tool to measure VTE risk, the medical records of all patients in the hospital from the year before who had hospital-acquired VTE were studied and compared with an equal number of patients who did not experience hospital-acquired VTE. Patients in the comparison group were matched to the VTE group for age, diagnosis, and gender. The risk assessment tool was used to determine the risk of each of the 75 patients who experienced VTE and the 75 patients who did not. The scores of both groups were compared, and the members of the group that experienced hospital-acquired VTE were found to have significantly higher scores on the risk assessment tool than patients who did not experience hospital-acquired VTE.

After the tool had been tested, the committee presented the tool to the nursing staff in a grand rounds format. Discussions were held to determine how best to implement the tool and where it should be placed so that the information regarding VTE risk would be shared with others. The nursing staff completed a mandatory online educational presentation on the risk of VTE in the hospital, which included risk factors for VTE, incidence and prevalence of VTE, mortality rates for patients who experience a pulmonary embolic event, and appropriate prophylaxis for patients at risk. During the educational program, the nursing staff identified concerns regarding how best to communicate risk to physicians so that appropriate prophylaxis could be ordered.

The committee took the concerns of the nurses to the medical staff during a medical staff meeting. The committee presented the research information and the development and testing of the risk assessment tool to the medical staff. The medical staff group decided it would be beneficial to place suggestions for prophylaxis at the bottom of the assessment tool based on risk level and place the tool and prophylaxis sheet on the front of the chart so that all rounding physicians could be aware of the patients' risk for VTE. The medical staff developed prophylaxis suggestions using the recommendations from the American College of Chest Physicians (ACCP) guidelines. Using a multidisciplinary approach, the nurses and physicians studied the compliance of nurses with the use of the assessment tool and the medical staff compliance with ordering appropriate prophylaxis for patients with identified risk and the overall number of episodes of hospital-acquired VTE.

The benefits of this program were thought to be significant by both the nursing and the medical staff members. Nurses felt empowered by their ability to recognize a problem, search for solutions, implement and test solutions, and share the solutions with the medical staff. The physicians were pleased with the nurses' ability to assess patients at risk. In addition, the physicians appreciated the convenience of using the suggested prophylaxis sheet to improve compliance with appropriate treatments for VTE risk. The hospital benefited from this program because hospital-acquired VTE can be expensive and nonreimbursable and present a risk management problem. Finally, and most importantly, patients benefited from this program when hospital-acquired VTE rates decreased after the implementation of the program.

This example is based on hospital evidence-based practice, which is of interest to nurse administrators and clinical nurse specialists. However, the same steps can be taken by nurse practitioners in community settings.

Examples of Evidence From DNP Capstone Projects

DNP capstone projects create new evidence of the effectiveness of practice interventions in specific groups of people. The purpose of the capstone project is to allow DNP students to expand their abilities as practice experts and clinical leaders by formally designing a program or interventional approach, implementing that approach in practice, and evaluating the approach for improved health outcomes or patient satisfaction.

A capstone project was undertaken by a student who worked as an advanced practice nurse in a pulmonology practice. Many of her patients had end-stage chronic obstructive pulmonary disease. The patients had difficulty getting to the practice office because of breathing problems. Often, patients could not get to the physician and waited until their breathing had deteriorated to the point where they were forced to call 911 to be taken to the hospital. The DNP student set up her own home visit practice for these patients. She worked in conjunction with a collaborative physician, a pharmacy, and a laboratory to provide all that patients needed at home. The student was able to get on insurance panels and Medicare so that she was able to bill and receive direct reimbursement for the home visits. Findings from this project included increased patient satisfaction with services, increased compliance with prescribed treatments, and fewer hospitalizations because of earlier interventions (Grissman, 2010).

Another DNP capstone project was performed by a hospital administrator. This student had responsibility for the operating room and found that a significant number of older adults had episodes of delirium or acute confusion after a surgical intervention. These episodes increased postoperative length of stay and often led to confusion and accompanying symptoms that could last for 1 year after surgery. The student developed a preoperative checklist to assess for possible risk factors that could be identified preoperatively that might indicate a higher risk for postoperative delirium. These risk factors included infection, dehydration, malnutrition, and metabolic disturbances. In addition, the student created an in-service for all preoperative and postoperative nurses to provide them with information concerning risks for postoperative delirium. During this in-service class, the nurses discussed nursing interventions that might assist older adults to avoid delirium. Among these interventions were frequent reorientation to time, place, and person; appropriate hydration; adequate pain management; and increased sensory stimulation with music or allowing family members to come into the postoperative recovery room to talk with the patient. Outcomes of this program were positive, and this student was asked by hospitals around the United States to come and speak to operating room staff to provide the same program and information.

Another DNP student talked with children 5 to 9 years old about obesity, diet, and exercise while they were at a summer camp that took place at a zoo. To increase interest among the children, the topics were related not only to human health but also to the health of the zoo animals. The children designed healthy snacks for elephants, kangaroos, and other animals as well as for themselves. They discussed and participated in exercises and designed exercises for animals at the zoo. This project had a very positive outcome; the children showed a greater knowledge of the importance of a proper diet and 60 minutes of exercise a day and were able to relate this information to the animals. Finally, the children discussed both animal and environmental aspects of health and how each of these was intertwined with the other. Children in the summer camp wrote stories about healthy eating and exercise for people and animals.

Finally, another DNP student noted in a literature review that African American women had about the same rates of breast cancer as white women but that African American women died more often from the disease. The research suggested that this increased level of mortality was due to later diagnosis and treatment in African American women, which could be due to a lack of understanding of the need for mammograms and breast examinations to improve early detection and treatment. The DNP noted that African American women go to the beauty shop regularly and that this was a place not only for hair care but also for meeting and discussion. The student was able to get a small grant to teach local hairdressers how to counsel their clients about the importance of breast health, mammograms, and breast examinations. The grant also paid the hairdressers a small stipend for this work. Outcomes of this program included a 35% increase in the number of mammograms for this group of women and a 50% increase in the number of these women who scheduled medical appointments for breast examinations.

These four examples of capstone projects are very different, but each of them enabled DNP students to use their knowledge and skill as practice experts to improve the health and well-being of a group of people in a formal way. Each of these students was able to publish the results of her capstone project so that others might use the information in program planning.

Developing and Assessing Clinical Guidelines

Clinical guidelines are developed to assist health-care professionals and patients make informed decisions about health promotion, disease prevention, and health interventions. Guidelines are established using the evidence of research, patient preference, and provider expertise. Guidelines represent the sum of knowledge known at a given time regarding treatment regimens, medications, or procedures and best practice for any given situation. Establishing guidelines for treatment assists in the delivery of effective and efficient health care that conserves the resources of the provider, the patient, and payers.

It is essential that guidelines accurately describe the quality of the evidence for each treatment or intervention contained in the guideline and the uncertainty that may underlie some recommendations. Using the guideline levels of recommendations is a way to ensure that the strength of the evidence for each aspect of a guideline is provided. Guidelines can be used by both the defense and the prosecution in legal cases to determine what the provider should have done or should have known regarding a patient, diagnosis, and treatment. Although variance among guidelines exists, guidelines created by nationally recognized entities such as the American College of Gynecologists are used most often in legal cases.

"Guidelines statements" are sometimes used to discuss differences in guidelines proposed by different clinical groups. For example, regarding DVT and PE, the American College of Chest Physicians (ACCP) and the American Association of Orthopaedic Surgeons (AAOS) have major differences in their respective guidelines for prevention in patients at risk. Among other differences, on one hand, the ACCP guidelines state that aspirin is an ineffective prophylactic measure for prevention of DVT or PE. On the other hand, the AAOS guidelines list aspirin as a first-line prophylactic measure for DVT and PE. Guideline statements are used to discern the differences in guidelines presented and the rationale for the differences. Providers must choose treatments based on their understanding of the guidelines and the guideline statements and on their own expertise and experience.

National guidelines can be found on several Web sites. One of the most complete Web sites is called the National Guideline Clearinghouse and was developed by the Association for Healthcare Research and Quality. This Web site can be found at http://www.guidelines.gov. At this site, guidelines are listed by disease, differentiating between physical and mental diseases, and therapeutics. Therapeutics is divided further into drug therapies, diagnostic therapies, and behavioral activities. The site also discusses guidelines for the use of complementary and alternative therapies. Elsewhere within this site, expert commentaries on guidelines and evidence-based research and guideline synthesis statements that discuss areas of disagreement between professional organizations can be found. The National Guidelines Clearinghouse site provides annotated bibliographies that support the listed guidelines and a place for the submission of new guidelines. Table 3-10 lists other Web sites that are useful when attempting to locate guidelines that have been developed by national organizations.

Table 3-10

Guideline Web Sites

Name of Site and Types of guidelines available	Web Address
National Heart and Blood Institute Asthma guidelines Obesity guidelines Cardiovascular guidelines Guidelines for cholesterol levels and the treatment of hypertension	*http://www.nhlbi.nih.gov/guidelines/index.htm*
Clinical practice guidelines from the American College of Physicians General guidelines for most diseases	*http://www.acponline.org/clinical_information/guidelines/*
American Urological Association Guidelines for diseases of the urinary tract	*http://www.auanet.org/content/guidelines-and-quality-care/clinical-guidelines.cfm*

Continued from page 146 Table 3-10

Guideline Web Sites

Name of Site and Types of guidelines available	Web Address
American Academy of Dermatology Guidelines for prevention and treatment of skin disease	http://www.aad.org/research/guidelines/index.html
American Academy of Orthopaedic Surgeons Guidelines for prevention and treatment of bone and joint diseases	http://www.aaos.org/Research/guidelines/guide.asp
Behavioral Health Recovery Management Guidelines for prevention and treatment of drug and alcohol addiction and mental health disorders	http://www.bhrm.org/guidelines/guidelines.htm
American Association of Respiratory Care Guidelines for prevention and treatment of pulmonary diseases	http://www.rcjournal.com/cpgs/
United States Preventive Taskforce Guidelines for screening and preventive services	http://www.ahrq.gov/clinic/uspstfix.htm

Although national guidelines are a good source of information and planning, each clinician or group of clinicians must develop guidelines for the patients they serve. Sometimes these guidelines closely follow national guidelines but contain subtle differences that are important for specific groups of patients. To be meaningful, guidelines should take into consideration cultural differences, patient preference, levels of insurance, gender, local resources, and other practice-specific requirements. For example, if a national guideline calls for a colonoscopy for people older than 50 years of age, what happens when the patient finds the preparation for the colonoscopy to be intolerable? Is it enough simply to recommend something when it is evident to the recommending provider that the patient will not comply with the recommendation? Perhaps adding a component to the guideline that allows for educating the patient on the dangers of not detecting colon cancer at an early stage and refining both the preparation for the colonoscopy and the procedure itself to be more acceptable to the patient would increase compliance. When the patient is unable to comply with guidelines, the provider should document the reasons for this inability in the chart. One of the most pressing issues in health care is that many guidelines can be met only in people with adequate health-care insurance. More specific methods for increasing compliance, especially for people without adequate access to health care through health insurance, should be added to guidelines to assist patients to remain healthy and treat diseases.

An important role for advanced practice nursing leaders is to know how to develop, implement, and evaluate sets of guidelines that are directly related to the nurse's setting. Individualized practice guidelines can be used as a benchmark for practice to create quality standards for care and evaluate treatments and clinical methodologies. Guidelines provide a consistent approach to increasingly complex medical care for patients and create a method to determine the success of a practice.

Advancing Your Knowledge

A group of nurse practitioners want to develop a guideline for the diagnosis and treatment of patients with diabetes in their practice. They have searched for and reviewed standard guidelines in order to create their own guideline for practice. They want to encourage patients to take part in their care, so the nurses are designing the guidelines so that patients can receive a guideline packet containing the guideline itself, diet education material, and a checklist to ensure they are doing what the guideline requires to keep track of their disease and treatment. The packet includes diagnostic procedures, medications, diet planning, and required referrals. Testing their guidelines, the nurses find that there is improved patient satisfaction and compliance with diagnostic testing, medications, diet, and referrals. After 1 year, the nurses find that there is a significant improvement in the numbers of diabetic patients who have blood sugar and hemoglobin A_{1C} levels within the norm, who have lost weight, and who are more compliant with medications and referrals.

1. Go to the National Guideline Clearinghouse at http://www.guidelines.gov and identify a guideline that pertains to your current practice. Evaluate the guideline for the specific group of patients or nurses you serve. How could the guideline be changed to reflect best practice for your group? How could compliance with the general guideline be improved?

Conclusion

Clinical scholarship focuses on integrating new knowledge from research into practice settings, testing and evaluating integration of knowledge, and standardizing the new knowledge in practice guidelines. Clinical scholarship is one method by which the DNP can improve and move nursing practice forward. Clinical inquiry is one area of clinical scholarship that allows for the development, testing, and application of new nursing knowledge.

Clinical scholarship includes not only findings from research or quality improvement programs but also nursing expert knowledge and experience and patient preference. The outcome of clinical scholarship is often the development of guidelines for practice. Guidelines already exist for many diseases and for health promotion and disease prevention activities. However, individual guidelines that reflect the culture and distinctive aspects of a given practice or area of practice are useful and increase coherence and compliance with the treatment plan generated by the guidelines.

Using the evidence of research requires that nurses, especially leaders in nursing such as the DNP graduate, have the skills to find, assess, and translate research into practice. Several types of research are well suited to practice applications. Translational research or taking what is discovered scientifically and translating the outcomes of that discovery into practice is one type of research that has been directly linked to DNP practice. Participatory action research is undertaken with the persons involved in the study as both researchers and participants. Coming to know a group, asking them how best to solve problems they are experiencing, and testing those solutions within the group are methods that could be used by the DNP-prepared nurse to resolve community and social issues that affect health and well-being.

The need to blend science, research, and practice within the discipline of nursing is one of the driving forces behind the development of the DNP. Working in multidisciplinary teams or in tandem with researchers, the DNP is valuable in the application and translation of research findings into the practice area and in the development of health-care guidelines that are practice-based and specific to a given population.

References

ABL Group. (1997). *Future search process design.* Toronto, ON: York University.

Agency for Healthcare Quality and Research. (2007). Closing the quality gap: A critical analysis of quality improvement strategies. Retrieved from http://www.ahrq.gov/clinic/epc/qgapfact.htm

Alexander, J., & Herald, L. (2010). The science of quality improvement: Developing capacity to make a difference. *Emerging Perceptions in Medical Care,* Dec;49 Suppl:S6-S20.

American Association of Colleges of Nursing. (2006). The essentials of doctoral education for advanced practice nurses. Retrieved from www.aacn.nche.edu

Atkins, S., & Murphy, K. (1993). Reflection: A review of the literature. *Journal of Advanced Nursing, 18,* 1188–1192.

Barker, A. (2009). Using patterns of knowing. In *Advanced practice nursing: Essential knowledge for the profession.* New York, NY: Jones & Bartlett Publishers.

Barnsteiner, J., Reeder, V., Palma, W., Preston, A.V., & Walton, K. (2010). Promoting evidence-based practice and translational research. *Nursing Administration Quarterly, 34*(3), 217–225.

Burns, N., & Grove, S.K. (2008). *Understanding nursing research* (4th ed.). New York, NY: Sauders Press.

Carper, B. A. (1978). Fundamental patterns of knowing in nursing. *Advances in Nursing Science 1*(1), *13–23.*

Cirocco, M. (2007). How reflective practice improves nurses critical thinking ability. *Gastroenterology Nursing, 30*(6), 405–413.

Cochrane Reviews. (2010). Retrieved from http://www2.cochrane.org/reviews/

Creswell, J.W. (1994). *Research design: Qualitative and quantitative approaches.* Thousand Oaks, CA: Sage Publications.

Duan, N., Braslow, J. T., Weisz, J. R., & Wells, K. B. (2001). Fidelity, adherence and robustness of interventions. *Psychiatric Services, 52*(4), 413.

Evanoff, B., Potter, L., Wolf, D., Dunagen, C., & Boxerman, S. (2006). Can we talk? Priority for patient care differences among healthcare providers. *Advances in Patient Safety, 1*(2), 139–143.

Flemming, K. (2007). The knowledge base for evidence-based nursing: A role for mixed methods research. *Advances in Nursing Science, 30*(1), 41–51.

Grimes, D. (1995). Over the counter oral contraceptives: An idea whose time has come. *Obstetrical and Gynecological Survey, 50*(6), 411–412.

Grissman, L. (2010). *Creating an advanced practice home visit practice for end stage COPD patients* (Unpublished Capstone Project). Florida Atlantic University, Boca Raton, FL.

Gross, D., & Fogg, L. (2001). Clinical trials in the 21st century: The case for participant-centered research. *Research in Nursing & Health, 24,* 530–539.

Hardin, S., & Kaplow R. (2005). Synergy for clinical excellence: An AACN synergy model for patient care. Washington DC: The American Association of Critical Care Nurses.

Holtzlander, L. (2008). Ways of knowing hope: Carper's fundamental patterns as a guide for hope research with bereaved palliative caregivers. *Nursing Outlook, 56*(1), 25–30.

John, C. (2008). *Framing learning through reflection within Carper's fundamental ways of knowing in nursing.* London, UK: Lancaster Press.

Kim, M. (2000). Evidence based nursing: Connecting knowledge to practice. *Chart, 97*(9), 4–6.

Kitson, A. L. (2007). What influences the use of research in clinical practice? *Nursing Research, 56*(4), S1–S4.

Kleinpell, R. (2008). Promoting research in clinical practice: Strategies for implementing research initiatives. *AACN Advanced Critical Care, 19*(2), 155–161.

Lauer, M. S., & Skarlatos, S. (2010). The meaning of translational research and why it matters. *Circulation, 121,* 929–933.

Lincoln, Y. S., & Guba, E. G. (1985). *Naturalistic inquiry.* Beverly Hills, CA: Sage.

Maloney, J., & Hahessy, S. (2005). Using reflection in everyday orthopedic nursing practice. *Journal of Orthopedic Nursing, 10*(1), 49–55.

Manthey, M. (2004). The practice of primary nursing. New York, NY: Creative Health Management.

McKenna, H., Cutliffe, J., & McKenna, P. (1999). Evidence based practice: Demolishing some myths. *Nursing Standard, 14*(16), 39–42.

Mikos-Schild, S., Endara, P., & Calvario, M. (2010). Journal clubs enlighten nurses, improve practice. *Nursing, 40*(10), 41–43.

Miller, W. (2010). Qualitative research findings as evidence: Utility in nursing practice. *Clinical Nurse Specialist, 24*(4), 191–193.

Minkler, M. (2000). Using participatory action research to build healthy communities. *Public Health Reports, 115,* 191–197.

National Academy of Sciences, National Academy of Engineering, and Institute Medicine. (2004). *Facilitating Interdisciplinary Research*. Washington, DC: National Academies Press.

Nightingale, F. (1869). *Nursing: What it is and what it is not.* Toronto, ON: Dover Publications.

Polit, D. F., & Beck, C. T. (2008). *Nursing research: Generating and assessing evidence for nursing practice* (8th ed.). Philadelphia, PA: Lippincott Williams & Wilkins.

Rogers, J. (2009). Transferring research into practice: An integrative review. *Clinical Nurse Specialist, 23*(4), 192–199.

Silva, J. (2011). Discover the power of intuition. Retrieved from http://www.silvaintuitionsystem.com/articles/intuition/intuition-quotes-and-intuition-theories/

Stetler, C. (2001). Updating the Stetler model of research utilization to facilitate evidence based practice. *Nursing Outlook, 49*(6), 272–278.

Tucker, S., Klotzbach, L., Olsen, G., Voss, J., Huus, B., Olsen, R., Orth, K., & Hartkopf, P. (2006). Lessons learned in translating research evidence on early intervention programs into critical care. *The American Journal of Maternal/Child Nursing, 31*(5), 325–331.

CHAPTER 4

EVIDENCE-BASED PRACTICE
Guidelines for Care

Objectives:

By the end of the chapter, students should be able to:

1. Define evidence-based practice, and explain how it is used to improve patient care and to bridge the knowledge to research to practice gap.
2. Describe the use of evidence-based practice in advanced practice nursing.
3. Find and assess evidence to be used in advanced nursing practice by:
   - Composing relevant and complete clinical questions.
   - Discussing where evidence can be found and distinguishing between different types of evidence.
   - Formulating evidence using systematic reviews of research literature.
   - Appraising research findings for significance and applicability in practice settings.
4. Use evidence as a foundation for practice decision making and translate findings of evidence into the practice setting.
5. Review critical thinking, and discuss the essential components of critical thinking as they relate to understanding and using evidence in the practice setting.
6. Discuss clinical guidelines and learn to:
   - Develop clinical guidelines.
   - Use clinical guidelines in practice.
   - Analyze evidence-based guidelines based on classification categories.

As nursing leaders contemplated the need for a clinical doctorate in nursing, one aspect of the motivation to create a doctor of nursing practice (DNP) degree was to educate and prepare advanced practice nurses in the acquisition, critique, and use of appropriate evidence in practice. In an effort to prioritize health, evidence-based practitioners adopted a process of lifelong learning that involves posing specific questions of direct practical importance to patients, searching objectively and efficiently for the current best evidence relative to each question, and taking appropriate action guided by evidence. This work is generally termed *evidence-based practice* (EBP). This chapter first defines EBP; it then discusses why EBP is important in advanced practice nursing, how to find and evaluate evidence, and how to use evidence in creating and evaluating guidelines for practice.

Foundations of Evidence-Based Practice

Evidence-based practice has become an increasingly important philosophy in nursing (Stiffler & Cullen, 2010). The basic definition of EBP for nurses includes three components: (a) research evidence, (b) nursing knowledge, and (c) patient preference. In 1998, DiCenso, Cullum, and Ciliska proposed a model of decision making that integrated research evidence, clinical expertise, patient's choices, and available assets. This model of integration is central to advanced nursing practice and forms the basis for practice.

EBP was described by Omery and Williams (1999) as a process whereby the nurse is able to explain or predict outcomes of actions. These authors stated that the evidence-based process is scientific and provides a practice discipline with the ability to anticipate and create meaningful interventions. Using this definition of EBP and the description of outcomes of using EBP supports the idea of systems thinking. The system of EBP creates a view of nursing care as a framework for improving healthy environments and developing a vision of a systematic method for creating nursing interventions and care based on evidence. However, in the area of advanced practice, additional attention must be paid to the cost-effectiveness of tests and treatments.

Burns and Grove (2009) discussed the aspect of cost-effectiveness as part of EBP. Evaluating the cost of care and the options for the most cost-effective care is an essential aspect of EBP and one of which the advanced practice nurse must be especially cognizant as he or she orders tests, prescribes medications, and offers other treatments in an autonomous manner. Polit and Beck (2006) posited that nurses who use evidence as the basis for practice are being professionally accountable to their patients. It might also be said that nurses who use EBP—with the added component of a cost focus—as the foundation for professional decision making are being professionally accountable to society in general.

The American Association of Colleges of Nursing (AACN) (2006) publication, "The Essentials of Doctoral Education for Advanced Practice Nurses," listed EBP (in the form of translation of research into practice, dissemination of new knowledge, and integration of new knowledge into everyday practice) as a key objective of DNP graduates (p. 11). Using evidence to solve practice problems and working within a multidisciplinary team to create improved patient outcomes are critical aspects of advanced nursing practice and can be enhanced through doctoral study. The DNP provides leadership in the area of EBP and is able to articulate the need for this type of nursing practice throughout all levels of health care. The AACN has developed the following objectives for the DNP graduate:

- Use analytical methods to appraise existing literature and other evidence critically to determine and implement the best evidence for practice.
- Design and implement processes to evaluate outcomes of practice, practice patterns, and systems of care within a practice setting, health-care organization, or community against national benchmarks to determine variances in practice outcomes and population trends.
- Design, direct, and evaluate quality improvement methodologies to promote safe, timely, effective, efficient, equitable, and patient-centered care.
- Apply relevant findings to develop practice guidelines and improve practice and the practice environment.
- Use information technology and research methods to:
  - Collect appropriate and accurate data to generate evidence for nursing practice.
  - Inform and guide the design of databases that generate meaningful evidence for nursing practice.
  - Analyze data from practice.
  - Design evidence-based interventions.
  - Predict and analyze outcomes.
  - Examine patterns of behavior and outcomes.
  - Identify gaps in evidence for practice.
- Function as a practice specialist or consultant in collaborative knowledge-generating research.
- Disseminate findings from evidence-based practice and research to improve health-care outcomes.

Linking Knowledge, Research, and Practice

Using evidence as the basis for practice requires nurses to bridge the theory-research-practice gap and base practice on research, other types of evidence, understanding of grand and middle range nursing theory, and patient preference and abilities. The DNP-prepared advanced practice nurse is the professional nurse best suited to bridge the theory-research-practice gap and use EBP in all health-care arenas, including hospitals, outpatient settings, and extended care. Learning to use the EBP model allows DNP graduates to integrate the knowledge from multiple levels of evidence into practice to solve problems, whether population based or individual, and improve care.

Creating the link between theoretical nursing knowledge, research, and practice is an important component of EBP. Testing theoretical concepts and propositions allows nurses to determine the evidence that is within the nursing domain or paradigm. The purpose of discipline-specific clinical inquiry is to improve and validate the profession of nursing and maximize the level of patient care and, more specifically, increase awareness of current clinical practice issues, develop and advance research competencies including becoming a consumer of research findings, empower nurses to participate collaboratively in multidisciplinary research or in research in coordination with nurses of other backgrounds, promote continuous quality improvement, close the gap between research and practice, and increase the visibility of nursing work. The DNP with expert clinical knowledge and an understanding of research is able to create an atmosphere in practice where research use is the norm.

Advancing Your Knowledge

S.F. is an advanced practice nurse with a DNP degree. He works in an outpatient practice setting with many patients who have drug and alcohol addiction. Because of the outpatient setting, he is unsure about how to work with these patients. Most of the patients with drug and alcohol problems are living on their own or with their families and function in society, but they feel they need help to overcome these habits. As S.F. reviews information about evidence-based practice, he finds the middle range *theory of self transcendence* (Reed, 2007). The concept of transcendence is that persons are able to expand self-boundaries and broaden their perspectives on life. A second concept in this theory is well-being; indicators of well-being include hopefulness, positive self-concept, satisfaction, and a positive perspective on life. Using this theory, S.F. finds research evidence that hopefulness and self-concept are often missing in people with drug and alcohol problems and that these people are often dissatisfied with their lives. S.F. discusses these concepts with a few of the patients and they agree that feelings of hopelessness and dissatisfaction are reasons for turning to drugs and alcohol.

S.F. creates a multidisciplinary team to meet with these patients as a group and individually, using story, individual discussion with the provider and a psychologist, and a behavior modification plan to stop thoughts of hopelessness and replace these with thoughts of gratitude and hopeful futures. At the same time, each individual meets with S.F. to develop a plan for withdrawal from alcohol or drugs and how to deal with cravings and relapses. S.F. institutes this plan in his practice with the help of a behavior modification specialist, an addiction specialist, and a psychologist. The success rate of this program exceeds the national success rate for this patient group, and S.F. develops and shares the findings of this experience in several nursing and addiction journals.

1. How did S.F. bridge the theory-research-practice gap in developing his program?
2. Did his method create a strong program? Why?
3. Describe an area of practice in which you might use a theory-guided approach to solving a problem, and then, using evidence from research studies, design and test a program in practice.

Outcomes as Evidence

The use of evidence alone does not always ensure positive outcomes in patient care. When nurses embrace the use of evidence-based interventions in practice settings, there are still questions to answer. What are the outcomes of EBP in a particular situation or with a particular population? How does using the different types of evidence as a basis for practice interventions influence patient outcomes, patient satisfaction, and improvements in health? The Agency for Healthcare Research and Quality (AHRQ) is a national organization that identifies health-care problems, funds evidence-based research, and tracks evidence-based outcomes. The AHRQ has identified outcomes research as important to determine the effect of a particular practice or intervention on the health and well-being of a subset of patients. For clinicians and patients, outcomes research provides evidence about the benefits, risks, and results of treatments so that clinicians and patients can make more informed decisions. One example of outcomes research provided by the AHRQ concerns the outcomes of hospitalization for pneumonia in older adults. The findings of this research revealed that many older adults with pneumonia can be treated effectively at home, which is preferred by patients and reduces the cost of care. In cases of disease in which a cure is impossible, outcomes research can provide information that allows patients to make choices that improve their quality of life and promote well-being. To support outcomes-based research and EBP in general, the AHRQ has created research funding initiatives in this area.

Research Funding to Support Evidence-Based Practice

In 2010, the AHRQ announced an award of $473 million in grants and contracts to support projects to help people make health-care decisions based on the best evidence of effectiveness. The projects support patient-centered outcomes research efforts in many areas, including health-care interventions in real-world settings, advanced use of research findings by diverse populations, development of effective patient registries and training, and career development for the next generation of researchers. Patient-centered outcomes research is designed to inform health-care decisions by providing evidence and information on the effectiveness, benefits, and harms of different treatment options. The evidence is generated from research studies that compare drugs, medical devices, tests, surgeries, or ways to deliver health care in real world settings.

The AHRQ has begun to require that all research receiving funding from the agency include translation activities so that the evidence found can be translated into changes or innovations in practice. Topics of interest for the AHRQ include research to reduce health disparities, research to improve positive health behaviors, and research to improve work conditions and reduce cost in health-care institutions. The AHRQ home page can be accessed at http://www.ahrq.gov/; a search box is available to review the work of the agency in different areas of quality and research.

As DNP-prepared nurses work in the area of outcomes research and EBP generally, and as they attempt to translate the findings of evidence into everyday practice settings to improve patient outcomes, it is important to have common definitions of EBP.

Definitions of Evidence-Based Practice

Many scholars and researchers have defined EBP. The first professional practice group to use the term *evidence-based practice* was physicians in the late 19th century (Sackett, Straus, Richardson, Rosenberg, & Hayes, 2000). The definition of EBP at that time focused solely on the findings of research and guideline development without consideration for practitioner intuition or knowledge concerning individual patients and patient preference. Despite initiating EBP, physicians became distrustful of it because they believed that it disregarded the art of diagnosis and treatment of each patient individually (Sackett et al., 2000). Since that time, the most used definition of EBP has been refined to become the current Institute of Medicine (IOM) definition:

"[EBP is] the conscientious, explicit, and judicious use of current best evidence in making decisions about the care of individual patients. The practice of evidence-based medicine means integrating individual clinical expertise with the best available external clinical evidence from systematic research" (IOM, 2001).

Evidence for practice comes from the following five sources of knowledge (Glanville, Schrim, & Wineman, 2000):

- Research
- Clinical experience
- Reasoning, authority
- Quality improvement data
- Patient's situation, experience, and values

Aside from the IOM definition, various formal and informal definitions for EBP exist, particularly as it applies to nursing. Newhouse, Dearholt, Poe, Pugh, and White (2009) proposed the following key assumptions for evidence-based practice:

1. Nursing is both a science and an applied profession.
2. Knowledge is important to professional practice, and there are limits to knowledge that must be identified.
3. Not all evidence is created equal, and there is a need to use the best evidence available.
4. Evidence-based practice contributes to improved outcomes.

These key assumptions describe the need for testing research evidence in the practice setting to create workable solutions to health-care problems that not only are effective but also affordable, reasonable, and acceptable to the patient. These assumptions also propose that nurses should understand the levels of research evidence that exist in order to use the highest level of evidence available for decision making (see Chapter 2). DNPs, through their advanced education, can combine research experience, organizational knowledge, an understanding of quality improvement and financial data, leadership, clinical expertise, and patient preference when making practice-based decisions.

Melnyk and Fineout-Overhold (2005) created a guide for nurses in the development and use of EBP. These authors conceptualized EBP as a process for the delivery of quality care. They attributed the expanding need for EBP to the multifaceted and complex clinical situations nurses and patients face in health care. Increasing complexity is part of the health-care picture because of longer life expectancy and increases in chronic diseases as well as the increasingly high cost of health care and the number of underserved individuals without access to health care. Melynk and Fineout-Overhold (2005) described EBP as a problem-solving approach that assists in clinical decision making. See Box 4-1 for an explanation of standards of care, which are often—but should not be—confused with EBP.

Evidence-Based Practice and Advanced Practice Nurses

EBP has become more prominent as a way to develop guidelines and tailor care as many health-care disciplines recognize the importance of evidence to all types of health-care decisions. Greater patient choice and complexity of care mean

Box 4-1

Standards of Care

Standards of care are developed using the findings of evidence and are often used in legal contexts. Standards of care are developed to define what is expected as a minimum standard of health-care practice for given situations in hospital care, disaster care, emergency department care, or primary care. These are measures against which practitioners and organizations are judged in the areas of ethical care and legal proceedings. Standards of care do not allow for the flexibility to determine individual needs because they differ from patient to patient. Standards set firm minimum benchmarks that should be met by all. Standards may focus on evidence but often are established by expert opinion or community practice standards without regard for evidence. By contrast, true evidence-based practice is more individualized to patient needs and desires and often creates a higher standard in practice settings.

In the legal context, a standard of care holds a person of exceptional skill or knowledge to a duty to act as would a reasonable and prudent person possessing the same or similar skills or knowledge under the same or similar circumstances. In other words, Nurse A has a duty to act as reasonable and prudent as Nurse B would in the same or similar circumstances. If Nurse A has acted differently, and harm has come to a patient, a jury or judge may find her to have been negligent in the care provided.

that many professionals practice as part of a team, and EBP has become a principle in the united commitment to best practice in all health-care disciplines.

In advanced practice nursing, EBP and evidence-based outcomes are important aspects of the quality and attention to individual wholeness for which the discipline is known. EBP includes consideration of internal and external influences in the patient's life and requires critical thinking to use the evidence to develop a plan of care. The American Academy of Nurse Practitioners (2007) created "Standards of Practice for Nurse Practitioners." Aspects of EBP included in these standards are the following:

- Nurse practitioners use the scientific process and national standards of care as a framework for managing patient care. This includes assessment of health status, diagnosis, development of a treatment plan, implementation of the treatment plan, and follow-up on the patient's condition.
- Nurse practitioners are responsible for patient and family education, facilitation of patient participation in self-care, promotion of optimal health, provision of continually competent care, facilitation of entry into the health-care system, and promotion of a safe environment.
- Advanced practice nurses must be aware of interdisciplinary and collaborative responsibilities, accurate documentation of patient status and care, responsibility as a patient advocate, quality assurance and continued competence, and research as a basis for practice.

The full document of standards for nurse practitioner practice can be found on the American Academy of Nurse Practitioners Web site at http://www.aanp.org/NR/rdonlyres/FE00E81B-FA96-4779-972B-6162F04C309F/0/Standards_of_Practice112907.pdf.

EBP guidelines propose specific care practices that are disease specific and adaptable to meet patient preference and nursing knowledge. EBP guidelines also provide details concerning where the evidence was gathered and the strength of the evidence. Using an evidence base to guide practice decision making is the underlying purpose of EBP guidelines.

The DNP is at the center of the practice and research axis and is able to meet the standards set by the IOM (2003) that call for a "restructuring of nursing" to allow for the delivery of patient-centered care in interdisciplinary teams that emphasize EBP. Not only is the DNP the appropriate practice-based professional to evaluate the research evidence, but also the DNP is in the best position to come to know the patient's values and desires related to health and well-being. Therefore, nursing has embraced EBP in the hospital, in primary care practices, and throughout community health-care settings.

By using evidence as the basis for practice decision making, nursing has progressed from using habit and usual practice as the foundation for disciplinary knowledge to a focus on EBP. EBP in nursing has three major components:

- Gathering, critiquing, and using the evidence of research to guide practice decision making
- Using the knowledge gained from practice experience to provide evidence

- Taking into consideration the patient's preference and desires as evidence to promote best practice

To advance the translation of evidence and evidence-based guidelines into everyday nursing practice, advanced practice nurses prepared at the DNP level should be able to evaluate evidence from many sources and use that evaluation to create guidelines for care. DNPs should be able to undertake translational research to test results from clinical studies and health-care guidelines in everyday clinical practice and health-care decision making. Translational research studies take evidence from research into the area of common practice where it can be refined to ensure that the best knowledge from available evidence becomes integrated into everyday nursing practice. To accomplish these goals, the DNP should remain aware of the three components of EBP—research evidence, nursing knowledge, and patient preference—and use these standards to evaluate and recommend best practice throughout the profession.

Advancing Your Knowledge

R.M. works as an advanced practice nurse in a practice with two physicians. Her patient is Mrs. P., a 40-year-old woman who complains of continuing abdominal pain. In reviewing Mrs. P.'s medical record, R.M. notes that she has been complaining of this dull achy cramping pain that comes and goes for several months. Today, Mrs. P. says the pain seems to be getting worse, and she has frequent bouts of diarrhea that alternate with bouts of constipation. During the constipation, the pain is worse. Mrs. P. does not have health insurance and is frightened that her condition might be something serious. She tells R.M. that she lost her job 4 months ago and has been unable to find employment even though she spends all day filling out applications. She has not been sleeping well and has a reduced appetite, although she has not lost weight since her last visit. She also tells R.M. that she has frequent headaches and has experienced some flutters in her stomach and chest. Mrs. P. has no family history of gastrointestinal problems or cancer; she is normal weight for her height; and she eats a healthy diet with fiber, fruits, and vegetables.

R.M. completes a thorough assessment of Mrs. P. Blood pressure is 110/68 mm Hg, temperature is 98.4°F, pulse is 76, and respirations are 16. The heart shows no murmur or rub. The lungs are clear. The skin is warm and dry without discoloration, the abdomen is soft without organ enlargement, bowel sounds are heard throughout, and there is no tenderness on palpation. An in-office electrocardiogram is normal. Hemoccult is negative for blood. Mrs. P. has blood drawn and her complete blood count and metabolic panel are within normal limits. Thyroid-stimulating hormone is 2.33 mIU/L.

R.M. knows from experience and intuitive knowledge that Mrs. P. is under a lot of stress. She knows Mrs. P. to be a type A personality and a person who has difficulty when her life seems out of her own control. The evidence mandates

Continued on page 162

Advancing Your Knowledge *Continued from page 161*

that a colonoscopy be ordered to rule out lesions or bleeding, but she knows that Mrs. P. cannot afford to pay for this procedure.

R.M. calls a gastroenterologist to whom she sends a lot of patients. They discuss the case and Mrs. P.'s inability to undergo a colonoscopy because of cost. R.M. and the gastroenterologist both believe that Mrs. P. has irritable bowel syndrome. They jointly develop a plan where Mrs. P. will acknowledge that she is refusing the colonoscopy and gastroenterology consult and undergo a trial of medical treatment including diet and pharmacological therapy for irritable bowel syndrome. A follow-up appointment is made for 10 days later to re-evaluate Mrs. P. R.M. also provides Mrs. P. with information on some health insurance programs that are affordable for people who are unemployed.

1. What types of knowledge does R.M use to develop this plan of care for Mrs. P.?
2. Did R.M. make the correct decisions for her practice? For the patient? For overall quality of care?
3. If R.M. had told Mrs. P. that if she did not agree to pay for the colonoscopy she would not be able to be a patient in the practice because of the liability, what might have happened to Mrs. P.?
4. How should R.M. use different kinds of evidence to proceed if Mrs. P. continues to have problems despite the treatment prescribed?
5. Why are different types of evidence needed to assess and treat many patients adequately?

Finding and Assessing Evidence for Use in Practice

An essential skill when creating EBP is the ability to evaluate the effectiveness of an intervention or practice in the clinical setting; this creates a new definition of translating science into practice. Translation has traditionally been thought of as taking what has been found in the "test tube" or at the "bench" and developing those findings into new therapies, whereas the newer definition of translational research is to take what has been found to be effective in any aspect of practice and use those findings in a broader clinical setting to determine whether they can be translated into common use. For example, if an educational program for patients with newly diagnosed hepatitis C is tested and demonstrates the ability to improve patient compliance with the medical regimen set out for them, translational research dictates translating that educational program into a larger number of practices to see if the increase in compliance continues. The ability to translate findings and evidence into general practice prepares the DNP with appraisal and evaluative skills to determine the effectiveness of outcomes of EBP in particular disease contexts and in general methods of practice.

Before learning to translate research evidence into general practice guidelines, it is necessary first to find and evaluate evidence. Research evidence is most often found in conference or journal presentations of research findings, integrative reviews, practice guidelines, quality improvement data, clinical experience, expert opinion, collegial relationships, pathophysiologic information, common sense, community standards, published material, and case studies There are four steps to collecting and appraising evidence to determine if it should be included in practice (Burns & Grove, 2009):

- Formulating a clinical question from which to generate practice
- Identifying appropriate evidence
- Completing a critical appraisal of the evidence
- Testing the evidence for use in a practice setting

Formulating Clinical Questions

The first step in beginning an evidence-based project is to formulate a complete clinical question. When beginning EBP inquiry regarding a practice issue, formulating an adequate question is essential because it outlines what information is needed and what groups are being compared. These EBP questions often arise out of questions about what are the best treatments, clinical implications of treatment plans, efficiency, cost, and best achievable outcomes. Effective clinical questions should have four components, which can be remembered as the mnemonic *PICO* (Newhouse, Dearholt, Poe, Pugh, & White, 2007):

- *P*—Patient: Describe as accurately as possible the patient or group of patients of interest.
- *I*—Intervention or diagnosis or observation to be studied: What is the main intervention, therapy, or observation to be considered? This can include an exposure to disease, a diagnostic test, a prognostic factor, a patient perception, or an intervention to influence predisposing risk factors for a disease.
- *C*—Comparison: Is there an alternative treatment to compare? Alternatives may include no disease, placebo, a different prognostic factor, or absence of risk factor.
- *O*—Outcome: What is the clinical outcome, including a time horizon if relevant?

Examples of appropriate PICO-based questions are as follows (Nursing Library and Information Resources, 2005):

- In patients with bronchitis, does prescribing an antibiotic or not prescribing an antibiotic reduce sputum production and number of sick days experienced?
- In children with frequent complaints of abdominal pain, how does psychological counseling compare with treatment with antihistamines on reduction in missed school days and reduction of pain levels?

- Does listening to tranquil music tapes played in surgical waiting rooms reduce anxiety among surgical patient family members?

Clinical questions generally address the following categories: diagnosis, therapy, harm or etiology, prognosis, prevention, and experience (qualitative). Examples of each of these types of questions are as follows (Nursing Library and Information Resources, 2005):

- *Diagnosis:* How to select a diagnostic test or how to interpret the results of a particular test. "What is the best test to use when attempting to diagnose thyroid disease?"
- *Therapy:* Which treatment is the most effective or what is an effective treatment given a particular condition. "In children with ear pain and fever, when should antibiotics be prescribed, and when is watchful waiting the best treatment?"
- *Harm or etiology:* Are there harmful effects of a particular treatment, or how can harmful effects be avoided. "In patients taking methotrexate for rheumatoid arthritis, what harmful effects might be experienced, and what testing should be done to monitor these effects?"
- *Prognosis:* What is the patient's likely course of a given disease, or what is the prognosis for the patient with treatment. "What is the likely course of hypertension if not controlled? What is the likely course if hypertension is partially controlled?"
- *Prevention:* How can a patient's risk factors be adjusted to help reduce the risk of disease. "What patient groups are at highest risk for poor outcomes if they contract influenza? How can the flu shot be provided to those most in need?"
- *Experience (qualitative):* Hopes to understand the clinical phenomena with emphasis on understanding the experiences and values of the patient. "What is the experience of having a child with autism? What are the most difficult aspects of this experience, and what could health-care providers do to alleviate these difficulties?"

After the clinical question has been formulated and approved by all members of the EBP team, the next step is to identify evidence that may answer the clinical question. There may be evidence that answers part of the question or answers a question similar to the one being asked but using a different population or setting.

Identifying Evidence

The second step in the four-step process is to identify evidence from articles and other resources that answer the question posed. Evidence can be found in (1) primary articles that present individual study results from the perspective of the researchers completing the study, (2) evidence summaries from systematic literature reviews, (3) integrative reviews, or (4) meta-analyses. Primary research articles are used to disseminate the findings of a particular research study and are usually written by the researcher or researchers who designed, implemented, and completed the study. Systematic reviews of the literature focus on a specific research question and identify, appraise, and evaluate all research literature relevant to this question. This type of review is designed to answer focused clinical questions and is an important source for developing EBP models (Stevens, 2001). An integrative review is broader in scope than a systematic review and does not always combine results in a focused manner the way a systematic review does (Stevens, 2001). Meta-analysis is a specific statistical method used to categorize and summarize data to provide an estimate of the effect of health-care variables (Mulrow, 1997). Evidence can also be derived from practice sources or from disciplined research performed by evidence-seeking nurses themselves and their colleagues. See Box 4-2 for two specific types of research well suited for advanced practice nurses when seeking sources of evidence.

Systematic Reviews as Evidence

Systematic reviews, also called *evidence summaries,* are important in identifying evidence for use in practice. The goal of the systematic review is to provide a reliable, scientifically derived base for clinical practice and provide a broader view of research findings than single research articles alone. Systematic reviews can resolve inconsistencies between conflicting research results and often combine studies with small and large samples into a single statement. One of the most important advantages of systematic reviews of research questions is that they increase the power and validity relationship between intervention and outcome (Stevens, 2001). Table 4-1 provides resources for finding systematic reviews.

Identifying Evidence From Practice Sources

In addition to research, there are three practice areas where evidence may be found. The first is from tradition, usual practice, or authorities in an area or from someone with specialized knowledge. The second is knowledge that comes from experience. The third is trial and error and assembled data. These practice

Box 4-2

Translational and Participatory Action Research

Translational research, as mentioned earlier in the chapter, takes the findings of research, applies them in the practice area, and evaluates the success of the intervention or innovation in practice. This type of analysis combines the three types of evidence—research, practice knowledge, and patient preference—to bridge the gap between traditional research and practice. Participatory action research is also very well suited to use by the DNP. This type of research combines the knowledge of the advanced practice nurse with the questions and proposals for change from community members to solve community problems.

Table 4-1

Finding Systematic Reviews on the Internet

Title of Database	Description	Web Address (URL)
United States Preventive Services Task Force Association for Health Research and Quality	Evidence synthesis and systematic evidence reviews	USPSFT Website *http://www.uspreventiveservicestaskforce.org/recommendations.htm*
The Cochrane Library	Systematic reviews updated regularly Database of Abstracts of Reviews of Effectiveness (DARE) Cochrane Controlled Trials Register Economic Evaluation Database of Health Technology Assessment Cochrane Methodology Register	*http://www.cochran.org/Cochran-reviews* This database is available only by subscription. Most universities and teaching hospitals have a subscription
Cumulative Index of Nursing and Allied Health Literature	Contains citations for systematic reviews	*http://www.ebscohost.com/cinahl/* This database is available only by subscription. Most universities and teaching hospitals have a subscription
The Joanna Briggs Institute for EBP and Midwifery	Systematic reviews that are freely available	*http://www.joannabriggs.edu.au/*
OVI Medline	To find systematic reviews in MEDLINE, do a subject search. Limit to human and English. Limit the search to EBP reviews	*http://www.nlm.nih.gov/bsd/pmresources.html*
National Quality Measures Clearinghouse	Sponsored by AHRQ. Structured, standardized abstracts containing information about measures and their development—useful for comparing attributes of two or more quality measures in a side-by-side comparison	*http://www.qualitymeasures.ahrq.gov/*
The Sarah Cole Hirsh Institute for Best Nursing Practice Based on Evidence	Affiliated with the Frances Payne Bolton School of Nursing at Case Western Reserve University. Systematic reviews are published in the open access publication *Online Journal of Issues in Nursing*	*http://fpb.case.edu/Centers/Hirsh/*

Source: Adapted from Nursing Library and Information Resources, Cushing Whitney Medical Library. (2005). Evidence-based practice: Asking the clinical question. Retrieved from http://www.med.yale.edu/library/nursing/education/clinquest.html

sources were discussed in detail in Chapter 3 but are reviewed here with specific examples for each type.

Evidence Gained From Tradition

Evidence gained from usual practice, tradition, authority, or someone with specialized knowledge is the first type of evidence used by nurses. An example of this type of evidence is the specialized knowledge a wound and ostomy nurse has to assist medical surgical nurses who are caring for a patient with a colostomy. The knowledge comes from the specialized training that the ostomy nurse has undertaken. From his or her training, a wound and ostomy nurse has learned to anticipate the physical and emotional issues that arise in the care of patients with a new colostomy. The nurse also uses knowledge gained from authorities in the area of ostomy care to anticipate skin breakdown or leakage of ostomy contents. Based on this knowledge, the ostomy nurse has at hand the appropriate equipment and educates the patient and significant others in how to deal with this issue and when to call for assistance. This nurse is able to instruct other nurses on best practice because of his or her expertise and learning in the area of ostomy care. Although the wound and ostomy nurse may be the "expert," he or she still remains current on new findings from research. The wound and ostomy nurse can pass knowledge, experience-based evidence, and findings from research studies to nurses at the bedside so that they can initiate effective and evidence-based practices and assist the wound and ostomy nurse in the teaching, coaching, and counseling of patients.

Evidence Gained From Clinical Experience

The second type of evidence available is clinical experience, which is based on observation, intuition, and hunch. This type of evidence often comes into use when the nurse simply "knows" that the status of a patient has changed without any physical evidence being present. This intuitive knowledge comes from being with the patient, coming to know the patient, and sensing subtle changes in physical signs and symptoms that are not yet measurable. This type of evidence is discussed by Benner (1982) as a tool used by expert nurses. Expert nurses intervene on the patient's behalf early in the course of physical changes to avoid more significant problems later when the physical signs and symptoms deteriorate and the patient's status becomes critical. An example of the use of this type of evidence is as follows:

An advanced practice nurse has a 27-year-old female patient for whom fatigue is the presenting complaint. The advanced practice nurse discusses signs and symptoms with the patient, assesses the patient's physical status, and because of an intuition does a urine pregnancy test that is positive. Although fatigue is a sign of early pregnancy, it is not often among the first in a list of differential diagnoses unless accompanied by other signs and symptoms of pregnancy. Using intuition enabled the advanced practice nurse to establish a diagnosis immediately and avoid expensive testing that would not have been useful. The diagnosis also provides the patient with the opportunity to make decisions about the pregnancy at early stages and begin to take appropriate measures to protect her own health and the health of her baby.

Knowledge Gained Through Trial and Error and Assembled Data

The third type of practice evidence used by nurses is trial and error. In this method, a problem is identified, and different solutions are tried to determine which one is most effective at solving the problem. For example, depression is a very common problem addressed in primary care settings. Patients who are prescribed antidepressants may require several trials to determine which antidepressant has the best result with the fewest side effects. The nurse practitioner may use the trial-and-error method to find the best antidepressant for the patient. From that time on, the nurse practitioner may use the antidepressant that worked best for this patient on other patients who present with depression and have similar age, gender, or other traits.

Assembled information, which includes benchmarks, quality assurance, and risk assessment data, is another type of practice-derived evidence that nurses use in practice situations. A "benchmark" in health care refers to an attribute or achievement that serves as a standard for other providers or institutions to emulate. For example, if 10 hospitals in an area meet the national benchmark of a 5% postoperative infection rate and 1 nearby hospital has a 10% postoperative infection rate, there is a problem, and there must be an investigation to gather evidence to determine the reasons and to strive to reduce the postoperative infection rate in the hospital to the benchmark rate.

Quality assurance data come from formal examinations of the outcomes of practice. These data can be provided from a health-care institution, an insurance company, or internal audits of individual practices. Quality assurance data provide the evidence of initiatives within health-care institutions to improve quality, such as fall prevention protocols, creating risk assessment protocols for deep vein thrombosis (DVT), or ensuring all patients are discharged with appropriate prescriptions and instructions for posthospital care.

Risk data provide sentinel event information, which the advanced practice nurse can use to develop questions about practice and identify evidence to improve routine practice. Risk data may point out process problems such as medication administration errors that can be corrected by education, new policies, or new equipment that can improve patient care and reduce adverse events.

Advancing Your Knowledge

G.R. is a DNP-prepared advanced practice nurse who works in the operating room of a hospital. He notices that there are many incidences of postoperative acute confusion among older patients undergoing hip or knee surgery. He also notices that patients are not screened in the preoperative area for risk factors for acute confusion, and postoperative nurses are unsure how to intervene with these patients except to sedate them. G.R. reviews the literature on acute confusion in older adults after surgery and creates a preoperative checklist for risk factors for acute confusion, including medications that can cause confusion, hydration, infection, dementia, and other factors that make a patient prone to postoperative acute confusion. G.R. gets permission from the hospital to conduct an in-service for all preoperative and postoperative nurses on the causes of and treatments for acute confusion after surgery. G.R. discusses appropriate interventions for this group, including placing the patient in a quiet corner to reduce sensory stimulation, providing frequent orientation, and allowing family members into the postoperative area. After the in-service and implementation of the risk assessment tool, identification of at-risk patients significantly increases, and the length of stay in the postoperative area related to acute confusion is significantly decreased.

1. Why would this experience be considered quality improvement rather than research?
2. What is the next step for G.R. after the outcomes of this project?
3. Why should DNP-prepared advanced practice nurses work within the hospital to improve care even when they are not hospital employees?

Identifying Evidence From Disciplined Research

Nurses also can identify evidence from performing disciplined research themselves. Many health-care settings now are implementing nursing research or evidence committees led by experienced nurse researchers. Staff nurses, regardless of their level of expertise or experience, can work together with nurse researchers to pose important practice-based questions, create well-designed studies, and use the findings from these studies to improve care. Translating the findings of research into practice is essential and an element that is often missing in the theory, research, and practice continuum. The inability of nursing to change practice based on the evidence of research findings has created the knowledge-practice gap. To decrease this gap, research knowledge and how to use that knowledge in practice are important aspects of the education of DNPs.

The DNP-prepared nurse is focused on practice and new evidence of the effectiveness of practice techniques, tests, medications, and treatments revealed on a daily basis. To identify and keep current in the area of new evidence, several e-mail alerts can be accessed daily. Table 4-2 lists the sites and addresses where registration for daily e-mails is possible.

Table 4-2

Daily Evidence and Research Alerts Available Online

Pri-Med Online	*http://www.pri-med.com/pmo/Home.aspx*
American Association of Nurse Practitioners Smart Brief	*http://www.smartbrief.com/aanp/index.jsp*
Physician's First Watch	*http://firstwatch.jwatch.org/*

Critical Appraisal of Evidence

The third step in the analysis of evidence is to appraise critically the evidence gathered to determine its validity and reliability. When reviewing the results of a literature search to find research articles on an identified topic, it is important to look at who wrote the article; their credentials; and any connection they have to a reputable organization, university, or health-care agency. It is important to find out who sponsored the research—was it a company that profits from the results, or was it a research agency that funds different types of research to improve knowledge and understanding of patient issues? When was this work published? Generally, the more recent a publication, the more timely and meaningful the results. However, there are older, seminal articles that are important as the seeds for understanding a health-related issue. Is the article from a peer-reviewed journal or publication? It is important to be sure that the sample size in the study and method of analysis for the data collected are adequate, that the information in the article is accurate, and that the results are not overgeneralized. Finally, has this work been quoted or paraphrased in other articles as having important findings? You can determine how often this work was cited and by whom using the Internet search engines that produced your literature review.

Evaluating Systematic Reviews and Meta-Analysis

To determine the quality and worth of a systematic review or meta-analysis, the reader must ask specific questions about the information provided in the review and whether that information is important to practice. Questions that should be used to evaluate systematic reviews include the following:

- Are the studies included in the systematic review of high scientific merit? Do the studies fall into level I, II, IIa, or III categories?
- Does the review state the methods used to find the other studies that are included in the review?
- Were results consistent from study to study?
- Are the study samples similar, and are they similar to patients in the practice for which the EBP is being studied?
- Were all clinical outcomes and benefits considered, including harms and benefits?
- How do the values of the patients studied in this review match with the practice for whom the EBP review is being done?

More information on evaluating and critiquing research literature is provided in Chapter 3.

Testing the Evidence

The fourth step is to devise a method of testing the evidence in practice. Stetler (2001) created a model for testing research findings in practice. The model uses the following six steps to test evidence in the practice area:

- *Preparation:* Identify the research literature on a given topic such as a clinical problem or an education issue.

- *Validate:* Determine which findings from research that you want to test in the practice setting.
- *Comparative evaluation:* Do the research findings fit with your population, environment, or problem? What adjustments might have to be made to test these findings in a particular situation? Is it feasible to use this research in a particular practice setting? What are the potential risks, what resources are required, and what is the readiness of the group who would implement the new research finding?
- *Decision making:* Should the findings be used now, should the project be put on hold until changes have been made in the practice area, or should the findings not be used at all because they do not meet the above-mentioned criteria?
- *Translation or application:* Determine how the new project should be applied and what implementation steps are needed. Implement the new practice with whatever adjustments have been made to meet the needs of the practice involved.
- *Evaluation:* Determine the impact of the new practice on providers, patients, staff, and outcomes.

An example might be to implement yoga practice for patients with migraine headache. In the preparation stage, it is determined that several research studies have identified yoga as a therapy that is beneficial to reduce migraine headaches. To validate these findings in practice, it is determined that a twice-weekly yoga program offered at a nearby wellness center might be helpful to patients with migraine headaches. After evaluation of patients with migraine in the practice, it is determined that only about half of these patients are able to participate in this yoga program because of cost and timing. It is determined that these patients should be called and encouraged to attend the yoga sessions to determine if they help to reduce migraine headaches. All of the patients identified agree to participate in the yoga sessions, and you ask each one to come in after 3 months of yoga to determine if the new practice is useful to this group. After 6 months, it is determined that yoga has reduced significantly the number of migraine headaches experienced by the group, and therefore yoga becomes a standard recommendation for all migraine patients.

Translating Evidence Into Practice

Research utilization is the ability to translate research findings into practice settings. Freshwater and Rolfe (2004) suggested that to bridge the gap between the discovery of evidence and the use of evidence in daily practice, nursing requires a paradigm of clinical research that focuses on the individual therapeutic encounter and translation of research findings into the practice arena.

When attempting to change practice (i.e., institute evidence into practice) or assist patients to change health behaviors, it is important to understand the change process. Although evidence of positive health behaviors may be known, assisting patients to make difficult changes in behaviors to move them to improved health and well-being is difficult. Examples of health-care behavior changes that can be difficult are smoking cessation and maintaining a healthy weight.

Change Process

Using evidence as a basis for practice requires changes in thinking and actions. Making changes in any aspect of clinical practice or asking patients to change health behaviors involves a change process that should be understood in order to make successful and meaningful change. Change, whether in the area of advanced nursing practice or asking a patient to make a health behavior change, is a process. Changes are not automatic and do not occur without a plan for implementation and evaluation of the success of the change. All persons involved in the change must be informed and agree to implement the change, or the change cannot be fully realized. In the case of a change in practice patterns, individuals who educate and advise patients and individuals who prescribe medications or order treatments are members of the change team. In the case of patients making a health behavior change, family members are also team members in facilitating and maintaining change.

For individuals attempting to institute change, it is important to understand that change is nonlinear; the people involved in the change should see the change as a challenge rather than a problem. This challenge can be to improve patient outcomes or to make personal healthy changes. Team members must feel empowered to voice concerns and discuss aspects of the change that do not seem to be working. Just because the leaders of the team tell people about the anticipated change does not mean it will happen smoothly. The leader of the team must listen to all team members.

Within a practice setting, stages can be recognized and used to manage needed changes and reduce resistance to the idea of change. Kern (2008) outlined one set of stages in the change process as follows:

- Preparation phase
  1. Contact stage: The earliest encounter a person has with the fact that change may take place or has already taken place. In the area of practice, this is the time when providers and others determine that new information is available regarding care for a diagnosis or a group of patients.
  2. Awareness stage: The person knows that a change is being contemplated. After obtaining and reading the available new evidence, the provider makes the decision to change the practice pattern in the area where new evidence exists.
- Acceptance phase
  1. Understanding stage: The person exhibits some degree of comprehension of the nature and intent of the change. The clinician must review all of the information necessary to make an evidence-based decision. The provider must make decisions at this point about what aspects of the evidence pertain to patients in the practice and the best way to meet the guidelines for care for these patients.

2. Positive perception: The person develops a positive view toward the change. After collecting and evaluating all of the evidence on a topic, the clinician must develop a practice change based on the findings of evidence and design the change as it best fits with the population under the clinician's care and the practice setting.

- Commitment phase
  1. Installation stage: The change is implemented and becomes operational. This is the time for a trial of the new evidence-based treatment to determine whether patients accept the recommendations and are willing to comply with the changes in the treatment and how office procedure might be affected by the change in practice. At this point, changes or adoption of new treatments or therapies can guide and inform effective strategies and enable a successful implementation process.
  2. Adoption stage: The change has been used long enough to demonstrate worth and a visible positive impact. During this stage, the practice performs an evaluation of the impact of the change and the progress that has been made toward the desired outcome. To perform this evaluation, the clinician should define the purpose of measurement, choose the aspects of the change to be evaluated, select specific indicators, and design specifications for the measures. Evaluation should compare baseline data with current data to determine whether the desired change has occurred and to measure success or failure.
- Institutionalization: The change has a long history of worth, durability, and continuity and has been formally incorporated into the routine operating procedures of the organization. During this phase, evaluation has occurred, and the entire practice is comfortable with the change. Patients expect this treatment as part of their health care plan and are comfortable with the benefits achieved through the implementation of the new treatment therapy.
- Internalization: People are highly committed to the change because it is congruent with their personal interests, goals, or value systems. The change has become a part of practice and is not regarded as new or a change but rather a normal treatment or therapy for this problem in practice.

Advancing Your Knowledge

L.G. has read about the overuse of antibiotics in children and adults and asks the clinical question: In adult patients, what are the signs and symptoms of upper respiratory bacterial infections compared with viral infections, and what is the best treatment for each type of infection to reduce symptoms and missed work days for this group? After a thorough review of the literature, her own nursing knowledge, and the preferences of her patients in getting well as quickly as possible, L.G. develops guidelines for her practice whereby patients

Continued on page 174

Advancing Your Knowledge *Continued from page 173*

who meet certain criteria receive an antibiotic, and others who meet different criteria receive supportive care and other treatments for viral infections. L.G. believes education is needed to be successful in implementing these new guidelines. L.G. creates a patient education sheet that outlines the differences between bacterial and viral infections, encourages patients to get a flu shot, and provides an outline of treatment for each type of infection and the problems with inappropriate treatment. L.G. also provides appropriate references to national organizations, such as the U.S. Centers for Disease Control and the National Institutes for Health, to allow patients to determine the background for her guidelines. She sends a copy of this guideline to each patient in the practice and posts the guidelines in each examination room and in the waiting room of the practice.

During the implementation of this guideline, there are a few patients who feel strongly that an antibiotic would be helpful to them. In these cases, L.G. carefully and patiently explains the reasons why an antibiotic would not help and provides the patients with the appropriate treatment. L.G. calls patients 2 days after their visit to be sure they are getting better on the treatments she has prescribed. After one season of flu, viral, and bacterial infection, patients are comfortable when L.G. tells them they do not need an antibiotic and are happy with the treatments she does prescribe. Overall, L.G. tracks patient visits and asks them about sick days from work. With the appropriate treatments, including flu shots and vitamins, patients state that they have fewer sick days than they have had in past years.

1. What aspects of the change process are evident in this scenario?
2. How did L.G. appropriately plan for and implement the change?
3. Is further follow-up needed for this change? If so, what could L.G. do to solidify the change?
4. Can you think of an example of a change that you have made in practice? What aspects of the change process did you use? How smooth was the change?

Changes to Patient Health Habits

When providers recommend a change in health habits to patients, such as smoking cessation, weight loss, or exercise, there is a specific change process that the patient and family go through. The stages of change model (Groth Marnat, 2009) illustrates that, for most people, a change in behavior occurs gradually, with the person moving from being uninterested, unaware, or unwilling to make a change (precontemplation); to considering a change (contemplation); to deciding and preparing to make a change. Genuine, determined action is then taken, and, over time, attempts to maintain the new behavior occur.

Relapses are almost inevitable and become part of the process of working toward lifelong change.

- *Precontemplation stage:* During the precontemplation stage, change is not even being considered. In the example of smoking cessation, smokers who are "in denial" may not see that the advice applies to them personally, or they may state that they are not ready to quit and need cigarettes to deal with their lives. Patients with high cholesterol levels may feel "immune" to the health problems that strike others. Sometimes people with high cholesterol believe that if they are not in pain or discomfort they do not need to take medication. Obese patients may have tried unsuccessfully so many times to lose weight that they have simply given up.
- *Contemplation stage:* During the contemplation stage, patients are beginning to think about making a change. Usually they are conflicted about trying to change a behavior, and they may think that changing behaviors might cause them to feel a sense of loss despite the perceived gain.
- *Preparation stage:* The preparation stage occurs after a decision to change has been made but before actually implementing the change. During this stage, preparations are made for the specific change. This is when patients and providers attempt to test the change by implementing small changes or trial changes. For example, sampling low-fat foods may be a move toward greater dietary modification.
- *Action stage:* The action stage is where change actually occurs. In the case of health behavior change, the provider must support and encourage patients as they attempt to stop smoking, lose weight, start cholesterol medication, or make any other change in health behaviors. For patients who want to quit smoking, the advanced practice nurse can encourage the patients to make a plan for quitting that would increase their chances of success. The plan should include what over-the-counter or prescription medications they will use, letting their friends and family know they have decided to quit and asking for their support, and finally determining when they smoke and what they will do instead of smoking at that time. It is important for providers not to react too quickly and to educate and listen to patients during this time.
- *Maintenance and relapse prevention:* Maintenance and relapse prevention involve incorporating the new behavior "over the long haul." Discouragement over occasional "slips" may halt the change process and result in the patient giving up. Most patients find themselves "recycling" through the stages of change several times before the change becomes truly established. If a patient contemplates a behavior change and then decides that he or she is not ready, the health-care provider must continue to encourage the patient to think about the change and the benefits of the change in the area of health. If a patient relapses to old habits during the maintenance stage, the provider should not voice frustration but rather continue to be

supportive and move the patient toward repeated actions that change behavior. Although this approach requires a time commitment from the health-care provider, it fosters improved patient outcomes, cost-effectiveness, and efficiency in care outcomes.

Critical Thinking Questions

1. Using the above steps for implementing change, how would you develop a smoking cessation guideline for a primary care practice?
2. How would you work with patients through each step of the change process? During the contemplation stage, how would you encourage patients to contemplate making a change? What is the role of the advanced practice nurse during the preparation and action phase of the change? How would you plan for the maintenance and relapse prevention stage?

Critical Thinking as a Component of Evidence-Based Practice

The ability to compile research evidence, nursing knowledge, and patient preference to create a framework for EBP and enable patients to make positive health-care behavior changes requires critical thinking skills. Critical thinking is the intellectually disciplined process that allows the advanced practice nurse to compile, analyze, and synthesize information in order to come to a conclusion about best practice and then to translate that knowledge into action (American Association of Colleges in Nursing, 1998). Knowledge is not a collection of facts, but rather an ongoing process of examining information, evaluating that information, and adding it to your understanding. Critical thinkers are able to keep an open mind, reflect and focus on deciding what to believe and how to act, and rethink their views as new knowledge emerges.

Rather than the mere acquisition and retention of information alone, critical thinking uses information and processing skills to guide behavior. Reflective reasoning, creativity, and divergent thinking are essential to critical thinking and EBP. Reflective reasoning allows for questions to be asked about whether assumptions are correct, whether one's ideas may be contrary to the evidence, or whether there are better explanations for a result than the one currently being used. Creativity allows nurses to consider multiple solutions to a problem, and divergent thinking permits analysis of various options before developing standards and guidelines for practice.

Paul, Binker, Jensen, and Kreklau (1990) developed a list of critical thinking strategies that are divided into three distinct categories. *Affective critical thinking strategies* are strategies that are based on feelings or judgments. *Macrolevel cognitive strategies* allow one to comprehend and use ideas in one view. *Microlevel cognitive strategies* are used to fine-tune critical thinking to a level where the outcome is usable. Table 4-3 lists the strategies and how they affect critical thinking.

Table 4-3

Critical Thinking Strategies

Strategies	How They Affect Critical Thinking
Affective	
Thinking independently	Critical thinkers use nursing knowledge and judgment along with experience to understand issues and possible solutions.
Developing insight into egocentricity or sociocentricity	Critical thinkers understand that one view of an issue is insufficient to understand the question from many different societal and cultural perspectives.
Fair-mindedness	Critical thinkers do what is best for the greatest number of people and are fair when allocating resources.
Exploring underlying feelings and thoughts, developing intellectual humility, and suspending judgment	Critical thinkers are able to listen to the ideas of others, suspending judgment until all facts are known and weighed. Critical thinkers do not think they know the answer before exploring the question.
Intellectual courage, integrity, perseverance, and confidence in reason	Critical thinkers have the ability to take a different path when the evidence shows that it is better, continuing to investigate evidence to move toward the best patient outcomes.
Macrocognitive Strategies	
Refining generalizations and avoiding oversimplifications	Critical thinkers are able to discern when evidence can or cannot be applied to different groups of people. *For example:* Studies that are completed on men may not apply to women, or studies using only one ethnic group may not apply to other ethnic groups. Oversimplification is using facts that point to a complex series of events and linking them to just one of those events. *For example:* Taking evidence that Asian American women who have higher education and are economically advantaged have lower rates of illegal drug use, one cannot conclude from these data that Asian American women have lower rates of illegal drug use.
Transferring insights to new contexts	Critical thinkers are able to develop new ways of seeing things and applying what they know. If an intervention to reduce obesity in elementary school children through an after-school exercise and outside play program is successful, it might be tried in the middle school to see if it can be successful there as well.

Continued on page 178

Continued from page 177 Table 4-3

Critical Thinking Strategies

Strategies	How They Affect Critical Thinking
Exploring, evaluating, and clarifying beliefs, arguments, or theories	Critical thinkers do not accept findings from research without evaluating the findings to determine if they truly demonstrate a significant piece of evidence. When evidence makes an assertion or an argument that something is correct or significant or that a study verifies a theoretical assumption, a critical thinker does not accept that without evaluating the evidence to determine whether it truly verifies these statements.
Developing criteria for evaluation and evaluating the credibility of sources of information	Critical thinkers develop formulas or criteria for evaluating evidence that are based on scientific and humanistic principles.
Creating and pursuing significant questions	Critical thinkers find that important questions that get at the "heart of the matter" must be developed. Using the PICO method of question development helps these questions to be meaningful.
Assessing solutions, actions, and policies	Critical thinkers assess possible solutions, actions, and policies to improve care from the information gathered.
Reading and listening critically	Critical thinkers are able to read and listen critically and sift through what is important and what is not.
Making interdisciplinary connections for discussion, clarification, and questioning beliefs	Health care is a multidisciplinary effort to provide needed care and treatment. Critical thinkers develop interdisciplinary connections to sustain their understanding and to seek clarification regarding beliefs and questions. This type of critical thinking strengthens the provider and the discipline of nursing as a whole.
Comparing and evaluating perspectives, interpretations, and theories	Critical thinkers are able to compare and evaluate the thoughts of others and determine how others interpret evidence and theoretical knowledge, which is essential to acquire a thorough understanding of issues and concepts.
Microcognitive Strategies	
Comparing and contrasting ideals with actual practice	Critical thinkers are able to compare and contrast ideas and evidence looking at all aspects of a problem, all types of evidence, and many different levels of findings.
Distinguishing relevant from irrelevant facts	Critical thinkers are able to evaluate evidence and to distinguish what is important to the findings and what is not. They also examine what aspects of a patient's preference are essential to the success or implementation of a plan of care.

Continued from page 178 Table 4-3

Critical Thinking Strategies

Strategies	How They Affect Critical Thinking
Noting similarities and differences	Critical thinkers are able to review evidence to determine its importance and to see patterns in research findings and areas where there are differences in findings. When there are groups of similar findings, the evidence is stronger than when there are multiple differences in the findings of research studies.
Making plausible inferences, predictions, or interpretations	Critical thinkers should be able to take information and develop conclusions and practice guidelines; this requires the ability to make plausible or true inferences from the research evidence. Once these inferences have been developed, predictions and interpretations of research findings can be used in the creation of guidelines.
Recognizing contradictions	Critical thinkers are able to see where there is opposition between two different groups and how to use the information that exists in the contradictions to determine how to use the evidence presented by both sides.
Exploring implications and consequences	Critical thinkers are able to translate the information obtained from evidence and develop guidelines for patient care. Within the guidelines created, it is imperative to determine and consider the implications of a treatment plan and the consequences that are possible for the patient, family, and provider.

Advancing Your Knowledge

T.T. is a cardiovascular clinical nurse specialist with a DNP degree. She works in a hospital setting. T.T. determines that her patients with heart failure require frequent admission to the hospital, and the stressors on the patient and family increase with each admission. T.T. begins a literature review to see what is known about readmissions for patients with heart failure. She finds several studies that point to the benefits of using an outpatient heart failure clinic to follow these patients and help them before they require hospitalization. She determines that this approach to reduction in hospitalization may be beneficial. She develops a business plan for this type of clinic, discusses the pros and cons with the hospital administration, investigates reimbursement rates with the chief financial officer, and determines space availability for such a clinic. The hospital agrees to try this type of clinic, and T.T. is asked to manage it along with her other duties. She hires one nurse practitioner to be the lead clinical person in the clinic and several allied health workers. She

Continued on page 180

Advancing Your Knowledge *Continued from page 179*

involves several cardiologists in this effort and the nurse manager of the cardiovascular floor at the hospital and several cardiovascular nurses. Working together with these professionals, T.T. develops a clinical guideline for the heart failure clinic. They develop a PICO-based question to determine the success of the clinic: Do patients who have been admitted to the hospital with heart failure within the last year benefit from being enrolled in a heart failure clinic? The clinic monitors the health status of the patients weekly and provides a place to answer questions and to call if symptoms occur. Has the advent of the clinic decreased admissions to the hospital for patients enrolled in the clinic compared with patients who are not enrolled in a heart failure clinic? Findings show a significant reduction in hospital admissions for the patients who are enrolled in the clinic.

1. What aspects of critical thinking did T.T. use in this plan?
2. Why is reducing hospitalizations a good idea for hospitals? Don't they lose patient days and therefore reimbursement?
3. Are you a critical thinker? Can you think of a program you might start in your practice or in a future practice that would improve patient outcomes and reduce costs?

The Johns Hopkins Nursing Evidence-Based Practice Model (Newhouse et al., 2007) proposes using a model that asks the advanced practice nurse to determine the clarity, accuracy, precision, and logic of questions being asked for critical thinking standards related to EBP. *Clarity* is used to determine if the nurse has a clear idea of the issue being examined and is able to provide an example. *Accuracy* refers to determining why we believe a thing to be true. Is it because we want to believe it is true because it is in our interest for it to be true, or is it because we have always believed it to be true? *Precision* asks for more information to be provided about the issue or if the issue can be compared with another intervention. *Logic* requires determination of the desired outcome and if that outcome makes sense (Newhouse et al., 2007, p. 23).

Critical thinking skills need to be used when developing an evidence base for practice. The challenge for DNP-prepared nurses is to embrace fully the concepts of critical thinking in practice and when working in an interdisciplinary team to develop evidence-based guidelines for practice. There are many examples of "practice as usual" that must be put aside to improve patient care and improve the efficiency of the health-care system. Persons with critical thinking skills will lead the way to evidence-based changes that benefit not only individuals but also the system as a whole.

Developing Clinical Guidelines

Often, the DNP-prepared nurse does not develop new evidence-based guidelines but rather evaluates guidelines that have been prepared by national expert groups or others for implementation into general practice. This section explores ways to develop, use, and analyze clinical practice guidelines. Clinical practice guidelines are systematically developed statements that assist advanced practice nurses to make decisions about appropriate health care for patients under any given circumstance (Kleinpell & Gawlinski, 2005). Evidence-based clinical practice guidelines can reduce the delivery of inappropriate care and support the introduction of new knowledge into clinical practice. In many cases, guidelines encapsulate the most current knowledge about best practices. Rigorously developed guidelines can translate complicated research findings into actionable recommendations for clinical care. Despite the enormous energies invested in writing guidelines, the quality of individual guidelines varies considerably (Shiffman et al., 2003).

Use of Clinical Guidelines

Clinical practice guidelines are evidence-based outlines of accepted management approaches, which may be disease, problem, or process specific. They are systematically developed statements that are used to assist practitioners and patients to make decisions about appropriate health care for specific clinical circumstances. In other words, guidelines are developed to aid the practitioner in pursuing the most appropriate health-care response for the clinical circumstances of a specific patient. Guidelines should be up-to-date in terms of science, highlight critical clinical information, and provide statements on common and accepted evidence-based medical practice. Applied at the individual level, guidelines are able to provide a set of standards and instructions that assist with problem solving. Guidelines can be individualized to patient preference and nursing knowledge and should be carefully documented in the patient record to understand the clinical reasoning for the individual changes. Using this approach, health care is delivered in an evidence-based outcome model.

Attributes of evidence-based clinical guidelines include the following (American Association of Orthopaedic Surgeons, 2009):

- Practice questions are defined, and decision options and outcomes are explicitly identified.
- The best evidence about prevention, diagnosis, prognosis, therapy, harm, and cost-effectiveness are explicitly identified, appraised, and summarized in ways that are most relevant to decision makers.
- Decision points are explicitly identified where the valid evidence needs to be integrated with individual clinical experience and patient values in deciding on a course of action.

Analysis of Clinical Guidelines

The IOM (1992) defined eight "desirable attributes" of clinical practice guidelines: validity, reliability and reproducibility, clinical applicability, clinical flexibility, clarity, documentation, development by a multidisciplinary process, and plans for review.

- *Validity:* Practice guidelines are valid if, when followed, they lead to the health and cost outcomes projected for them. A prospective assessment of validity would consider the substance and quality of the evidence cited, the means used to evaluate the evidence, and the relationship between the evidence and recommendations.

- *Reliability and reproducibility:* Practice guidelines are reproducible and reliable (1) if, given the same evidence and methods for guidelines development, another set of experts produces essentially the same statements, or (2) if, given the same clinical circumstances, the guidelines are interpreted and applied consistently by practitioners (or other appropriate parties).
- *Clinical applicability:* Practice guidelines must be applicable to practice settings using available staff and services.
- *Clinical flexibility:* Practice guidelines should be flexible to meet the needs of individual patients and patient populations.
- *Clarity:* Practice guidelines should be clear and understandable to the reader.
- *Documentation:* Practice guidelines should be developed using evidence from research that is clearly documented.
- *Development by a multidisciplinary process:* Practice guidelines should cross practice boundaries so that all clinicians involved in patient care are included in the guidelines.
- *Plans for review:* The IOM has also created a system to determine the strength of evidence in evidence-based guidelines. These levels are provided in guidelines from expert panels or from professional associations such as the American College of Chest Physicians or the American Society of Anesthesiologists. These levels are presented in Table 4-4.

Table 4-4

Levels of Evidence for Analyzing Evidence-Based Guidelines

- Class I recommendation: Conditions for which there is evidence or general agreement that a given procedure or treatment is useful and effective.
- Class II recommendation: Conditions for which there is conflicting evidence or a divergence of opinion about the usefulness or efficacy of a procedure or treatment.
- Class IIa recommendation: Weight of evidence or opinion is in favor of usefulness and efficacy.
- Class IIb: Usefulness or efficacy is less well established by evidence or opinion.
- Class III: Conditions for which there is evidence or general agreement that the procedure or treatment is not useful or effective and in some cases may be harmful.
- Class A: There is good evidence to support the usefulness of this treatment.
- Class B: There is fair evidence to support the usefulness of this treatment.
- Class C: There is poor evidence to support this procedure, but recommendations may be made on other grounds.
- Class D: There is fair evidence that this procedure should not be used.
- Class E: There is good evidence that this treatment or procedure should not be used and may be harmful.

Source: Institute of Medicine. (2001). Glossary of EBM terms. Center for Evidence-Based Medicine. Retrieved from http://www.cebm.net/index.aspx?o=1025

Using only clinical guidelines to diagnose and treat patients is inappropriate. EBP consists of three distinct areas of knowledge: the area of clinical evidence, which includes clinical guidelines; the nurse's intuition and knowledge of the patient; and the patient's preference. For example, a guideline may call for a magnetic resonance imaging (MRI) examination, but the advanced practice nurse knows that the patient has no insurance and is out of work and cannot afford MRI. The patient also states that he cannot pay his monthly bills and could never afford MRI. The advanced practice nurse may use another, less expensive modality to diagnose the patient or may use history and physical assessment to develop a plan for the patient.

Sometimes, different professional groups disagree in guideline recommendations. For example, the American College of Chest Physicians guidelines for DVT prophylaxis states that aspirin is insufficient for anticoagulation in patients at risk for DVT. However, the American Association of Orthopaedic Surgeons states that aspirin is an adequate anticoagulant in persons at risk for DVT from orthopedic surgery. This disagreement makes following guidelines confusing. Developing an EBP framework that takes all aspects of evidence into consideration helps to guide decision making in all aspects of care.

The Australian National Health and Medical Research Council (1999) developed guidelines for the development of clinical practice guidelines. These guidelines are unique among clinical guidelines because they focus on patient quality of life. The Australian National Health and Medical Research Council stated that the development of clinical guidelines should focus on outcomes, including quality-of-life outcomes. The following is a list of the attributes that this council suggested should guide the development of clinical guidelines:

- Clinical guidelines should be based on the best available evidence and should include a statement about the strength, quality, and relevance of the evidence used. Strength refers to the level of evidence found for each aspect of care within the guideline, quality refers to the methods used to minimize bias, and relevance refers to the extent that findings can be applied in other settings.
- The process of guideline development should be multidisciplinary and should include consumers; this increases the likelihood that guidelines would be adopted and used.
- Guidelines should be flexible and adaptable to varying local conditions and should include evidence relevant to different target populations and clinical settings. Cost constraints and values and preferences of patients should be considered when creating clinical guidelines.
- Guidelines should be developed with resource constraints in mind. They should incorporate an economic appraisal, which may be helpful for choosing among treatment options.
- Guidelines are developed to be disseminated and implemented, taking into account their target audiences. They should be disseminated so that practitioners and consumers become aware of them and use them.

- The implementation and impact of guidelines should be evaluated.
- Guidelines should be reviewed and revised regularly as new knowledge and technologies emerge.

Broad acceptance of guidelines is always more likely if the process by which the guideline is developed is transparent and explicit. Experts in the EBP arena recognize how difficult it is to develop a guideline when the quality of the literature is not high (e.g., no randomized controlled clinical trials or case control series) and acknowledge that in such instances, expert opinion plays a supplementary role.

The American Heart Association developed a checklist for writing clinical guidelines from a review of the evidence. This checklist identifies the requirements that should be met to produce acceptable and usable guidelines for clinical practice (see Box 4-3). See also Box 4-4 for examples of clinical guidelines in use.

Translating Established Evidence-Based Clinical Practice Guidelines Into Practice

The goals of clinical guidelines are to identify all treatment options and possible outcomes; weigh the benefits against the risks and costs; and, in the broadest context, factor in logistics, ethical, economic, societal, and legal considerations.

Box 4-3

American Heart Association Checklist for Clinical Guidelines

Writing Guideline Recommendations

- Write all recommendations in complete sentences.
- Write separate recommendations that apply to specific clinical objectives.
- Write recommendations that are practical in the real-world setting.
- Describe the patients to whom the recommendation applies.
- Use unambiguous language and clearly defined terms when writing recommendations.
- Write recommendations in terms of active or positive actions rather than passive or negative actions (e.g., class I recommendation to perform a test or give a treatment that is useful or effective rather than a class III recommendation not to perform or give it).
- When there are areas of uncertainty or controversy, include this information in the recommendation.
- Quantify benefits, harms, and time frames as much as possible.
- Write recommendations that incorporate data on patient preferences, when applicable.
- Specify subpopulation variability and exceptions in the recommendations. List the exceptions whenever possible.
- Include flexibility in applying the recommendations, where applicable.

Source: American Heart Association. Circulation Web site. Retrieved from http://circres.ahajournals.org/

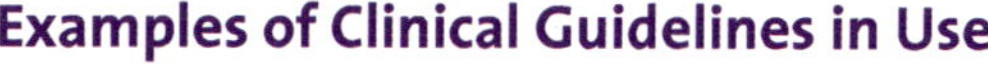

Box 4-4

Examples of Clinical Guidelines in Use

Clinical Guideline 1

Clinical guideline 1 is an example of a guideline presented by the United States Preventive Services Task Force (USPSTF).

The evidence base for the updated guidelines was a systematic review of published evidence of the efficacy of five screening modalities in lowering breast cancer mortality rates. These modalities include film mammography, clinical breast examination (CBE), breast self-examination (BSE), digital mammography, and magnetic resonance imaging (MRI).

Other evidence reviewed by the USPSTF included two studies commissioned by the task force, a systematic evidence review targeting six questions concerning the benefits and harms of screening, and a decision analysis using population modeling techniques to determine anticipated health costs and outcome benefits of screening every year versus every 2 years and of starting and ending mammography screening at various ages.

Specific recommendations of the USPSTF and the accompanying strength of recommendations were as follows:

- The USPSTF recommends against routine screening mammography in women 40 to 49 years old. Based on patient context, including patient values concerning specific benefits and harms, individual decisions should be made regarding starting regular, biennial screening mammography before age 50 years (grade C recommendation).
- Women 50 to 74 years old should undergo biennial screening mammography (grade B recommendation).
- Current evidence is insufficient to determine additional benefits and harms of screening mammography in women 75 years or older (I statement).
- In women 40 years or older, current evidence is insufficient to determine the additional benefits and harms of CBE beyond screening mammography (I statement).
- The USPSTF recommends against clinicians teaching women the technique of BSE (grade D recommendation).
- Current evidence is insufficient to determine additional benefits and harms of either digital mammography or MRI versus film mammography as screening modalities for breast cancer (I statement).

The accompanying updated evidence review on breast cancer screening looked at published studies identified from a search of Cochrane Central Register of Controlled Trials and Cochrane Database of Systematic Reviews through the fourth quarter of 2008, MEDLINE January 2001 to December 2008, and bibliographies of identified articles. Also reviewed were Web of Science searches and Breast Cancer Surveillance Consortium for screening mammography data.

Inclusion criteria for studies were randomized controlled trials with breast cancer mortality outcomes for screening effectiveness and studies of varying designs and multiple data sources regarding harms. The reviewers found that for women 39 to 49 years old, mammography screening was associated with a 15% decrease in breast cancer

Continued on page 186

Box 4-4

Examples of Clinical Guidelines in Use *Continued from page 185*

mortality rates (relative risk 0.85; 95% credible interval 0.75 to 0.96; 8 trials). Data are lacking for women 70 years or older.

Radiation exposure from mammography is low, and adverse experiences are common but transient and do not alter screening practices. The estimated rate of overdiagnosis from screening ranges from 1% to 10%. Overdiagnosis comes from mammograms where there are areas that the radiologist is uncertain about or where there are false-positive findings. Compared with older women, younger women have more false-positive mammography results and additional imaging but fewer biopsies. Trials of CBE are ongoing. In trials of BSE, benign biopsy results increased, and there were no decreases in mortality rates (Barclay, 2009).

1. How would you evaluate this guideline? What level of evidence was used for each recommendation?
2. How do these recommendations fit within your practice or personal experience?
3. How have other groups, such as the American College of Obstetricians and Gynecologists, responded to these recommendations?
4. How would you adapt these recommendations to your practice?
5. How might women in a practice react to these changes?
6. How would you measure the outcome of implementing these recommendations into a practice setting?

Clinical Guideline 2

Clinical Guideline 2 contains recommendations from the Agency for Healthcare Research and Quality (AHRQ) as guidelines for clinicians to use in treating patients who use tobacco.

Recommendation: All patients should be asked if they use tobacco and should have their tobacco use status documented on a regular basis. Evidence has shown that clinic screening systems, such as expanding the vital signs to include tobacco use status or the use of other reminder systems such as chart stickers or computer prompts, significantly increase rates of clinician intervention. (Strength of evidence = A)

Recommendation: When a tobacco user is identified and advised to quit, the clinician should assess the patient's willingness to quit at this time. (Strength of evidence = C)

Recommendation: All physicians should strongly advise every patient who smokes to quit because evidence shows that physician advice to quit smoking increases abstinence rates. (Strength of evidence = A)

Recommendation: Minimal interventions lasting less than 3 minutes increase overall tobacco abstinence rates. Every tobacco user should be offered at least a minimal intervention, whether or not he or she is referred to an intensive intervention. (Strength of evidence = A)

Box 4-4

Examples of Clinical Guidelines in Use

Continued from page 186

Recommendation: There is a strong dose-response relationship between the session length of person-to-person contact and successful treatment outcomes. Intensive interventions are more effective than less intensive interventions and should be used whenever possible. (Strength of evidence = A)

Recommendation: Person-to-person treatment delivered for four or more sessions appears to be especially effective in increasing abstinence rates. If feasible, clinicians should strive to meet four or more times with individuals quitting tobacco use. (Strength of evidence = A)

Recommendation: Treatment delivered by various types of clinicians increases abstinence rates. All clinicians should provide smoking cessation interventions. (Strength of evidence = A)

Recommendation: Proactive telephone counseling, group counseling, and individual counseling formats are effective and should be used in smoking cessation interventions. (Strength of evidence = A)

Recommendation: Smoking cessation interventions that are delivered in multiple formats increase abstinence rates and should be encouraged. (Strength of evidence = A)

Recommendation: Tailored materials, both print and Web-based, appear to be effective in helping people quit. Clinicians may choose to provide tailored self-help materials to patients who want to quit. (Strength of evidence = B)

Recommendation: All patients who receive a tobacco dependence intervention should be assessed for abstinence at the completion of treatment and during subsequent contacts. (1) Abstinent patients should have their quitting success acknowledged, and the clinician should offer to assist patients with problems associated with quitting. (2) Patients who have relapsed should be assessed to determine whether they are willing to make another quit attempt. (Strength of evidence = C)

Recommendation: Two types of counseling and behavioral therapies result in higher abstinence rates: (1) providing smokers with practical counseling (problem-solving skills or skills training) and (2) providing support and encouragement as part of treatment. These types of counseling elements should be included in smoking cessation interventions. (Strength of evidence = B)

Recommendation: The combination of counseling and medication is more effective for smoking cessation than either medication or counseling alone. Whenever feasible and appropriate, both counseling and medication should be provided to patients trying to quit smoking. (Strength of evidence = A)

Recommendation: There is a strong relationship between the number of sessions of counseling and counseling combined with medication and the likelihood of successful smoking cessation. To the extent possible, clinicians should provide multiple counseling sessions, in addition to medication, to patients who are trying to quit smoking. (Strength of evidence = A)

Continued on page 188

Box 4-4

Examples of Clinical Guidelines in Use *Continued from page 187*

Recommendation: Motivational intervention techniques appear to be effective in increasing a patient's likelihood of making a future quit attempt. Clinicians should use motivational techniques to encourage smokers who are not currently willing to quit to consider making a quit attempt in the future. (Strength of evidence = B)

Recommendation: Clinicians should encourage all patients attempting to quit to use effective medications for tobacco dependence treatment except where contraindicated or for specific populations for which there is insufficient evidence of effectiveness (i.e., pregnant women, smokeless tobacco users, light smokers, and adolescents). (Strength of evidence = A)

Recommendation: Sustained-release bupropion is an effective smoking cessation treatment that patients should be encouraged to use. (Strength of evidence = A)

Recommendation: Nicotine gum is an effective smoking cessation treatment that patients should be encouraged to use. (Strength of evidence = A)

Recommendation: Clinicians should offer 4-mg rather than 2-mg nicotine gum to highly dependent smokers. (Strength of evidence = B)

Recommendation: Varenicline is an effective smoking cessation treatment that patients should be encouraged to use. (Strength of evidence = A)

Recommendation: The nicotine inhaler is an effective smoking cessation treatment that patients should be encouraged to use. (Strength of evidence = A)

Recommendation: The nicotine lozenge is an effective smoking cessation treatment that patients should be encouraged to use. (Strength of evidence = B)

Recommendation: Nicotine nasal spray is an effective smoking cessation treatment that patients should be encouraged to use. (Strength of evidence = A)

Source: Agency for Healthcare Research and Quality. (2008). Treating tobacco use and dependence 2008 Update. Retrieved from http://www.ahrq.gov/path/tobacco.htm

Source: *http://www.uspreventiveservicestaskforce.org/recommendations.htm*

Taking the findings of an evidence review and making practice recommendations from this evidence requires a specific set of skills for the DNP-prepared advanced practice nurse. Evidence-based clinical practice guidelines can reduce the delivery of inappropriate care and support the introduction of new knowledge into clinical practice. However, translation is important because it is the primary reason for an evidence-based review. Rigorously developed guidelines can translate complicated research findings into actionable recommendations for clinical care.

The process begins with the group or individual summarizing all of the findings and developing a set of valid and reliable clinical recommendations. Transformation of evidence into practice recommendations or guidelines begins after consensus is reached on the best research evidence, nursing knowledge, and patient preference for a given issue. After all of the research has been summarized,

Table 4-5

Guideline for Treatment of Diabetic Patients

1. All patients with a fasting blood sugar greater than 126 are considered to be diabetic.
2. All patients with a nonfasting blood sugar greater than 200 are considered to be diabetic.
3. All patients with a fasting blood sugar greater than 110 should be tested for diabetes using a glucose tolerance test.
4. After a diagnosis is made, all patients receive the following educational information:
   - Foot care instructions
   - Need for yearly ophthalmology visit
   - Need for yearly dental visit
   - Need for blood work and urine testing every 3 months for hemaglobin A_{1C}, urine protein/albumin levels
5. Medications for new diabetics are based on blood sugar levels and include the following:
   - Metformin (with normal creatinine)
   - Sulfonylureas
   - Insulin
   - Saxagliptin (Onglyza)
   - All diabetic patients should be on an angiotensin-converting enzyme (ACE) inhibitor or angiotensin receptor blocker (ARB) unless contraindicated

a list of findings is established that reflects the research summary. When this list is complete, a guideline is developed. The guideline may focus on health promotion and risk assessment or assessment for the presence of disease and treatment of disease. Table 4-5 provides an example of a practice guideline for diabetics.

Clinical guidelines often come from national expert groups and are then translated into individual practice use by the advanced practice nurse and other health-care team members. Carefully reviewing guidelines and collecting data on outcomes in an individual practice from guideline use is a step toward determining the efficacy of any guideline in practice.

Adapting a set guideline into individual practice requires the clinician to make connections between the population in the practice and the population for which the guideline was developed. These connections may be financial, ethnic, or geographic and can significantly change the ability of the guideline to be effective in this population. After the group or clinician adapts the guideline to individual practice needs, the final step is to implement the guideline and activate the steps in practice. Applying the guidelines requires clinicians to continue to use judgment, patient preferences, and information in each decision that is made regarding guideline implementation.

To implement new guidelines in practice, knowledge of how to effect change is essential. All members of the team should be alerted to any intended changes to be made. Having a meeting of all individuals affected by the change provides an opportunity to point out flaws in the implementation plan or the guideline itself that can be corrected before implementation. If the implementation is marred by problems, it is less likely to be successful and unlikely to gain the full cooperation of all team members. Generally, a small test of the intended change helps to determine whether and how each member of the health-care team and the patient would be affected by the contemplated change. All members of the team involved in the change should understand their role in the change process, who is the leader in this process, and where to go for assistance in the change.

Advancing Your Knowledge

T.K. has decided to implement the guidelines from the United States Preventive Services Task Force for breast cancer screening into her primary care practice. Reviewing the guidelines, T.K. decides to offer a baseline mammogram to patients 40 to 49 years old but not to implement yearly mammograms until age 50. This recommendation is not only supported by research evidence but also would reduce health-care costs. She plans to discontinue mammograms in women after age 75, which also is supported by the evidence and would reduce health-care costs for patients. Because, in T.K.'s experience, women often are the first to find lumps in their breasts by doing breast self-examination, she plans to continue to teach it to patients and to encourage a monthly breast self-examination. However, she plans to advise patients that a lump is not always cancer and that a lack of lumps does not mean that there is no cancer. This practice is cost neutral, and she plans to track the patients who perform breast self-examinations to determine if any problems arise. To foster these changes, T.K. does a short in-service for office staff members on the changes in protocol so that they can understand and support the changes made. A flyer is posted in the patient waiting room outlining the changes, and a letter is sent to each of T.K.'s female patients older than 40 to inform them about the change and provide the supporting evidence for the change.

1. In your opinion, has T.K. made good choices for breast health based on the evidence?
2. Is it acceptable that she continues to teach breast self-examination to her patients?
3. What is the best course of action for T.K. if a 45-year-old patient wants a yearly mammogram?
4. What would you add to T.K.'s new plan for breast health? Why?

Conclusion

Advanced practice nurses use evidence to make patient assessment, diagnosis, and treatment decisions. Understanding the individual elements that make up an evidence-based decision is critical to making the best decisions and obtaining the best outcomes for patients and families. Systematic review of the literature is one of the best ways to obtain evidence because such reviews look at many different studies on a topic and compare results. Being able to appraise research critically and determine the validity and reliability of research studies is another important aspect of EBP.

Critical thinking is vital to EBP nursing and contributes substantially to patient outcomes. The development of critical thinking skills prepares advanced practice nurses with skills, habits, and attitudes to support EBP. Critical thinking assists the advanced practice nurse to determine what evidence is important and provides a process for translating evidence into the practice setting.

Guidelines, whether created by the advanced practice nurse or by expert groups, are useful in obtaining and using the best evidence in practice. Once guidelines have been developed, the DNP-educated nurse is charged with translating the findings of evidence, patient values and preference, and nursing knowledge into practice. For this type of action to be successful, the person instituting the new actions should be aware of the change process.

References

Agency for Health Research and Quality (2010). HHS awards $473 million in patient-centered outcomes research funding. Retrieved from http://www.ahrq.gov/news/press/pr2010/recovryawpr.htm

American Academy of Nurse Practitioners. (2007). Standards of practice for nurse practitioners. Retrieved from http://www.aanp.org/NR/rdonlyres/FE00E81B-FA96-4779-972B-6162F04C309F/0/2010StandardsOfPractice.pdf

American Association of Colleges of Nursing (2006). The essentials of doctoral education for advanced nursing practice. Retrieved from http://www.aacn.nche.edu/publications/position/DNPEssentials.pdf

American Association of Colleges of Nursing. (1998). *The essentials of baccalaureate education in nursing practice*. Washington, DC: Author.

American Association of Orthopaedic Surgeons. (2009). Position statement: Evidence based guidelines. Retrieved from http://www.aaos.org/about/papers/position/1178.asp

Australian National Health and Medical Research Council. (1999). A guide to the development, implementation and evaluation of clinical practice guidelines. Retrieved from http://www.nhmrc.gov.au/_files_nhmrc/file/publications/synopses/cp30.pdf

Barclay, L. (2009). USTSPF issues new breast cancer screening guidelines. *Annals of Internal Medicine, 151,* 716–726, 727–737, 750–752.

Benner, P. (1982). From novice to expert. *American Journal of Nursing, 82*(3), 402–407.

Burns, N., & Grove, S. (2009). *The practice of nursing research: Conduct critique and utilization* (5th ed.). New York, NY: Elsevier.

DiCenso, A., Cullum, N., & Ciliska, D. (1998). Implementing evidence-based nursing: Some misconceptions. *Evidence Based Nursing, 1*(10), 38–39.

Freshwater, D., & Rolfe, G. (2004). Deconstructing evidence based practice. London, UK: Routledge Press.

Glanville, R., Schrim, V., & Wineman, M., (2000). Using evidence-based practice for managing clinical outcomes in advanced practice nursing. *Journal of Nursing Care Quality, 15*(1), 1–11.

Groth-Marnat, D. (2009). *Handbook of psychological assessment* (5th ed.). New York, NY: John Wiley & Sons.

Institute of Medicine. (1992). *Guidelines for clinical practice: From development to use.* Washington, DC: National Academy Press.

Institute of Medicine. (2001). Glossary of EBM terms. Retrieved from http://ktclearinghouse.ca/cebm/glossary/

Institute of Medicine. (2003). Patient safety: Achieving new standards of care. Retrieved from http://www.addictioninfo.org/articles/11/1/Stages-of-Change-Model/Page1.html First Accessed on November 9, 2011.

Kern, M. (2008). Stages of change model. Retrieved from http://www.addictioninfo.org/articles/11/1/Stages-of-Change-Model/Page1.html Accessed on November 9, 2011

Kleinpell, R., & Gawlinski, A. (2005). Assessing outcomes in advanced practice nursing practice: The use of quality indicators and evidence-based practice. *AACN Clinical Issues: Advanced Practice in Acute and Critical Care, 16*(1), 43–57.

Melnyk, M. B., & Fineout-Overholt, E. (2005). *Evidence-based practice in nursing and healthcare: A guide to best practice.* Philadelphia, PA: Lippincott Williams & Wilkins.

Mulrow, C. (1997). Systematic reviews: critical links in the great chain of evidence. *Annals of Internal Medicine, 126,* 389–391.

Newhouse, R. P., Dearholt, S., Poe, S., Pugh, L. C., & White, K. (2007). *Johns Hopkins nursing evidence-based practice: Model and guidelines.* Indianapolis, IN: Sigma Theta Tau International Press.

Newhouse, R. P., Dearholt, S., Poe, S., Pugh, L. C., & White, K. (2009). Evidence based practice: A practical approach to implementation. *Journal of Nursing Administration, 35*(1), 35–40.

Nursing Library and Information Resources, Cushing Whitney Medical Library. (2005). Evidence-based practice: asking the clinical question. Retrieved from http://www.med.yale.edu/library/nursing/education/clinquest.html

Omery, A., & Williams, R. P. (1999). An appraisal of research utilization across the United States. *Journal of Nursing Administration, 29(*12), 50–56.

Paul, R., Binker, A., Jensen, K., & Kreklau, H. (1990). *Critical thinking handbook: A guide for remodeling lesson plans in language arts, social studies and science.* Rohnert Park, CA: Foundation for Critical Thinking.

Polit, D., & Beck, C. (2006). *Nursing researching: Generating and assessing evidence for nursing practice.* New York, NY: Lippincott.

Reed, P. (2007). Toward a nursing theory of self-transcendence: deductive reformulation using developmental theories. *Advances in Nursing Science, 13*(4), 64–77.

Sackett, D. L., Straus, W. S., Richardson, W. S., Rosenberg, W. M., & Hayes, R. B. (2000). *Evidence-based medicine: How to practice and teach EMB.* London, UK: Churchill-Livingstone.

Shiffman, R., Shekelle, P., Overhage, J. M., Slutsky, J., Grimshaw, J., & Deshpande, A. (2003). Standardized reporting of clinical practice guidelines: A proposal from the conference on guideline standardization. *Annals of Internal Medicine, 139*(6), 493–498.

Stetler, C. (2001). Updating the Stetler model of research utilization to facilitate evidence-based practice. *Nursing Outlook, 49*(6), 272–278.

Stevens, K. (2001). Systematic reviews: The heart of evidence based practice. *AACN Clinical Issues: Advanced Practice in Acute and Critical Care, 12*(4), 529–538.

Stiffler, D., & Cullen, D. (2010). Evidence-based practice for nurse practitioner students: A competency based teaching framework. *Journal of Professional Nursing, 26*(5), 272–277.

CHAPTER 5

Mary E. Bishop, DNP, RN
Rose O. Sherman, EdD, RN, FAAN

ORGANIZATIONAL AND SYSTEMS LEADERSHIP FOR QUALITY IMPROVEMENT

Objectives:

By the end of the chapter, students should be able to:

1. Identify leadership competencies and skills expected of doctor of nursing practice (DNP) graduates.
   - Present transformational leadership theory as a potential framework for DNP leadership practice.
   - Present the concept of systems thinking as a key component to effective leadership.
2. Analyze the business of health care and the changes that may occur that would affect DNP leadership in practice management settings.
   - Describe current quality and patient safety initiatives.
   - Provide an overview of quality indicators that affect the financial reimbursement of organizations and providers.
   - Analyze the trends in public reporting of quality data and the impact on the health-care delivery system.
3. Describe the components of a healthy work environment.
   - Provide examples of how DNP leaders can create healthy workplaces and engage staff.
4. Present an overview of complexity and chaos theory as a framework to understand change in today's health-care environment.
5. Analyze the role of the DNP leader in promoting change and describe the process of innovation.

This chapter presents an overview of the key components of organizational and systems leadership for quality improvement and systems thinking. It is important that nursing has leaders who can role model the needed competencies to meet organizational needs. Nursing leaders today are asked to administer large budgets, manage large groups of diverse staff, coordinate care for patients, and represent nursing at multidisciplinary meetings. Nurses who are prepared with a doctor of nursing practice (DNP) degree can help fill these critical positions with important leadership expertise in areas such as risk assessment, collaboration, systems thinking, and financial acumen. With their advanced knowledge and education, DNP graduates are well positioned to function as leaders and pioneers in health-care systems today and in the future.

In his groundbreaking book *The Innovator's Prescription,* Christensen (2009) suggested that today's health-care system screams for disruptive innovation, which he defined as a process or product introduced at the bottom of the market that ultimately displaces established competitors. Introducing new innovation is challenging. Rogers (1995), in his work on the diffusion of innovation, noted that implementing innovation is a difficult process even when a new idea may have obvious advantages. The development of the DNP grew from discussions held by the American Association of Colleges of Nursing (AACN, 2002) with supporters stating ways that nurses in practice environments could help reform health care. The lack of leadership content and focus in advanced practice programs was identified as a weakness. There was a need to provide leadership education to help advanced practice nurses influence policy and system changes. The AACN (2006) document "The Essentials of Doctoral Education for Advanced Nursing Practice" addressed the critical need for organizational and systems leadership competence. DNP graduates are expected to have the expertise to assess organizations, identify systems issues, and facilitate organization-wide change in practice delivery.

The Institute of Medicine (IOM, 2010) report *The Future of Nursing: Leading Change, Advancing Health* included a recommendation that nurses be prepared and able to lead change to advance health. The report noted that strong leadership is critical if the vision of a transformed health-care system is to be realized. Nurse leaders must be prepared to serve as full partners with other health professions across the continuum of delivery of high-quality care. Challenges found in the health-care system today provide unprecedented opportunities for DNP nurses to assume leadership responsibilities and to reduce costs, while improving health outcomes.

This chapter first delves into the concept of leadership development. The chapter continues with discussions of health-care reimbursement and its effect on DNP leadership, quality and patient safety initiatives and reporting, components of a healthy work environment, and complexity and chaos theory. The chapter concludes with a discourse on the role of the DNP in leading change and in the process of innovation.

Leadership Development

The Council on Graduate Education in the Administration of Nursing (2010) defined *leadership* as the process of influencing others toward the attainment of one or more goals. Leadership can be either formal or informal. Formal leaders have designated leadership titles within their organizations, associations, or societies. Informal leaders, who usually do not have designated titles, can be a powerful force in influencing the actions and perceptions of others. DNP graduates are expected to be leaders in their organizations in either a formal or an informal capacity. Leadership is not confined only to one's organization; DNP nurse leaders are qualified to lead in diverse capacities, including as members on governing boards of health-care organizations (Curran & Totten, 2010), as consultants for health policy development, and in the establishment of nurse-managed care services. To achieve these expectations, it is essential that DNP-prepared nurses recognize the importance of personal mastery in developing leadership competencies.

Leadership development is an ongoing journey that requires continual reassessment of the knowledge and skills needed to guide organizations and individuals in increasingly complex environments (Porter O'Grady & Malloch, 2011). The context of leadership has shifted dramatically over the past 2 decades with rapid technological change and the rise of the worldwide Web as a major avenue for communication. Tapscott and Williams (2010) described in their book *Macrowikinomics* how the newly networked professional communities and individuals are using mass collaboration to revolutionize not only the way we work but also how we live, learn, create, and care for each other. Prominent in their discussion are the ways that Web sites such as PatientsLikeMe (http://www.patientslikeme.com/) promote a change in the way patients see their role in the health-care system and how treatment options and outcomes can be shared more rapidly in a collaborative community. Nevertheless, although the context of leadership has changed, the behaviors, actions, and practices of good leadership remain the same.

Kouzes and Posner (2010), in an analysis of their 30 years of work with thousands of executives globally, proposed the following 10 fundamental truths about leadership and becoming an effective leader:

- Truth 1—You make a difference
- Truth 2—Credibility is the foundation of leadership
- Truth 3—Values drive commitment
- Truth 4—Focusing on the future sets leaders apart
- Truth 5—You can't do it alone
- Truth 6—Trust rules
- Truth 7—Challenge is the crucible for greatness
- Truth 8—You either lead by example or you don't lead at all
- Truth 9—The best leaders are the best learners
- Truth 10—Leadership is an affair of the heart

These 10 truths can serve as a foundation for DNP leaders in developing their leadership values, attitudes, and beliefs to guide their practice. Leadership style is also an important component of leadership practice. Transformational leadership is an evidence-based leadership style that promotes healthy work environments and better patient outcomes.

Transformational Leadership

Historically, there have been many different theories to explain leadership emergence, the nature of the leader, and the consequences of leadership (Bass & Bass, 2008). In nursing, transformational leadership theory has received the greatest attention because it has been a key ingredient in nursing departments that achieve Magnet Hospital designation, a benchmark of nursing excellence (Wolf, Triolo, & Ponte, 2008). The theory of transformational leadership was introduced by Burns in 1978. He described transformational leadership as occurring when "two or more persons engage with others in such a way that the leader and followers raise one another to high levels of motivation and morality" (Burns, 1978).

Transformational leadership is characterized by the following four core components (Bass & Riggio, 2006, pp. 5-7):

1. *Idealize influence:* Transformational leaders behave in ways that allow them to serve as role models for their followers. The nurse leader exemplifies outstanding professional practice and sets high standards for the staff.
2. *Inspirational motivation:* Transformational leaders behave in ways that motivate and inspire those around them by providing meaning and challenge to the work of their followers. The nurse leader is able to inspire staff with a vision of the future and engage staff in laying out goals and ways of reaching them.
3. *Intellectual stimulation:* Transformational leaders stimulate their followers' efforts to be innovative and creative by questioning assumptions, reframing problems, and approaching old situations in new ways. The nurse leader creates a climate of continuous learning that seeks ways to provide growth and development opportunities. Nurses are encouraged to voice their innovative ideas about improving care.
4. *Individualized consideration:* Transformational leaders pay special attention to each individual follower's needs for achievement by acting as a coach or mentor. A transformational nurse leader knows his or her individual staff member's career aspirations and is often in a position to guide individuals to invaluable mentoring opportunities.

This theory of leadership was the first to identify the importance of followers in achieving high work performance. Burns was influenced in his thinking about leadership by Maslow's hierarchy of needs (Maslow, 1954). Most organizations focus their energies on motivating employees by meeting their basic needs, which Burns described as a transactional leadership approach—good behavior is rewarded, and perceived negative behavior is punished.

Burns suggested that higher order needs, such as self-esteem and self-actualization, should be a focus of leaders. Transformational leadership has the potential to motivate followers to achieve these higher level needs. There is increasing evidence in the nursing literature to support the ideas proposed by Burns. Weberg (2010) reviewed the nursing research examining the impact of transformational leadership. Transformational leadership was found to be significantly related to staff satisfaction, well-being, decreased burnout, and reduced levels of overall stress in staff nurses. The IOM (2010) report on the future of nursing included a call for a style of nursing leadership that involves working with others as full partners in a context of mutual respect and collaboration. DNP-prepared nurses interested in building high-performance teams and organizations need to commit to developing transformational leadership qualities.

Advancing Your Knowledge

D.R., DNP, CNE-BC, has just assumed a chief nursing officer position in a large metropolitan medical center. She considers herself to be a transformational nurse leader and looks forward to engaging the staff in moving the medical center toward Magnet designation. Her predecessor was neither visible nor available to staff members and had a transactional leadership style. D.R. has told her leadership team and the staff that she has a transformational leadership approach. They are deeply skeptical based on their past experiences.

1. What initial steps should D.R. take as a DNP nurse leader to build a transformational leadership culture?
2. What barriers can D.R. expect to face based on the prior leadership culture?
3. What short-term and long-term goals should D.R. establish on her journey toward a transformational leadership culture?

Leadership Competencies for DNP Nurse Leaders

Montgomery and Porter-O'Grady (2010) observed that because DNP graduates are expected to take practice leadership roles in their settings, it is necessary to include in the educational process activities that challenge self-perceptions and expectations. The IOM (2010) report included a chapter on transforming leadership in nursing. The report recommended that being a full partner in reforming health care would require nurses to develop new leadership competencies and skills.

The American Organization of Nurse Executives (AONE, 2005) developed a set of leadership competencies that can serve as a foundation for DNP leaders to understand what is needed to manage the business of health care, promote quality, create healthy work environments, and serve as a change agent. The competency categories include the following:

- *Communication and relationship building:* Ability to influence others, work with diverse groups, manage community relationships
- *Knowledge of the health-care environment:* Ability to advocate for policy changes, knowledge of risk and quality management

- *Leadership:* Ability to manage change, systems thinking
- *Professionalism:* Use of evidence-based practice, active in professional organizations
- *Business skills:* Understanding health-care financing, thinking strategically

The above-listed competencies describe skills common to nurses in executive leadership positions regardless of organizational setting. Although all nurse leaders share these competency domains, the emphasis on specific competencies may vary depending on the leader's organization and position.

The AONE competency domains reinforce that leadership is both an art and a science. The art of leadership involves managing relationships with individuals and influencing their behaviors. The science of leadership is recognizing that numerous opportunities exist for nurses in leadership positions to question current leadership practices and to ask themselves questions: "What is the evidence for my leadership intervention?" or "Am I using strategies here that will lead to the best outcomes for staff and patients?" The use of evidence-based practice helps leaders to make more effective leadership decisions based on research and knowledge instead of traditions, hunches, advice of colleagues, or outdated leadership information. One of the most significant challenges that nurse leaders face in the health-care environment is how to manage the conflict that often occurs when individuals have divergent values, beliefs, and attitudes. Guiding individuals and teams past their day-to-day problems, conflicts, and communication issues toward a goal of high performance takes leadership skill (Sherman & Pross, 2010). One suggested approach to address this situation is called *carefronting*.

Carefronting

Carefronting is an important new competency for DNP-prepared nurse leaders to help resolve conflict and create healthy work environments. Augsburger (1981), a professor of pastoral care and counseling, coined the term *carefronting* to refer to the skill of caring enough about oneself, others, and desired goals to confront inappropriate behavior responsibly while offering the opportunity for change. Carefronting is the act of inviting, not demanding, another to change through conflict, a way to unite caring and candor in relationships (Kupperschmidt, 2006a). Carefronting encompasses the following tenets (Kupperschmidt, 2006b, 2008):

- *Truthing it: A simplified speech style. Truthing it* encompasses the willingness and ability to listen deeply, empathetically, and accurately to ensure understanding of others' points of view. *Truthing* also encompasses speaking simply, "I want to hear you accurately," and speaking honestly, "I want to share my feelings and attitudes with you; I want to be heard; I care about our relationship."
- *Owning anger: Let both your faces show.* Anger is both a positive, self-affirming emotion and a demand. When one feels ignored or rejected, the normal response is anger: "I am a person of worth. I demand that you recognize and respect me." Each person, regardless whether the context is

a practice or educational setting, is responsible for choosing how he or she responds and reacts to others when conflicts occur.

- *Inviting change: Careful confrontation.* Carefronting invites change but does not demand it. Inviting change means focusing feedback on the behavior, not the person; on observations, not conclusions; on descriptions, not judgments; and on ideas and alternatives, not advice and answers. Inviting change encompasses clear, simple descriptions and observations couched in concern and caring. Change is invited carefully, gently, constructively, and clearly.
- *Giving trust: A two-way venture.* Trust connects and integrates all human emotions. Trust, essential in work relationships, is grounded in authentic self-disclosure. Trust confronts openly, frankly, respectfully, and responsibly—trusting that the other person will assume his or her responsibility to be equally honest and frank. Such trust releases demands and accepts apologies.
- *Ending blame: Forget whose fault the conflict is.* Confrontation that endeavors to place blame inevitably evokes resistance and resentment. Carefronting ends the blame game, leading to the real questions: What is the respectful thing to do now? Where do we go from here? When do we start to discuss the conflict? If not now, when? If not us, who cares enough about our goals, such as patient safety? Who will end blame and work toward the professional practice we deserve?
- *Getting unstuck: The freedom to change. Getting unstuck* means owning responsibility for one's part in the conflict and refusing to waste time in assigning blame, accepting accountability for the present conflict, and focusing on what can be shared.
- *Peacemaking: Getting together again.* Nurse leaders who are peacemakers are caring people who dare to be truly present in conflict situations, listening and caring for all stakeholders. Peacemakers care enough to confront and drop the demands of the past. Peacemakers are nurse leaders who value others and who have rediscovered that the values that shape their decisions must be lasting values consistent with the values of the profession.

Carefronting is an alternative to traditional conflict resolution. The use of carefronting is especially important in health-care environments where team synergy and interdependence are required for high-quality and safe patient care. The essentials for DNP education emphasize the need for advanced practice nurses to become systems thinkers in their leadership practice.

Advancing Your Knowledge

C.S., DNP, ARNP, manages a large primary care practice group. Several of the younger nurse practitioners and physicians have become impatient with the

Continued on page 202

Advancing Your Knowledge *Continued from page 201*

slow implementation of electronic health records in the group. Some of the more seasoned practitioners are resistant to using electronic records, and the time frame for full implementation has been pushed back several times at their request. The ability and skills of C.S. to lead this diverse group are now being questioned. She recognizes that she dislikes and avoids conflict. She has tried to accommodate the desires of practitioners who have been with the practice for years and have large patient caseloads. She realizes that retaining the younger practitioners and smooth functioning of the practice require a different leadership strategy.

1. As a DNP nurse leader, how could C.S. use carefronting to manage this situation better?
2. How would you as a DNP nurse leader manage the conflict in this diverse practice group?
3. What recommendations would you have for C.S. about ways to seek input from members of the practice group about her leadership strengths and weaknesses?

Systems Thinking for Leaders

In his provocative book, *The World Is Flat,* Friedman (2005) challenged leaders to examine trends in the global environment that ultimately will influence every sector of life in the United States as we know it. Friedman's message was that leaders must continue to learn how to learn, remain curious and innovative, and stay attentive to the forces in the environment that are creating global flattening. At the time this book was written, many nurse leaders believed that in contrast to other industries, delivery of health care would always be local. This perception has changed with the rise in medical tourism and outsourcing of certain aspects of health care. The ability of DNP nurse leaders to see the systems and patterns of interdependency within and surrounding their organizations is vital to effective leadership.

The concept of systems thinking was popularized by Senge (1990) in his book, *The Fifth Discipline*. In this work, Senge observed that from an early age, we are taught to break apart problems and complex tasks to make them more manageable. In doing this, he suggested that we pay an enormous price by losing the intrinsic sense of connection to the larger whole. All organizations and human endeavors are interconnected systems. Traditionally, leaders have focused on solving isolated problems in a system without considering patterns and the invisible fabric of the whole. Senge defined systems thinking as the fifth discipline in a learning organization (the other four being personal mastery, building a shared vision, team learning, and the ability to create mental models). The language of systems thinking is circular rather than linear. Douglas and Kerfoot (2008) proposed that using the big picture approach, leaders should realize that relationships and context are just as important as the details in a situation. Historically, health-care leaders have lost sight of the bigger picture and have acted as though independent actions could be taken without affecting anything else.

In a report from the World Health Organization (Savigny & Tagheed, 2009), "Systems Thinking for Health Systems Strengthening," the authors argued that a stronger systems perspective among the designers, implementers, stewards, and providers of funds of health care is critical to strengthening the overall health-care system globally. They proposed that every health-care delivery system should have the following building blocks as part of the system:

1. Service delivery
2. Health workforce
3. Information
4. Medical products, vaccines, and technologies
5. Financing
6. Leadership and governance

Viewing health care from a systems perspective, the DNP nurse leader seeks to understand the nature of the relationships among the building blocks, the spaces between the blocks and what happens there, and the synergies emerging from interactions among the blocks. Ultimately, all health interventions have system level effects. A systems thinking approach helps to mitigate negative effects by modifying interventions and potentially avoiding unintended consequences. A DNP nurse who is seeking to open a new practice needs to consider not only the health-care needs in the community but also the environmental, social, economical, and political forces that shape the community and the nature of the relationships.

Advancing Your Knowledge

J.T., DNP, RN, owns and manages a highly successful, quality-driven home-care agency with an excellent community reputation. J.T. recently learned that a well-respected Magnet Hospital in his community is opening a home-care service line. Many of his current referrals come from case managers in this facility. Several of his most experienced nurses have applied for positions with the hospital to work as part of its home-care staff. J.T. is unsure what the impact will be on his business but is very concerned. He is determined to seek information and plan a strategy using a systems thinking approach.

1. As a DNP nurse leader, how should J.T. evaluate the building blocks of his health-care environment?
2. What could some of the outcomes of this change mean to J.T.'s business?
3. What proactive measures could J.T. take to mitigate the negative effects on his home-care agency?

The Business of Health Care and Its Effect on Leadership

The business of health care today can be broken down into two major areas of concern: cost and quality. As health-care providers, most advanced practice nurses begin their professional careers expecting to provide high-quality, safe, cost-effective patient care. Once in the working world, they realize that health-care systems are very complex and fraught with problems of access, waste, and inequitable resources, making the provision of quality health care—especially cost-effective high-quality care—challenging. DNP-prepared leaders have the necessary skills and knowledge to design and implement programs of care delivery that significantly influence health-care outcomes. In their role as change agents, DNPs have the potential to transform health-care delivery by becoming leaders in the clinical arenas, establishing standards and policies, and meeting the needs of the diverse health-care systems of today.

This section focuses on quality and patient safety initiatives from different legislative bodies, reimbursement, and the reporting of quality indicators. These initiatives require leadership to create success in implementation and outcomes. For DNP-prepared advanced practice nurses, understanding these initiatives and using leadership skills to create a commitment to these initiatives or a "buy in" from other health-care professionals is essential to achieve and meet goals for positive patient outcomes and financial stability.

Quality Initiatives and Patient Safety

Over the past 2 decades, studies began to quantify the incidences of injuries and threats to patient safety in health-care organizations (Leape, 1994). Additionally, investigations of adverse drug reactions revealed the surprising frequency of medication-related harm (Leape, Bates, Cullen, & Gallivan, 1995). As the number of avoidable adverse outcomes and events became public, health-care organizations and individual practitioners became motivated to change their thinking and their behaviors to reduce adverse outcomes to patients.

In 1999, concerns over patient safety reached a tipping point when the IOM published *To Err Is Human: Building a Safer Health System.* This report indicated that more than 98,000 deaths a year occurred because of medical errors in hospitals. Medical errors were defined as "the failure of a planned action to be completed as intended or the use of the wrong plan" (IOM, 1999, p. 6). This first phase documented the "serious and pervasive nature" of the nation's overall quality problem (IOM, 1999, p. 6).

This first report and the accompanying media coverage prompted the U.S. Congress to allocate millions of dollars for research on the quality and safety of health care. The IOM produced a follow-up report emphasizing how the health-care system and related policy environment must be transformed to "close the chasm between what we know to be good quality care and what actually exists in practice" (IOM, 2001, p. 6). The follow-up report, *Crossing the Quality Chasm: A New Health Care System for the 21st Century* (2001), recommended the need to address the way health professionals were educated and paved the way for developing a blueprint for reform in health professions education. These two reports were the stimulus for the current quality initiatives, emphasizing a systems approach to identifying and correcting failures in the organizations of the health-care systems, rather than blaming individual clinicians for mistakes and injuries to patients.

Defining Quality

The word *quality* means so many things to many different people. To patients, it may be compassionate care from a nurse, whereas health-care providers may view quality as the efficient delivery of care. The IOM (2001) defined quality as "the degree to which health services for individuals and populations increase the likelihood of desired health outcomes and are consistent with current professional knowledge" (p. 6). The IOM described this definition as the beginning of reform for the broken health-care system. An acronym was developed to present the components of quality from the IOM basic definition. The acronym *STEEEP* stands for the fact that all health care should be safe, timely, effective, efficient, equitable, and patient-centered:

- *Safe:* Patients should not be harmed by the care that is intended to help them.
- *Timely:* Unnecessary waits and harmful delays should be reduced.
- *Effective:* Care should be based on sound scientific knowledge.
- *Efficient:* Care should not be wasteful.
- *Equitable:* Care should not vary in quality because of patient characteristics.
- *Patient-centered:* Care should be responsive to individual preferences, needs, and values.

The authors of *Crossing the Quality Chasm* created 10 basic rules of health care, reflecting each of the six STEEEP elements and calling them guides to the redesign of the current health-care system (IOM, 2001):

- Care based on continuous healing relationships
- Customization based on patient needs and values
- The patient as the source of control
- Shared knowledge and the free flow of information
- Evidence-based decision making
- Safety as a system property
- The need for transparency
- Anticipation of needs
- Continuous decrease in waste
- Cooperation among clinicians

The IOM recognized the need for health-care professionals to acquire specific skills relating to quality of care during their professional educational training. The blueprint for educational reform, *Health Professions Education: A Bridge to*

Quality, was developed by an interdisciplinary team of experts at a Health Professions Summit in 2003 (Greiner & Knebel, 2003). In this report, the committee recommended the following overarching vision for all programs and institutions engaged in the education of health professionals: "All health care professionals should be educated to deliver patient-centered care as members of an interdisciplinary team, emphasizing evidence-based practice, quality improvement approaches, and informatics" (Greiner & Knebel, 2003, p. 3).

The committee proposed the following set of five core skill sets that all health clinicians should possess, regardless of their discipline, to meet the needs of the 21st-century health-care system (Greiner & Knebel, 2003, pp. 45-46):

- *Provide patient-centered care:* Identify, respect, and care about patients' differences, values, preferences, and expressed needs; relieve pain and suffering; coordinate continuous care; listen to, clearly inform, communicate with, and educate patients; share decision making and management; and continuously advocate disease prevention, wellness, and promotion of healthy lifestyles, including a focus on population health.
- *Work in interdisciplinary teams:* Cooperate, collaborate, and integrate care in teams to ensure that care is continuous and reliable.
- *Employ evidence-based practice:* Integrate best research with clinical expertise and patient values for optimal care, and participate in learning and research activities to the extent feasible.
- *Apply quality improvement:* Identify errors and hazards in care; understand and implement basic safety design principles, such as standardization and simplification; understand and measure continually quality of care in terms of structure, process, and outcomes in relation to patient and community needs; design and test interventions to change processes and systems of care, with the objective of improving quality.
- *Use informatics:* Communicate, manage knowledge, mitigate error, and support decision making using information technology.

To improve care, health-care workers need to acquire more than just the professional knowledge related to their discipline. These five essential skills sets can be used by the DNP leader to change a system of care positively. Knowledge of the culture of an organization at the site of care delivery, an understanding of quality improvement tools, use of evidence-based interventions, and an understanding of how to manage change are essential for the DNP leader to affect the health-care environment in a positive way. With the expansion of the five skill domains in 2006 to include the area of patient safety, the leaders of the Quality and Safety Education for Nurses (QSEN) outlined six skill domains with associated requisite knowledge, skills, and attitudes identified as competencies for each of these domains (Cronenwett, Sherwood, Barnsteiner, Johnson, & Mitchell, 2007): patient-centered care, teamwork and collaboration, evidence-based practice, quality improvement, safety, and informatics. The overall goal for the QSEN project is to meet the challenge of preparing future nurses who will have the knowledge, skills, and attitudes necessary to improve the quality and safety of the health-care systems within which they work.

In many ways, these six skill domains for quality are the foundational values of the nursing profession. DNP leaders can enhance their effectiveness by learning more about these competencies and using the accompanying templates for clinical evaluations of the professional nursing staff. Emphasizing these skill domains and accompanying competencies through continuing education can enhance the effectiveness of the staff and accelerate change in the health-care workplace.

Acquisition of these competencies comes through two basic approaches to quality improvement: general and specific (Stanhope & Lancaster, 2004). Promoting quality with an emphasis on developing core competencies for health-care professionals is part of a general approach to improving quality through curricular revisions in educational institutions and programs. Identifying and addressing quality issues and implementing continuous quality improvement are examples of specific approaches. Preparing DNP leaders who are experts in translating research in practice, evaluating evidence, and applying and implementing viable clinical innovations to change practice will enable nurses to improve quality outcomes for all patients. DNP leaders build on the foundation of past experiences. Using the leadership skills and competencies outlined in this chapter, DNP leaders can make an impact on the quality of health care.

Quality Indicators

Quality indicators are based on empirical evidence and are measures of health-care quality in various provider settings. These indicators can be defined as a policy, protocol, standard, guideline, assessment measure, or other evaluation tools that show there is reason to believe measures are in place to ensure provision of a high level of care (Mackey & McNeil, 2002). As nursing moves from clinical practices based on tradition to an evidence-based practice approach, the DNP leader has the skill sets to implement and assess changes to improve outcomes. In "The Essentials of Doctoral Education for Advanced Nursing Practice," the AACN (2006) stated that "DNP graduates must understand principles of practice management, including conceptual and practice strategies for balancing productivity and quality care" (p. 4). Additionally, "they must be able to assess the impact of clinical policies and procedures on meeting the health needs of the patient population with whom they practice" (p. 4). DNP graduates must also "be proficient in quality improvement strategies and sustaining changes at the organizational and policy levels" (p. 4). Evaluating practice changes is essential to improve outcomes.

Several clinical outcomes are used to evaluate system outcomes, including inpatient quality indicators, nurse-sensitive quality indicators, and pay for performance. The DNP-prepared nurse must be competent in all aspects of quality indicators to provide patient-centered care that is both cost-effective and quality-focused.

Inpatient Quality Indicators

There are several sources of quality indicators that make use of readily available hospital inpatient Medicare administrative data. These inpatient quality indicators include core measures, the Agency for Healthcare Research and Quality (AHRQ) quality indicators, and Hospital Consumer Assessment of Healthcare Providers and Systems (HCAHPS). Each of these quality indicators is reported publicly and is described in this section.

Core Measures: A set of care processes called *core measures* were developed by The Joint Commission to improve the quality of health care by implementing a national, standardized performance measurement system. The core measures represent the results of evidence-based research and include input from multiple stakeholders (care providers, consumers of health care, and professional organizations); a validation phase; and alignment of patient care indicators among organizations such as the Centers for Medicare and Medicaid Services (CMS), National Quality Forum (NQF), and Institute for Healthcare Improvement. These indicators have been shown to reduce the risk of complications and prevent recurrences. Core measures help hospitals improve the quality of patient care by focusing on the actual results of care. Hospitals across the United States are measured and compared by The Joint Commission with all other accredited institutions on their performance in these core measures. There are 33 core measures altogether, in four categories (acute myocardial infarction, community-acquired pneumonia, congestive heart failure, and surgical care improvement project). Under each category, key actions are listed that represent the most widely accepted, evidence-based care process for appropriate care in that category.

The Joint Commission started requiring its accredited hospitals to report performance data for core measures in 2002. In 2003, federal law tied the hospital Medicare inpatient prospective payment system (IPPS) annual payment to the reporting of designated quality measures. Hospitals that do not participate in voluntary reporting received reduced Medicare payments. In the future, it is planned to reduce payments to hospitals that are not achieving high thresholds for each core measure indicator.

Agency for Healthcare Research and Quality Quality Indicators: The AHRQ Quality Indicators measure four aspects of inpatient care: inpatient quality indicators, prevention quality indicators, patient safety indicators, and pediatric quality indicators. *Inpatient quality indicators* provide a perspective on hospital quality of care using hospital administrative data. These indicators reflect evidence-based processes of quality care inside hospitals and include inpatient mortality for certain procedures and medical conditions; use of procedures for which there are questions of overuse, underuse, and misuse; and volume of procedures for which there is some evidence that a higher volume of procedures is associated with lower mortality.

Prevention quality indicators review hospital admissions that evidence suggests could have been avoided, at least in part, through high-quality outpatient care. Prevention quality indicators assess the quality of the health-care system as a whole and especially the quality of ambulatory care in preventing medical complications. As a result, these measures are of the greatest value when calculated at the population level and when used by public health groups and other organizations concerned with the health of populations. These indicators serve as a screening tool rather than as definitive measures of quality problems. They can provide initial information about potential problems in the community that may require further, more in-depth analysis.

Patient safety indicators also reflect quality of care inside hospitals but focus on potentially avoidable complications and iatrogenic events. Patient safety indicators are a set of measures for adverse events that patients experience as a result of exposure to the health-care system. These events are likely amenable to prevention by changes at the system or provider level. Widespread consensus exists that health-care organizations can reduce patient injuries by improving the environment for safety—from implementing technical changes, such as electronic medical record systems, to improving staff awareness of patient safety risks. Clinical process interventions also have strong evidence for reducing the risk of adverse events in a patient related to hospital care.

Pediatric quality indicators reflect quality of care inside hospitals and identify potentially avoidable hospitalizations among children. Development of quality indicators for pediatric patients involves many of the same challenges associated with the development of quality indicators for adults. These challenges include the need to define carefully indicators using administrative data, establish validity and reliability, detect bias and design appropriate risk adjustment, and overcome challenges of implementation and use.

Hospital Consumer Assessment of Healthcare Providers and Systems (HCAHPS): In 2002, the CMS in partnership with the AHRQ developed HCAHPS, which is the first national standardized publicly reported survey of patients' perspectives of hospital care. The intent of the HCAHPS initiative is to provide a standardized survey instrument and data collection methodology for measuring patients' perspectives on hospital care. Although many hospitals have collected information on patient satisfaction, before HCAHPS, there was no national standard for collecting or publicly reporting patients' perspectives of care information that would enable valid comparisons to be made across all hospitals. The survey asks discharged patients 27 questions about their recent hospital stay, including critical elements related to communication with health-care providers, responsiveness of staff members, pain management, discharge information, cleanliness, communication about medicines, and if they would recommend the hospital. Since July 2007, hospitals subject to the IPPS annual payment update provisions must collect and submit HCAHPS data to receive their full IPPS annual payment update. The survey produces comparable data on the patient's perspective on care that allow objective and meaningful comparisons between hospitals on domains that are important to consumers; this has created the incentive for hospitals to improve their quality of care. Public reporting serves to enhance public accountability in health care by increasing the transparency of the quality of hospital care.

Core measures, AHRQ quality indicators, and HCAHPS are publicly reported. Despite widespread dissemination of the core measures, safety goals, and related quality guidelines, there is significant variation in the results across providers. Reasons for this variation are complex and may include differences in guideline familiarity, resistance to the use of the evidence-based recommendations, and variation in the infrastructure of documentation systems to ensure that recommended care is provided and documented. Hospital characteristics, such as physician leadership and organizational support, also appear to contribute to the consistent use of evidence-based processes of care. DNP leaders play an important role in ensuring compliance and keeping abreast of changes and updates to quality indicators and the reporting requirements. Recognizing the challenges in undertaking quality improvement, DNP leaders need to focus on improvements in practice and health-care delivery to ensure that care is safe, timely, effective, efficient, equitable, and patient-centered.

Overall, health-care quality measurement is in the midst of a revolution because of the desire to create a health-care system that is more patient-centered, accountable, and cost-effective. As an adjunct to the Patient Protection and Affordable Care Act, the U.S. Department of Health and Human Services established national quality goals and a mechanism to track their progress. The NQF is working on more consensus-endorsed measures to support the transformation of the health system, with the highest priorities being the development and endorsement of measures to address appropriate resource use and effective care coordination.

Nurse-Sensitive Indicators

Nurse-sensitive indicators reflect the process, structure, and outcomes of nursing care. *Process* includes various aspects of care, such as assessment, restraints, and job satisfaction of registered nurses. *Structure* refers to the supply, competency, and education of the nursing staff. *Patient outcomes* are the measures that improve if there is a greater quality or quantity of nursing staff. Examples of outcome indicators include falls, falls with injury, pressure ulcers, and IV infiltrations.

Reporting and comparing nurse-sensitive outcomes with a national database is a requirement of the Magnet Hospital recognition program. One such database is the National Database of Nursing Quality Indicators (NDNQI), which is the proprietary nursing quality measurement program of the American Nurses Association (ANA). NDNQI collects and reports data from more than 1500 hospitals in the United States on 18 nursing-sensitive indicators with a wide variety of comparison options. Using NDNQI data, participants can compare their unit-specific measures with other facilities of similar size, specialty, or geographic location for quality improvement purposes. The CMS has determined that by 2013, all acute care hospitals will voluntarily report eight nurse-sensitive indicators to the CMS through a national database such as NDNQI.

Advancing Your Knowledge

C.W., DNP, RN, is the vice-president for patient care services in a large metropolitan medical center. Nate Wilson, a state legislator, requests an appointment with her. He has reviewed the medical center's HCAHPS, a national survey that asks patients about their experiences during a recent hospital stay. He had planned to have his cardiac bypass surgery in C.W.'s medical center but is very concerned about the scores on HCAHPS. He notes that the scores on communication and pain control were lower than he expected. He also expresses concern that only 58% of patients would definitely recommend the hospital to others. C.W. is aware that the medical center HCAHPS scores need to improve, but they are similar to other hospitals in her geographic area.

1. How should C.W. as a DNP-prepared nurse leader respond to these concerns about quality?
2. What strategies would you recommend to raise patient perceptions about nursing communication and pain management?
3. How would you inform and involve staff in developing strategies to improve HCAHPS scores?

Using Quality Indicators

Following the initial reports from the IOM, the volume and breadth of studies focused on improving health care increased. Over time, the AHRQ, The Joint Commission, and the CMS and many private organizations began to publish quality indicators for identifying, monitoring, comparing, and publicly reporting the performance of health-care organizations. Many state and national initiatives are under way to mandate or induce health-care organizations to disclose publicly information on organizational performance and physician outcomes. The term *report cards* refers to information sources and tools designed to enable health-care consumers to compare quality of care and other characteristics of health plans or providers. On the Web site of the AHRQ, there is a national directory of more than 200 report cards listing outcomes and quality for various health-care organizations. The AHRQ (http://www.ahrq.gov/) stated that use of these report cards can influence quality in at least three ways, as follows:

- Informed choices make it more likely that consumers will obtain high-quality health care for themselves and their family members.
- The collective effect of many informed choices may stimulate quality improvement among providers. That is, providers may be motivated to improve as a way to protect or enhance their market share.
- Public reports that affect the public image of providers by identifying them as high-quality or low-quality providers may encourage them to improve the quality of care they provide to protect or enhance their reputations.

Consumers have been slow to use comparative performance reports to make health-care choices. Measures of quality are frequently misinterpreted. Misunderstanding takes many forms. For example, some hospital reports include length of stay (LOS) or readmissions as performance indicators. Longer LOS and higher readmission rates are intended to indicate poor performance, yet many consumers view these as measures of access and interpret them in the opposite way—viewing a longer LOS or higher readmission rates as indicators of high-quality care. Other measures are beyond the scope of understanding of lay consumers. Reporting on measures such as administration of angiotensin-converting enzyme inhibitors assumes a higher level of clinical knowledge and understanding than most consumers have. Finding ways to make public reporting more relevant and useful to consumers is part of an overall strategy to improve health care.

Pay for Performance

Pay for Performance (P4P) is a nationwide trend in both private and government-sponsored health-care programs to measure efficiency and increase the transparency of medical costs, reduce resource use, and improve quality to move forward the concept of value in health care (AHRQ, n.d.[b], 2011). Providers under this arrangement are rewarded for meeting pre-established targets for delivery of health-care services. P4P is a fundamental change from fee-for-service payment, also known as *value-based purchasing*. This payment model rewards physicians, hospitals, medical groups, and other health-care providers for meeting certain performance measures for quality and efficiency. Disincentives, such as eliminating payments for negative consequences of care (medical errors) or increased costs, have also been proposed.

P4P can engage providers and change behaviors by encouraging providers to participate in quality improvement to reduce unnecessary variation in the practice of care. P4P programs reward hospitals, physicians, nurse practitioners, and other providers with both financial and nonfinancial incentives based on performance on select measures. The use of standardized and actual costs is considered essential to creating a balanced, fair, comprehensive comparison of health-care provider performance as part of P4P. These performance measures can cover various aspects of health-care delivery, including clinical quality and safety, efficiency, patient experience, and health information technology adoption.

The IOM report *Preventing Medication Errors* (2006a) recommended incentives through increased payments from insurance carriers so that patient safety goals are aligned with the profitability of hospitals, clinics, pharmacies, insurance companies, and manufacturers. A second IOM report, *Rewarding Provider Performance: Aligning Incentives in Medicare* (2006b), stated that the existing payment systems do not reflect the relative value of health-care services in important aspects of quality, such as clinical quality, patient-centeredness, and efficiency, and they do not recognize or reward prevention and the treatment of chronic conditions. This report also recommended P4P programs as an opportunity to align incentives with performance improvement.

Sponsors of P4P programs include government agencies, employers, health-care providers, health insurance plans, and a variety of quality coalitions. A multitude of payers have introduced P4P programs, including the government's Physician Quality Reporting Initiative (PQRI) and e-prescribing programs. Select private payers also provide bonuses to practices for using technology, and most have programs in which providers are asked to report on quality indicators. Health-care reform legislation introduces a penalty that begins in 2015 for Medicare providers who do not participate in PQRI (IOM, 2006b). Penalties beginning in 2012 were already in place for Medicare providers who do not use e-prescribing.

Seeking to improve quality and avoid unnecessary health care costs, the CMS has various P4P initiatives in offices, clinics, and hospitals. Hospitals that do not meet a threshold for patient quality are subject to reductions in reimbursement. This rule, which became effective in 2008, reduced payments for certain hospital-acquired medical complications, such as the 28 "never events." *"Never events"* are defined as adverse events that are serious, largely preventable, and of concern for the purpose of public accountability (NQF, 2006). These events include patient falls with injury, hospital-acquired infections, venous thromboembolism, and stages 3 and 4 decubitus ulcers.

Private health payers are considering similar actions; the Leapfrog Group (a voluntary program aimed at mobilizing employer purchasing power) is exploring how to provide support to its members who are interested in ensuring that their employees do not get billed for "never events." Physician groups involved in the management of complications have voiced objections to these proposals, observing that some patients develop infections despite application of all evidence-based practices known to avoid infection and that a punitive response may discourage further study and slow the dramatic improvements that have already been made (Infectious Diseases Society of America, Society for Healthcare Epidemiology of America, & Association for Professionals in Infection Control and Epidemiology in America, 2006). These groups also express concern over the validity of quality indicators, patient and physician autonomy and privacy, and increased administrative burdens. However, statements by professional medical societies generally support incentive programs to increase the quality of health care.

Advancing Your Knowledge

A.C., DNP, CNS, is an oncology clinical nurse specialist in a large academic medical center. She has recently been evaluating quality performance data on her oncology patient population, and she found that her medical center has an infection rate on central line catheters that exceeds national benchmarks. In

Continued on page 214

Advancing Your Knowledge *Continued from page 213*

reviewing the reimbursement implications, she learns that the medical center will potentially lose $8000 on the care of each oncology patient who develops a central line infection. A.C. has been working on new protocols to improve care. Practice changes are needed in both the insertion and the care of the lines for oncology patients. Many interdisciplinary team members need to be educated.

1. As a DNP nurse leader, how can A.C. create a sense of urgency with interdisciplinary team members about the reimbursement issues?
2. How could A.C. design an evaluation strategy to measure improvements in patient outcomes?
3. How should DNP leaders such as A.C. monitor and interpret national benchmarks that could affect their organizational reimbursement?

Patient Safety Initiatives

Patient safety has been defined by the IOM as the prevention of harm to patients (Aspden, Corrigan, & Wolcott, 2004). Emphasis is placed on the system of care. The health-care delivery system must work to (1) prevent errors; (2) learn from the errors that do occur; and (3) build on a culture of safety that involves health-care professionals, organizations, and patients (Clancy, Farquhar, & Sharp, 2005). Patient safety practices have been defined as practices that reduce the risk of adverse events related to exposure to medical care across a range of diagnoses or conditions (AHRQ, n.d.[a]). Practices that have sufficient evidence to be included in the category of *patient safety practices* include, but are not limited to, the following (Shojania, Duncan, & McDonald, 2001):

- Appropriate use of prophylaxis to prevent venous thromboembolism in patients at risk
- Use of perioperative beta blockers in appropriate patients to prevent perioperative morbidity and mortality
- Use of maximum sterile barriers while placing central IV catheters to prevent infections
- Appropriate use of antibiotic prophylaxis in surgical patients to prevent postoperative infections
- Asking that patients recall and restate what they have been told during the informed consent process to verify their understanding
- Continuous aspiration of subglottic secretions to prevent ventilator-associated pneumonia
- Use of pressure-relieving bedding materials to prevent pressure ulcers
- Use of real-time ultrasound guidance during central line insertion to prevent complications
- Patient self-management with warfarin (Coumadin) to achieve appropriate outpatient anticoagulation and prevent complications

- Appropriate provision of nutrition, with a particular emphasis on early enteral nutrition in critically ill patients and surgical patients to prevent complications
- Use of antibiotic-impregnated central venous catheters to prevent catheter-related infections

Many patient safety practices, such as use of simulation laboratories for education, bar coding, computerized physician order entry, and resource management, have been considered as possible strategies to avoid patient safety errors and improve health-care processes. Although researchers have explored these areas, innumerable opportunities remain for further research. DNP-prepared nurses are well equipped to lead implementation of the science developed by researchers. The enhanced knowledge that the DNP has acquired can enhance patient safety and quality outcomes by translating research into new models of care.

Another organization focused on patient safety is the NQF, which is a nonprofit organization that aims to improve the quality of health care for all Americans through fulfillment of its three-part mission: (1) setting national priorities and goals for performance improvement, (2) endorsing national consensus standards for measurement and public reporting, and (3) promoting the attainment of national goals through education and outreach programs (NQF, 2010b). The NQF was created in 1999 by a coalition of leaders in the public and private sectors in response to the recommendation of the Advisory Commission on Consumer Protection and Quality in the Health Care Industry. In its 1998 final report, the commission concluded that an organization such as the NQF was needed to promote and ensure patient protection and health-care quality through measurement and public reporting. Today, the NQF receives funding from both public and private sources, including grants from foundations, corporations, and the federal government. In 2009, the U.S. Department of Health and Human Services awarded a contract to the NQF to help establish a portfolio of quality and efficiency measures that would allow the federal government to identify more clearly how and whether health-care spending is achieving the best results for patients and taxpayers (NQF, 2010b).

The NQF (2010a) attempted to bring clarity to the multiple definitions of patient safety with its report, "Standardizing a Patient Safety Taxonomy." This standardized framework for classifying patient safety data and taxonomy defines *harm* as the impact and severity of a process of care failure as well as temporary or permanent impairment of physical or psychological body functions or structure. The origins of the patient safety problem are classified in terms of type (error), communication (failures between patient or patient proxy and practitioners, practitioner and nonmedical staff, or among practitioners), patient management (improper delegation, failure in tracking, wrong referral, or wrong use of resources), and clinical performance (before, during, and after intervention).The types of errors and harm are classified further regarding domain, or where they occurred across the spectrum of health-care providers and settings. The NQF framework identifies the root causes of harm in the following terms:

- *Latent failure:* Involves failures from decisions that affect the organizational policies, procedures, or allocation of resources
- *Active failure:* Direct contact with the patient
- *Organizational system failure:* Indirect failures involving management, organizational culture, protocols or processes, transfer of knowledge, and external factors
- *Technical failure:* Indirect failure of facilities or external resources

A small component of the taxonomy is devoted to prevention or mitigation activities. These mitigation activities can be universal (implemented throughout the organization or health-care settings), selective (within certain high-risk areas), or indicated (specific to a clinical or organizational process that has failed or has high potential to fail). The NQF endorsed 34 safe practices in the 2009 update of the "Safe Practices for Better Healthcare and 28 Serious Reportable Events (SRE)."(National Quality Forum, 2009). The Safe Practices, SREs, and NQF-endorsed patient safety measures are important tools for tracking and improving patient safety performance in health care.

Significant gaps remain in the measurement of patient safety. There is a recognized need to expand available patient safety measures beyond the hospital setting to include entities across the continuum of health care. To fill these gaps and to develop a more robust set of safety measures, the NQF is soliciting patient safety measures to fill gap areas and to address environment-specific issues with highest potential leverage for improvement, such as health-care–associated infections, cultures of safety, and hospital standardized mortality rates.

An essential role of the DNP leader is "to direct care policies, programs and protocols that are organized, monitored, and continuously improved by expert clinicians" (AACN, 2005, p. 3). DNP leaders are positioned to identify and implement nursing interventions that influence health-care outcomes in the direct care of patients or to provide administrative leadership for practice changes to improve patient safety.

Health-Care Spending

Health-care spending is a major national concern and requires leadership from all of the sectors involved in the health-care debate, including government, health-care professionals, insurers, and the public. Health-care professionals need leadership in attempting to influence health-care funding and support evidence-based options to improve population-based care. Improvements in health-care quality and positive patient outcomes are a means to reduce health-care spending. Sisko et al. (2009) projected that spending is expected to increase 6.2% annually, reaching $4.4 trillion in 2018. Although spending is high, the United States has consistently ranked low compared with other developed nations in many areas of quality of care and health access.

Under the current payment system, individual providers, hospitals, and other entities are paid for services they provide to patients. Criticism has been levied that this payment system has led to a lack of integration of care leading to overtreatment of patients and duplication of services. Under the Patient Protection and Affordable Care Act of 2010, the Medicare program received authorization to contract with accountable care organizations (ACOs). ACOs are networks of providers that could include hospitals, physicians, nurse practitioners, and other health team members that work together to promote care integration, improve the quality of health services, and reduce the costs for a defined patient population (Robert Wood Johnson Foundation, 2010). An ACO is a payment and delivery reform model that ties provider reimbursements to quality metrics and reductions in the total cost of care for an assigned population of patients. A group of coordinated health-care providers forms an ACO and provides care to a group of patients.

The ACO may use a range of different payment models, such as capitation or fee-for-service with shared savings. The ACO is accountable to the patients and the third-party payer for the quality, appropriateness, and efficiency of the health care provided. According to the CMS, an ACO is "an organization of health care providers that agrees to be accountable for the quality, cost, and overall care of Medicare beneficiaries who are enrolled in the traditional fee-for-service program who are assigned to it." (CMS, 2011) The Congressional Budget Office has estimated that ACOs could save $5 billion in the first 8 years (Robert Wood Johnson Foundation, 2010). Public reporting of cost and quality information is a key way that ACOs are held accountable for their performance.

The ACO concept is new, and models are expected to evolve over time. Potential ACOs include integrated health delivery systems, such as Kaiser Permanente; multispecialty practice groups; physician-hospital organizations; independent practice associations; and virtual physician/provider organizations. Devers and Berenson (2009) pointed out that beneficiary reaction to ACOs will be very important. If ACOs are tightly managed and seen as reinvented health maintenance organizations (HMOs), there could be political reactions. If beneficiaries find that ACOs make the health-care system easier to navigate, they will be positively received.

ACOs differ from older health-care delivery models such as HMOs. The goals of ACOs are to reduce costs while improving population health, whereas HMOs were designed to reduce individual health-care costs and place the burden and risk of health-care costs on the provider. The critical tools that ACOs possess are the ability to measure both clinical and financial performance and, ultimately, to hold provider systems accountable for both cost and quality for assigned patient populations, while providing primary care providers with opportunities to meet goals through a broader system of care providers beyond the physician. For example, an ACO may have a physical therapist, home health nurses, and a psychologist on staff to meet the needs of patients.

In contrast to HMOs, ACOs are designed to minimize barriers to entry for both patients and providers. ACOs have adopted a patient-attribution or patient-responsibility methodology rather than acquiring patient enrollment. The ACO is designed to be a very flexible model that allows for different configurations of providers to come together in different organizational and legal contexts.

DNP-prepared nurse leaders in group practice and hospital settings are in an excellent strategic position to help plan these new ACOs and redesign the delivery system. There is strong evidence that access to quality care could be substantially improved by increasing the use of registered nurses and advanced practice nurses in primary, long-term, and transitional care. In some states, however, there are still regulatory barriers to allowing nurses to practice to the full extent of their education. The IOM (2010) highlighted the critical need for providers in primary care with demand expected to increase. Hansen-Turton and Ritter (2008) found in their research that nearly half of all managed care organizations in the United States refused to credential and reimburse nurse practitioners as primary care providers. Expansion of advanced practice nursing scope of practice and reimbursement for services should be a key part of ACO planning.

The DNP leader plays a pivotal role in improving health-care quality and reducing costs. Nursing leaders can partner with other health-care disciplines to create cultures that view challenges in care delivery as opportunities for interdisciplinary systematic improvements. DNP leaders can assist staff to move quality initiatives from theory into practice. Continuous quality improvement is based on the concept that improvement comes from building on knowledge, and DNP leaders are well equipped to assist others to apply this knowledge in the shared quest for improved patient quality and outcomes.

Healthy Work Environments

Quality patient care is a goal that health-care professionals strive to achieve on a daily basis. A growing body of evidence suggests that factors in the hospital work environment can have positive or negative effects on patient outcomes and quality care (Aiken, Clarke, Sloane, Sochalski, & Silber, 2002). Work environments that are referred to as *healthy* are important for the overall health of both registered nurses and the patients under their care. Healthy work environments can be characterized by a high level of trust between leadership and employees, by employees who treat each other in a respectful manner, and by a climate where employees feel safe both emotionally and physically (Shirey, 2006). These environments are healing and empowering environments where there are high levels of staff engagement.

Healthy work environments are empirically linked to positive patient satisfaction, improved recruitment and retention, increased job satisfaction, work engagement, and lower levels of job stress (Aiken et al., 2002). Several studies have shown that job resources, such as social support from colleagues and leadership, performance feedback, skill variety, autonomy, and learning opportunities, are positively associated with engagement (Bakker, Schaufeli, Leiter, & Taris, 2008). These job resources act as an intrinsic motivational factor as they foster growth, learning, and development of registered nurses and are extrinsically motivational as they help to achieve the organizational goals. The possibility of a positive work environment exists when there is an active state of interdependence among the organization, the leaders and directors, and the employees (Manion, 2009). When nurses learn ways to manage the stress in the workplace, they experience greater vigor, absorption, and dedication in their interactions with their patients and families and are more likely to be proud of their work, which leads to greater job satisfaction and improved patient outcomes.

This section focuses on the healthy work environment as a part of the system to create the best possible patient care. The DNP can foster a healthy work environment in his or her area of practice, leading to improved health-care quality.

Creating and Promoting Healthy Workplaces: A Shared Responsibility

The landmark IOM report entitled *To Err Is Human: Building a Safer Health System* (1999) changed the perception of patient safety. By exposing the dangers patients face when they enter the current health-care system, the IOM used its powerful influence to call for a focus on error prevention in a just culture, instead of individual punishment. In *Crossing the Quality Chasm: A New Health System for the 21st Century*, the IOM (2001) attacked the dysfunctional processes of the U.S. health-care system, citing pervasive poor communication, a punitive climate, and decisions made by sole individuals. The IOM called for a redesign of the way health-care providers communicate, anticipate, and modify patient risk. Institutions should evaluate the effectiveness of the changes by focusing on team performance, data-driven analysis of system failures, and continuous process improvement (IOM, 2001).

A healthy work environment provides a foundation to support efforts to improve safe patient care. Safe patient care is directly and positively linked to the quality of work environments of staff nurses. The consequences of an unhealthy health-care work environment include work-related accidents, high absenteeism, high turnover, poor patient outcomes, stress, and increased health-care litigation (Whitehead, 2006).

For many years, the phrase "healthy work environment" has been used to describe proposed changes to the workplace of health-care providers. *Healthy* means productive, able to give quality care, satisfying, and able to meet personal needs. By definition, a *healthy work environment* is a work setting in which policies, procedures, and systems are designed so that employees are able to meet organizational objectives and achieve personal satisfaction in their work (Disch, 2002). Shirey (2006) defined healthy work environments as supportive of the whole human being, patient-focused, and joyful. A healthy work environment has organizational cultures, systems, and management practices that support employee health and wellness goals. Often, the words "healthy work environment" are interchanged with a healing work environment. Ideally, healthy work environments should have the infrastructures to create sanctuaries of healing (Kerfoot & Ivy, 2004) as the healing environment must also extend to the staff members providing the care to patients.

Increasingly, professional organizations and state and national commissions are challenging nurses, leaders in acute care, and health care organizations to improve the practice environment for bedside nurses to improve patient safety and job satisfaction and retention of nurses. In an effort to promote healthy work environments, numerous nursing organizations and professional groups have developed programs to guide health-care organizations in their efforts to improve working conditions for registered nurses. An understanding of a healthy work environment is essential for the DNP leader so that others can be inspired to be involved in the shared mission for change.

Organizing Nursing's Influence: Responses to Create Healthy Work Environments

Organizations such as American Association of Critical-Care Nurses (AACN), The Joint Commission, IOM, AONE, American Association of Colleges of Nursing, Nursing Organizations Alliance, Center for American Nurses, and American Nurses Credentialing Center have identified and established criteria for healthy, professional, excellent, effective, and rewarding work environments. No matter what adjective is used to describe changes to the work environment, common to all the lists of attributes provided by the organizations is the focus on structures, policies, systems, and programs that reflect the perspective and domain of nurses in leadership roles.

The standards established by five of these organizations—Nursing Organizations Alliance, AONE, AACN, American Nurses Credentialing Center (ANCC) Magnet Recognition Program, and Center for American Nurses—provide a road map for creating a healthy practice environment where there is interdisciplinary communication, mutual respect, and a focus on the patient as the center of health care. Each organization has a different focus and membership, but there is one common thread: transformation of the health-care work environment.

Nursing Organizations Alliance

The Nursing Organizations Alliance began in 2001 when two nursing organization coalitions, the National Federation for Specialty Nursing Organizations and the Nursing Organizations Liaison Forum, united to form a stronger voice for nurses. The mission of the Nursing Organizations Alliance is "to increase nursing's visibility and impact on health through communication, collaboration and advocacy" (Nursing Organizations Alliance, n.d.). Given the mission of this organization and its links with numerous nursing organizations, the Nursing Organizations Alliance is in a position to foster partnerships among nursing organizations to support nursing's agenda for quality health care for the American public.

The Nursing Organizations Alliance believes that a healthful practice or work environment is supported by the presence of the elements shown in Table 5-1.

Table 5-1

Nine Principles of Healthy Work Environments

Principle	Elements
1. Collaborative practice culture	Respectful collegial communication and behavior Team orientation Presence of trust Respect for diversity
2. Communication-rich culture	Clear and respectful Open and trusting
3. Culture of accountability	Role expectations are clearly defined Everyone is accountable
4. Presence of adequate numbers of qualified nurses	Ability to provide quality care to meet patient needs Work and home life balance
5. Presence of expert, competent, credible, visible leadership	Serve as an advocate for nursing practice Support shared decision making Allocate resources to support nursing
6. Shared decision making at all levels	Nurses participate in system, organizational, and process decisions Formal structure exists to support shared decision making Nurses have control over their practice
7. Encouragement of professional practice and continued growth and development	Continuing education and certification are supported and encouraged Participation in professional associations is encouraged Information-rich environment is supported
8. Recognition of value of nursing's contribution	Reward and pay for performance Career mobility and expansion
9. Recognition of nurses for their meaningful contribution to the practice	Provide recognition

Source: Nursing Organizations Alliance. (2004). http://www.nursing-alliance.org/

These nine elements are fostered and incorporated into the work of individual member organizations of the Nursing Organizations Alliance. Self-assessment tools have been developed by the AONE to accompany the nine elements of the healthful practice work environment of the Nursing Organizations Alliance (Nursing Organizations Alliance, n.d.). The nine principles and elements include the following:

- Collaborative practice culture
- Communication-rich culture
- Culture of accountability
- Presence of adequate numbers of qualified nurses
- Presence of expert, competent, credible, visible leadership
- Shared decision making at all levels

- Encouragement of professional practice that continues growth and development
- Recognition of the value of contribution nursing
- Recognition of nurses for their meaningful contribution to practice

American Organization of Nurse Executives

The AONE is the national organization of nurses who design, facilitate, and manage care (AONE, n.d.). The AONE has more than 7000 members and is recognized as the voice of nursing leadership in health care. Since 1967, the organization has provided leadership, professional development, advocacy, and research to advance nursing practice and patient care, promote nursing leadership excellence, and shape public policy for health care. The AONE serves its members by providing vision and actions for nursing leadership to influence legislation and public policy related to nursing and patient care issues, offering educational programs that advance professional practice, and facilitating research that advances improvement in nursing administration practices (AONE, 2009).

The AONE 2010–2012 Strategic Plan includes objectives to provide a positive, safe, and healthful practice environment. These objectives support evidence-based leadership development that builds a culture of active nurse engagement; advocates to secure the resources needed from the federal government to ensure an adequate and diverse nursing workforce in the future; promotes the collaboration between nursing and other health professionals to create positive, safe, and healthful practice or work environments; and serves as a catalyst for change (AONE, 2009).

In response to the growing realization that the solution to the widespread shortage of nurses must include substantial innovation in the nursing work environment, AONE (2003) published a study titled *Healthy Work Environments: Striving for Excellence*. This study highlighted various approaches hospitals used to strengthen the nursing work environment and important common threads running through the multifaceted efforts under way. It is evident from this study that the impact of the nursing shortage generated a new openness to nursing innovation and related organizational change within many hospitals in the United States. The wide range of work environment initiatives described in this report testifies to the enormous amount of creative energy that was unleashed to address opportunities for improvement and change.

The study suggests that six critical factors are essential for achieving an excellent work environment. Each of these success factors is briefly described (AONE, 2003):

1. *Leadership development and effectiveness:* The leader is a trusted coach and advisor. There are processes for evaluating and improving leadership effectiveness at all levels.
2. *Empowered collaborative decision making:* Nurse empowerment, combined with multidisciplinary decision making, is essential. Effective teamwork and interdisciplinary decision-making processes are core competencies.

3. *Work design and service delivery innovation:* The capacity for continuous organizational learning and process improvement is a critical competency. There is frontline staff involvement in work redesign.
4. *Values-driven organizational culture:* Individuals in the organization understand and embrace organizational values, finding their work meaningful. There is a process of cultural change addressing leadership styles, staff empowerment, workforce relationships, customer focus, accountability, and quality communication.
5. *Recognition and reward systems:* There is a positive and supportive work environment with appreciation for the work of individuals who are high performers or have made special contributions.
6. *Professional growth and accountability:* The organization provides well-defined and supported career development and clearly defined performance standards and patient outcome measurements.

The standards are listed in Table 5-2.

American Association of Critical-Care Nurses

The AACN recognizes the important relationships of quality of work environment, excellence in professional nursing practice, and patient outcomes. The AACN is strategically committed to using its resources and influence to create work and care environments that are "safe, healing, humane, respectful of the rights, responsibilities, and needs of all people—including patients, their families and nurses" (AACN, 2005). In January 2005, the AACN published national standards for establishing and sustaining healthy work environments (AACN, 2005).

The six standards that represent evidence-based and relationship-centered principles of professional performance are as follows:

- *Skilled communication:* Nurses must be as proficient in communication skills as they are in clinical skills.

Table 5-2

Principles and Elements of a Healthful Work Environment

- Collaborative practice culture
- Communication-rich culture
- Culture of accountability
- Adequate numbers of nurses on staff
- Competent, credible, visible leaders
- Shared decision making
- Encouragement for professional practice and continued growth
- Recognition of the value of nurses' contribution
- Recognition of nurses' contributions to practice

Source: American Organization of Nurse Executives: Healthy Work Environments Striving for Excellence. (2003). http://www.mcmanis-monsalve.com/files/publications/healthy_work_environments_full.pdf

- *True collaboration:* Nurses must be relentless in pursuing and fostering true collaboration.
- *Effective decision making:* Nurses must be valued and committed partners in making policy, directing and evaluating clinical care, and leading organizational operations.
- *Appropriate staffing:* Staffing must ensure the effective match between patient needs and nurse competencies.
- *Meaningful recognition:* Nurses must be recognized and must recognize others for the value each brings to the work of the organization.
- *Authentic leadership:* Nurse leaders must embrace the imperative of a healthy work environment, authentically live it, and engage others in its achievement.

The standards put forth by the AACN complement and support the ANA Code of Ethics for Nurses, the IOM recommendations for core competencies, and the elements of a healthy work environment as written by the Nursing Organizations Alliance (AACN, 2005). The standards do not address education or credentialing but rather focus on systemic behaviors that establish and sustain healthy work environments. The standards are designed to be used to engage in meaningful dialogue between health-care workers and their leaders about the realities of their unique work environment. Critical elements required for successful implementation accompany each standard. Working together as collaborative partners, health-care workers and leaders can make decisions on the depth and breadth of implementation. The standards are listed in Table 5-3.

American Nurses Credentialing Center: Magnet Recognition Program

In the early 1980s, the American Academy of Nurses conducted research to identify which hospitals attract and retain registered nurses in their employment and to identify factors that are associated with these successful health-care

Table 5-3

Standards for Establishing and Sustaining Healthy Work Environments

- *Skilled communication:* Nurses must be as proficient in communication skills as they are in clinical skills
- *True collaboration:* Nurses must be relentless in pursuing and fostering true collaboration
- *Effective decision making:* Nurses must be valued and committed partners in making policy, directing and evaluating clinical care, and leading organizational operations
- *Meaningful recognition:* Nurses must be recognized and must recognize others for the value each person brings to the work of the organization
- *Authentic leadership:* Nurse leaders must fully embrace the imperative of a healthy work environment, authentically live it, and engage others in its achievement

Source: American Association of Critical-Care Nurses. (2005). *AACN standards for establishing and sustaining healthy work environments: A journey to excellence.* Aliso Viejo, CA: Author.

facilities. From this study, McClure, Poulin, Sovie, and Wandelt (1983) coined the term *Magnet Hospitals* in recognition of the fact that these facilities contained characteristics that attracted registered nurses like magnets. The Magnet Recognition Program was developed by the ANCC 3 years after the original study. The program is voluntary and recognizes environments that attract professional nurses and acknowledge nursing excellence and the role professional nurses play in quality, safe patient care.

The newest Magnet Model, introduced in 2008, serves as a "road map" (ANCC, 2008) to help hospitals and health-care organizations achieve Magnet recognition. The Magnet Model requires hospitals to demonstrate nursing excellence in patient, nurse, and organizational results. The overarching theme of the Magnet Model is "Global Issues in Nursing and Health Care" (ANCC, 2008). The Magnet Model focuses on five areas, as follows (ANCC, 2008):

- *Transformational leadership:* Strong nurse leaders have the vision, knowledge, and influence to guide their team where it needs to go, not just where it wants to go.
- *Structural empowerment:* Strong nurse leaders create an environment where the hospital's mission and vision come to life, and all nurses are encouraged to achieve desired results.
- *Exemplary professional practice:* Nurses practice, work together, communicate, and develop professionally to achieve the highest quality of care for patients and the community.
- *New knowledge, innovations, and improvements:* Nurses take the lead in research efforts and have an ethical and professional responsibility to contribute new findings, evidence, and quality improvement to the nursing profession.
- *Empirical outcomes:* Strong nursing structures and processes are in place to achieve good outcomes, but nurses go further to show results and the impact of those results. Empirical outcomes move beyond what nurses do and how they do it to focus on the question: "What difference have you made?"

ANCC Magnet Recognition is the highest and most prestigious international distinction a health-care organization or hospital can receive for nursing excellence and outstanding patient care. There are many benefits associated with Magnet Recognition. A growing amount of research reveals that Magnet status has a positive impact on nursing quality care, patient outcomes, the work environment, and nurse recruitment and retention (Aiken, 2002). Magnet Hospitals are international models for nursing care. Other hospitals look to Magnet organizations for ways to improve patient results, reduce hospital stays, and attract and keep the most qualified nursing staff.

Center for American Nurses

The Center for American Nurses is a national professional nursing organization that educates, equips, and empowers registered nurses to create healthy work environments. The Center for American Nurses offers evidence-based solutions and powerful tools to navigate workplace challenges, optimize patient outcomes, and maximize career benefits (Center for American Nurses, 2008). Established in 2003, the Center for American Nurses partners with individuals and organizations to develop resources, strategies, and tools to help nurses manage evolving workforce issues and succeed in their careers. In an effort to provide nurses with the strategies and resources for their professional and personal growth, the Center for American Nurses has organized its work into a document entitled, "The Workforce Ecosystem" (Center for American Nurses, 2008). "The Workforce Ecosystem" describes how the tools of the Center for American Nurses can empower nurses in professional actions to create healthier work environments. The elements of the workforce ecosystem that offer evidence-based solutions and powerful tools to navigate workplace challenges, optimize patient outcomes, and maximize career benefits include the following:

- *Staffing:* Refers to job assignments, including the volume of work assigned to individuals, the professional competencies required for particular job assignments, the duration of experience in a particular job category, and work schedules
- *Workflow design:* Pertains to on-the-job activities of health-care workers, including interactions among workers and the nature and scope of the work
- *Personal and social factors:* Refers to individual and group factors such as stress, job satisfaction, and professionalism and skills that may be underdeveloped among nurses, such as financial literacy
- *Physical environment:* Includes aspects of the workplace such as light, esthetics, and sound
- *Organizational factors:* Refers to structural and process aspects of the organization as a whole, such as the use of teams, divisions of labor, shared beliefs, and an increasing leadership capacity among nurses

This approach offers a holistic view of the nurse from both a personal and a professional perspective. The framework assists nurses in self-advocacy in their work environments. The services and strategies of the Center for American Nurses support nurses at all levels of experience who are striving to improve their practice environments and promote excellence in patient care and who want to meet their personal and professional goals (Center for American Nurses, 2008).

Essential Elements of Healthy Work Environments

If one were to examine the attributes of health-care facilities that have healthy work environments, the following four major attributes would come to light (Heath, Johanson, & Blake, 2004):

1. The employees are treated with respect and fairness with concern and value for each individual being foremost and a sense of being a work family.
2. There is trust and respect between management and employees. Employees are empowered through shared decision making to be risk takers, to make decisions, and grow both personally and professionally.

3. An organizational culture supports communication and collaboration in decision making at all levels of the organization.
4. Decisions are made not solely based on financial impact, but rather are based on the impact to the mission and the members of the organization.

These four elements are consistent with the standards set forth by the various organizations discussed earlier in this chapter. The following discussion is a compilation of the four attributes identified by Heath et al. (2004) and the five initiatives for healthy work environments outlined earlier in this chapter.

Collaboration and Teamwork

The quality of health care depends on each member of the team communicating effectively to coordinate care and resolve differences. Health-care workers who work in isolation run the risk of working with incomplete information and incorrect perceptions of the patients' needs. Research findings suggest that poor collaboration and teamwork among health-care workers is significantly related both to medical errors and to staff turnover (Maxfield, Grenny, McMillan, Patterson, & Switzler, 2005). Poor colleague relationships with conflict, aggression, and the resulting lack of communication can lead to decreased effectiveness, lack of concentration, and decreased work performance (Manojlovich & Laschingrer, 2002).

There are two attributes of effective and healthy working relationships: collaboration and teamwork. Collaboration is a complex process requiring intentional knowledge sharing and joint responsibility for patient care. Teamwork underscores the importance of communication, trusting relationships, and the collegial support needed to create a healthy work environment.

Although there always is some level of interpersonal conflict at work, how the conflict is handled is what matters. Conflict that is handled constructively can lead to improvement in practice, greater innovation, and creativity. It is crucial to identify the causes and explore the effects of conflict. Conflict has its roots in differences in values, culture, and beliefs. Constructive discussion of these differences can build bridges for ongoing dialog and communication. Understanding and identifying the sources of conflict and positive and negative aspects of conflict is the first step. Nurse leaders can effectively manage conflict by employing several strategies, including negotiation, mediation, and effective communication.

Autonomy and Accountability as Part of a Healthy Work Environment

In a healthy work environment, autonomy, accountability, and shared decision making occur at all levels. Nurses participate in system, organizational, and process decisions and have control over their practice in caring for their patients. Registered nurses must be involved in making decisions about the care of the patients if they are to serve as a patient advocate (ANA, 2001). There is a significant gap between what nurses are accountable for and their ability to make decisions (AACN, 2005). Autonomy and decision making do not imply independence, but rather the right and responsibility to use clinical judgment within the context of one's professional practice.

Within the context of the health-care organization, all members of the health-care team should understand and articulate their boundaries based on their practice discipline and their individual knowledge. When boundaries are clearly defined and appropriately supportive of the professional discipline, health-care workers understand their level of authority and autonomy (Koloroutis, 2004). The outcome of autonomy is accountability. Workplace accountability involves taking ownership of one's work and the outcomes. There are six primary elements that assist leadership to establish accountable practice:

1. Establish clear direction
2. Align people, process, and systems
3. Engage staff
4. Lead the way
5. Monitor progress
6. Review and evaluate results

When these elements are achieved, there are defined levels of responsibility, authority, and accountability for each member of the health-care team (Koloroutis, 2004). A professional nurse has effective control over his or her individual practice, an attribute that has been linked to increased status, respect, and recognition (Kramer & Schmalaberg, 2003). Lack of accountability can lead to errors or lapses in judgment. The consequences of these errors are often punitive rather than corrective. Staff members learn to exhibit less responsibility and accountability because of fear of retribution and punishment. Studies have revealed that just cultures, where mistakes and errors are evaluated as learning opportunities, boast increased responsibility, autonomy, and accountability of staff (Gorzeman, 2008).

Control of Practice

Control of nursing practice within a health-care organization is demonstrated by a model of shared decision making. In the report *Keeping Patients Safe: Transforming the Work Environment of Nurses,* the IOM (2004) stated that nursing staff members who provide direct care should be involved, engaged, and empowered in decisions about patient care and how the care is delivered. The shared governance model is an organizational structure in which clinical nurses have a voice in determining aspects of nursing practice, standards, and quality of care. The advantages of shared governance are twofold: It empowers nurses to use their clinical knowledge and expertise to develop, direct, and sustain their own professional practice, and it allows nurses to network with colleagues, collaborating among units and departments (Unruh, 2005). Control of practice also includes the use of professional practice councils to address practice concerns and creating policies and procedures based on evidence-based practices. Providers of direct care who are involved in hiring decisions and development of staffing models become stakeholders in their practice.

Appropriate Staffing

Staffing is defined as the number and competency of the staff. Administrative decisions about staffing are largely based on three factors: (1) the containment of health-care costs, (2) the complexity of patients requiring care, and (3) the desired level of quality of care. The increasing complexity of hospitalized patients, the shortage of qualified nurses, and declining reimbursements have added to the difficulties associated with achieving high-quality care. A top cause of dissatisfaction of registered nurses with their work environment is inadequate staffing (Buerhaus, Staiger, & Auerbach, 2009). According to the AACN (2005), inadequate staffing is listed as one of the most harmful threats to patient safety and to the well-being of nurses. Poor staffing leads to an overwhelming workload that leaves little time for nurses to complete their assignments or provide the caring aspects of nursing. Low registered nurse staffing levels and poor organizational climates have been found to put nurses at risk for needle-stick injuries (Aiken et al., 2002). After adjusting for hospital characteristics, Aiken et al. (2001) reported that an increase of one patient per nurse was linked to a 23% increase in the likelihood of burnout and a 15% increase in the likelihood of job dissatisfaction.

The goal of staffing should be to match the needs of the patients to the competence of the staff. Health-care organizations must recognize the need for proper staffing and engage registered nurses through shared governance to make informed decisions on staffing for each facility. The Joint Commission monitors staffing and its effectiveness as related to adverse events. The Joint Commission requires that the leaders of health-care organizations report any adverse outcomes that were the result of inadequate staffing to the governing body of The Joint Commission organization.

Authentic Leadership

The evidence in the literature clearly supports the key role of leadership in creating healthy work environments. The AACN identified authentic leadership as a key element for healthy work environments. Authentic leadership has been described as the glue that holds a healthy work environment together (Shirey, 2006). The AACN proposed that leaders who are in a position of responsibility are authentic leaders if they speak the truth and are worthy of trust, reliance, and belief. In the book, *True North: Discover Your Authentic Leadership* (George, Sims, & Gergen, 2010), an authentic leader is described as a leader who brings people together around a shared purpose and empowers others to step up as authentic leaders. Authentic leaders lead by their own expectations, serving others rather than leading for success or recognition. An authentic leader is described as an individual in a position of responsibility who is genuine, trustworthy, reliable, and believable (George et al., 2010).

This description is consistent with the AACN definition of the term *authentic* (AACN, 2005).

According to George et al. (2010), authentic leaders have five key characteristics or abilities: (1) understand their own purpose, (2) practice solid values, (3) lead with heart, (4) establish enduring relationships, and (5) practice self-discipline. The more an authentic leader stays true to his or her core values, the more authentic his or her views are. Authentic leaders have defined their purpose and passion in life and practice their values by basing their decisions on them. They are open to close personal relationships, getting to know the life stories of the people with whom they work, and practice self-discipline that develops their personal energies. They act with courage and have high degrees of emotional intelligence. Authentic leaders are anchored by their deep sense of self; they know where they stand on important issues, values, and beliefs and convey who and what they represent by their actions (Avolio & Gardner, 2005). Authentic leadership shares common attributes with other forms of leadership, such as transformational or servant leadership, including self-awareness and commitment to service. Becoming an authentic leader is a journey of personal growth and commitment.

Professional Development

The nursing profession is obligated to provide adequate and competent nursing care. Licensure determines competency on entry to the profession. Sufficient time for orientation and support for ongoing education and clinical advancement are desirable qualities of healthy work environments. Nursing professional development goes beyond orientation in that it is a lifelong process of active participation by nurses in learning activities. Such activities assist nurses in developing and maintaining continuing competence, enhancing professional practice, and supporting achievement of their career goals. Nursing professional development builds on the educational and experiential bases of nurses across their professional careers with the ultimate goal of ensuring the quality of health care to the public (ANA, 2001). In Magnet accredited facilities, considerable focus is placed on orientation, lifelong learning, and the educational preparation of the professional nurse.

Nurse Recognition

Reward and recognition, whether formal or informal, create motivation and job satisfaction. Employee recognition is not just a nice thing to do for people. Most of us want to feel appreciated; we never outgrow this need. Inwardly, we need others to help us feel valued. When you recognize people effectively, you reinforce the actions and behaviors you most want to see people repeat. Recognition of the values and meaningfulness of one's contribution to an organization is a fundamental human need and essential to professional and personal development (AACN, 2005). Employee recognition is a communication tool that reinforces and rewards the most important outcomes people create for the organization.

An effective employee recognition system is simple, immediate, and powerfully reinforcing. Employee recognition programs are designed to promote respect, communication, excellence, innovation, and teamwork through the recognition of staff in meeting the vision and mission of the organization. The top motivator for job performance is recognition of a job well done.

Adequate Support

The challenge of providing safe, reliable, efficient, timely, quality care is compounded by the increasing acuity levels of patients, shorter patient stays, the nursing shortage, budget cuts because of declining reimbursement, and increasing technological complexity. Adding to these stressors is an increasing diversity of the patient populations, an ever-expanding range of new therapies and medications, and new patient safety indicators that must be incorporated into practice. In many hospitals, registered nurses do not have enough support at the bedside to provide the needed care. Hospitals cannot stay with the status quo of exhorting staff to work harder; they must establish new models of care. Effective interprofessional teamwork and collaboration are of utmost importance for the transformation of bedside care on medical and surgical units. A promising new model for transforming care on medical and surgical units has emerged through a collaboration of the Robert Wood Johnson Foundation and the Institute for Healthcare Improvement. The model is called *Transforming Care at the Bedside* (TCAB) (Robert Wood Johnson Foundation, 2008).

TCAB, a national program, engages leaders at all levels of the organization to:

- Improve the quality and safety of patient care on medical and surgical units
- Increase the vitality and retention of nurses
- Engage and improve the patients' and family members' experience of care
- Improve the effectiveness of the entire care team

TCAB is not a traditional quality improvement program; the primary characteristic that sets it apart is its focus on engaging frontline staff and unit managers to develop innovations and exemplary care models on medical and surgical units to improve outcomes for patients and staff members. At the present time, hundreds of hospitals in the United States and internationally are implementing TCAB strategies on medical and surgical units to provide registered nurses with the needed support to provide excellent care (Baker, Whittington, Resar, Griffin, & Nolan, 2010).

Staff Engagement

To provide quality care, registered nurses must be engaged in their practice. *Work engagement* is a positive, fulfilling, affective, motivational state of work-related well-being that is the antithesis of job burnout (Schaufeli & Bakker, 2003). It goes deeper than just being satisfied with one's job role. Work engagement is a personal and professional commitment to both the job and the organization. There are three related components to engagement: vigor, dedication, and absorption (Schaufeli, Salanova, Gonzalez-Roma, & Bakker, 2002). *Vigor* refers to high levels of mental resilience and energy, along with the willingness to invest effort and persistence while working. *Dedication* is a strong involvement in one's work while experiencing feelings of enthusiasm, significance, inspiration, pride, and challenge. *Absorption* refers to the undivided concentration, immersion, and happy engrossment in one's work where time goes by quickly (Bakker et al., 2008). Engaged employees are physically energized, emotionally connected, mentally focused, and spiritually alighted with a purpose beyond their own self-interest (Loehr & Schwartz, 2003).

Burnout is the erosion of work engagement. Maslach and Leiter (2008) defined burnout as "the index of disassociation between what people are and what they have to do. It represents an erosion in values, dignity, spirit and will—an erosion of the human soul" (p. 17). The characteristics of burnout are exhaustion, cynicism, and ineffectiveness, which are the opposite of work engagement. Individuals who feel burnout experience both physical and psychological manifestations that result in decreased productivity and ineffectiveness (Maslach & Leiter, 2008). Several studies conducted by Aiken et al. (2002) linked lower levels of burnout to acute care work environments that provide job autonomy, control over practice environment, and good nurse-physician relationships.

There is increasing empirical evidence that opportunities to recover from work such as vacations and other respites decrease burnout (Fritz & Sonnentag, 2006). A study of registered nurses and work engagement found that nurses who psychologically detached from work-related demands during short respites showed a higher increase of work engagement when they returned (Kuhnel, Sonnetag, & Westman, 2009).

Healthy work environments that support engagement are essential to provide patient safety and maintain financial viability. Significant relationships exist between job satisfaction and job engagement. If one is more satisfied with his or her job, one is also more engaged (Simpson, 2009). Work engagement is a shared responsibility of the manager and the employee, both supported by the leadership of the organization.

Role of DNP Leaders in Creating Healthy Work Environments

The DNP leader is uniquely prepared to bridge the gap between research and practice by bringing to the health-care work environment strengths and talents beyond clinical expertise. DNP leaders can be innovative and creative in fostering healthy work environments by doing the following:

- Supporting and encouraging health professional interdisciplinary practice and education
- Maintaining work environments that provide for professional nurse involvement in decision making for patient care delivery that incorporates workforces at all levels of the organization

- Understanding the complexities of care delivery, which is essential for any changes to be made
- Creating a patient work environment that encourages not only recruitment but also retention of the workforce through improved collaboration and shared decision making

Advancing Your Knowledge

C.J., DNP, ARNP, is the executive director of a large retirement community that includes both assisted living and a nursing home care facility. He values staff engagement and has tried to create a healthy work environment. He recently conducted a practice environment scale survey and was surprised to learn that his nursing staff reported feeling very disengaged and dissatisfied with their work environment.

1. What steps should C.J. take next as part of his assessment of staff engagement and satisfaction?
2. How should the results of the assessment be communicated to staff members?
3. What strategies would you recommend to C.J. to involve staff members in an improvement plan?

Organizational and Systems Change

The American Association of Colleges of Nursing (2006) DNP essentials addressed the need for DNP graduates to be prepared with sophisticated expertise in assessing organizations, identifying systems issues, and facilitating organization-wide changes in practice delivery. Porter-O'Grady and Malloch (2010) observed that the issue in most organizations is not the capacity to innovate but rather the skills to coordinate, integrate, and facilitate the innovation. Historically, health-care systems have been viewed using a reductionistic paradigm in which the system is considered the sum of its parts. Nurse leaders currently are embracing the view of complexity science, in which systems are recognized as being composed of diverse, interconnected, adaptive agents. Wheatley (2005) pointed out the need for organizations to embrace an adaptive, flexible, self-renewing, resilient, and continuous learning approach. For this to happen, leaders need to recognize that their organizations are complex adaptive systems in which order can emerge.

Health-Care Organizations as Complex Adaptive Systems

Complexity science is the study of complex adaptive systems, the relationships within these systems, how they are sustained, how they self-organize, and how outcomes emerge (Wheatley, 1992). Complex adaptive systems sometimes evolve in unpredictable ways. Concepts from chaos theory are integral to understanding complex adaptive systems. Chaos in complex adaptive systems is not random, although sometimes it may appear so. Complex adaptive systems have distributive control across the system rather than centralized control. The outcomes in a complex adaptive system cannot be fully understood just by understanding all the individual parts. They are nonlinear systems in which leaders may be unable to predict accurately the effect of a change by the size of input in the system. The meteorologist Lorenz coined the term *butterfly effect*, a key component to chaos theory, to explain how a seemingly insignificant change in the environment can have a huge weather impact (Zimmerman, Lindberg, & Plsek, 1998). These concepts illustrate the importance of why leaders need to understand systems theory. Seemingly small changes in a system can have unexpected impact. Complex adaptive systems are history dependent. They are shaped and influenced by where they have been. Failure to respect the history of both an organization and its culture can be detrimental to the health and well-being of any individual organization or group of organizations as they work together.

The application of concepts of complex adaptive systems to health-care environments has been driven by the work of Lindberg and other members of the Plexus Institute. Key leadership principles generated by this institute that apply to complex adaptive systems include the following (Zimmerman et al., 1998):

- The power to generate change resides not only at the top but also is distributed among all members of an organization, and so is the power to prevent change.
- It is not the individual that is the most critical but the relationships among individuals.
- All people are agents affecting and being affected by each other; no one can stand outside the system, and that includes leaders. Perceptive leaders realize their behavior is only one factor affecting the system.
- All people can act locally only, and that includes leaders.
- In complex systems, detailed planning from the top is best replaced by minimum specifications and appropriate autonomy for individuals to self-organize.
- What an organization can accomplish cannot be understood without first understanding its history.
- Among the factors that affect organizational creativity are information flow, diversity, connectivity, power differentials, and anxiety. Most organizations have too little information flow and diversity and too much difference in power.

Zimmerman and Dooley (2001) proposed that health-care organizations are ideal settings to use the principles of complex adaptive systems. Organizations within and across health care are increasingly interdependent. Restructuring in health care often occurs across very short time frames. However, the actual implementation of change that accompanies restructuring is often frustratingly slow and unpredictable. Zimmerman and Dooley (2001) argued that improvements in the overall health-care system would be facilitated by the metaphor of the system as a living organism, rather than the system as a machine. Porter-O'Grady and Malloch (2011) proposed that to be effective in the 21st century, leaders must take the responsibility to see and to live "systemness." This means that leaders look for opportunities in their organizations to improve coordination, teamwork, shared learning, and shared responsibility.

Promoting Change

Senge (1990) observed that people do not resist change, but rather they resist being changed. This resistance occurs because when humans are asked to make major changes in their lives, everything is called into question—from their relationships with others to their work and status in the organization. Wheatley (2005) noted from her work with organizations that leaders who have led organizations through change often find that the most important changes made are personal.

Lewin developed a model that is still considered a classic for understanding organizational change (Schein, 1995). His model, known as *unfreeze—change—refreeze,* describes three stages in the change process. According to Lewin, the first step in changing behavior is to unfreeze the existing situation or status quo. The status quo is considered to be the equilibrium state. Unfreezing is necessary to overcome both individual and group resistance. To do this effectively, Lewin suggested that the driving and restraining forces that could negatively affect movement toward change need to be made clear. For example, many organizations in the health-care arena over the past 5 years have implemented electronic medical records. The introduction of electronic medical records required the unfreezing of behaviors of many health professionals and often evoked considerable resistance. Lewin's second stage in the change process is the change or movement itself. During this stage, building commitment is important. The third step in the change model is the refreezing of behavior to ensure that it is sustained. Applying this model to the example of the electronic medical record, staff would be given a target date for full implementation with no option to return to a paper record.

Although we live in a world where change is constant, it can be very difficult for nurse leaders to promote the type of system changes that are necessary. One frequently cited example is the relative lack of innovation that has occurred during the past 50 years with nursing care delivery models (Kimball, Joynt, Cherner, & O'Neil, 2007). Kotter, a professor at the Harvard Business School, is the most well-known contemporary thinker on change management. Kotter (1996) proposed the following eight-step process for introducing change:

1. *Create a sense of urgency:* For an individual or group to embrace the need for change, a sense of urgency must be created. This involves honest dialogue about what the threats could be if change is not implemented.

2. *Form a powerful coalition:* Managing change is not enough; you must also lead it. This involves obtaining a commitment from key people in the organization and building a change coalition.
3. *Create a vision for change:* People need a clear vision about what the goals of the change are. This involves creating a "vision" speech that is repeated often.
4. *Communicate the vision:* You will be watched closely for both verbal and nonverbal messages about the vision. Tie everything back to the vision and lead by example.
5. *Remove obstacles:* Barriers to change need to be removed. People need to be rewarded and recognized for making the change happen.
6. *Create short-term wins:* Nothing succeeds like success. Look for small target projects that create early wins in the change process.
7. *Build on the change:* Do not declare victory too early. Each success should provide an opportunity to build on what went well and look for areas of improvement.
8. *Anchor the changes in the organizational culture:* To make any change permanent, it must become part of the core culture. The story needs to be told, and the change needs to be embedded in policies, procedures, hiring processes, and reward programs.

Advancing Your Knowledge

J.S., DNP ARNP, is the practice manager of a large nurse-managed health center affiliated with a college of nursing at a prestigious state university. She recently met with the dean who informed her that the affiliation agreement with the college would be discontinued in 10 months. The university president is concerned about both liability issues and costs to the college during the economic downturn. J.S. is confident that the clinic will be successful as a freestanding clinic and is positioned to become a federally qualified health center. The staff members of the clinic are quite concerned about the change in identity for the clinic and the loss of their status as university employees.

1. Using Kotter's process for introducing change, how should J.S. create a sense of urgency with the staff to begin the formation of a new clinic identity?
2. What are some possible ideas for a vision for change?
3. What are obstacles that the clinic could encounter in the change process?
4. What early wins could be created?

Conclusion

This chapter has presented an overview of the key components of organizational and systems leadership for quality improvement and systems thinking. With advanced knowledge and education, DNP graduates are well positioned to function as leaders and pioneers in the health-care systems of the future. Leadership development is an ongoing process, and DNP graduates need to be lifelong learners. The health-care environment is a complex adaptive system that changes rapidly. With changes anticipated from ongoing health-care reform legislation, the business model for health care may look very different in the future. Consumers are likely to be much more involved in their own care, and their concerns about quality and safety are likely to increase. Projected health-care workforce shortages will require that leaders adopt a transformational leadership style and build healthy work environments. Innovation will be a necessity for system survival. Nurse leaders who view their organizations as complex adaptive systems will be the most successful in driving the changes needed as we move into the future.

See Table 5-4 for a list of Web resources.

Table 5-4

Web Resources

Agency for Health Care Research and Quality	*http://www.ahrq.gov*
American Association of Colleges of Nursing	*http://www.aacn.nche.edu/*
American Association of Critical-Care Nurses	*http://www.aacn.org/*
American Association of Nurses	*http://www.nursingworld.org/*
American Organization of Nurse Executives	*http://www.aone.org/*
American Nurses Credentialing Center	*http://www.nursecredentialing.org/*
Association for Professionals in Infection Control and Epidemiology	*http://www.apic.org*
Center for American Nurses	*http://centerforamericannurses.org/*
Center for Medicare and Medicaid	*http://www.cms.gov*
Hospital Compare Care	*http://www.hospitalcompare.hhs.gov/*
Institute for Healthcare Improvement	*http://www.ihi.org/*
National Association for Healthcare Quality	*http://www.nahq.org*
National Database of Nursing Indicators	*http://www.nursingquality.org/*
National Quality Forum	*http://www.qualityforum.org/*
Nursing Alliance Organization	*http://www.nursing-alliance.org/*
Patient Safety Institute	*http://www.ptsafety.org/*
Plexus Institute	*http://www.plexusinstitute.org/*
Quality and Safety Education for Nurses	*http://www.qsen.org*
Robert Wood Johnson Foundation	*http://www.rwjf.org/*
Shared Governance	*http://www.sharedgovernance.org/*
The Joint Commission	*http://www.jointcommission.org/*

References

Agency for Healthcare Research and Quality. (2011). Home Page. Retrieved from http://www.ahrq.gov/

Agency for Healthcare Research and Quality. (n.d.[a]). Patient safety network. Retrieved from http://psnet.ahrq.gov/glossary.aspx#

Agency for Health Care Research and Quality. (n.d.[b]). Talking quality. Retrieved from http://www.talkingquality.ahrq.gov/content/reportcard/search.aspx

Aiken, L. H. (2002). Superior outcomes of magnet hospitals: The evidence base. In M. McClure & A. Hinshaw (Eds.), *Magnet Hospitals revisited: Attraction and retention of professional nurses* (pp. 61–81). Washington, DC: American Nurses Publishing.

Aiken, L., Clarke, S., Sloane, D., Sochalski, J., Busse, R., Clarke, H., & Schamian, J. (2001). Nurses' reports on hospital care in five countries. *Health Affairs, 20*(3), 43–53.

Aiken, L., Clarke, S., Sloane, D., Sochalski, J., & Silber, J. (2002). Hospital nursing staff and patient mortality, nurse burnout and job dissatisfaction. *Journal of the American Medical Association, 288*(16), 1987–1993.

American Association of Colleges of Nursing (2002) AACN adopts a new vision for the future of nursing education and practice. Retrieved from http://www.aacn.nche.edu/news/articles/2004/dnp-release

American Association of Colleges of Nursing. (2006). The essentials of doctoral education for advanced nursing practice. Retrieved from http://www.aacn.nche.edu/DNP/pdf/Essentials.pdf

American Association of Critical-Care Nurses. (2005). *AACN standards for establishing and sustaining healthy work environments: A journey to excellence.* Aliso Viejo, CA: Author.

American Nurses Association. (2001). *Code of ethics with interpretive statements.* Washington, DC: Author.

American Nurses Credentialing Center. (2008). Magnet Recognition program. Retrieved from http://www.nursecredentialing.org/Magnet/ProgramOverview.aspx

American Organization of Nurse Executives. (2003). Healthy work environments: Striving for excellence. In McManis and Monsalave Associates Retrieved from http://www.mcmanis-monsalve.com/

American Organization of Nurse Executives. (2005). AONE nurse executive competencies. Retrieved from http://www.aone.org/resources/leadership%20tools/PDFs/AONE_NEC.pdf

American Organization of Nurse Executives. (2009). AONE advocacy and policy. Retrieved from http://www.aone.org/advocacy/index.shtml

American Organization of Nurse Executives. (2010). AONE guiding principles for future patient care delivery. Retrieved from http://www.aone.org/resources/leadership%20tools/guideprinciples.shtml

American Organization of Nurse Executives. (n.d.). 2010-2012 Strategic plan. Retrieved from http://www.aone.org/membership/about/pdfs/AONE_2012.2014.Graphic.FINAL.pdf

Aspden, P., Corrigan, J., & Wolcott, J. (2004). *Patient safety: Achieving a new standard for care.* Washington, DC: National Academies Press.

Avolio, B. J., & Gardner, W. L. (2005). Authentic leadership development: Getting to the root of positive forms of leadership. *Leadership Quarterly, 16,* 315–338.

Baker, N., Whittington, J. W., Resar, R. K., Griffin, F. A., Nolan, K. M. (2010). *Reducing costs through the appropriate use of specialty services*. IHI Innovation Series white paper. Cambridge, MA: Institute for Healthcare Improvement.

Bakker, A., Schaufeli, W., Leiter, M., & Taris, T. (2008). Work engagement: An emerging concept in occupational health psychology. *Work and Stress, 22*(3), 187–201.

Bass, B. M., & Bass, R. (2008). *The Bass handbook of leadership: Theory, research and management applications.* New York, NY: Free Press.

Bass, B. M., & Riggio, E. G. (2006). *Transformational leadership* (2nd ed.). Mahwah, NJ: Lawrence Erlbaum Associates.

Buerhaus, P., Staiger, D., & Auerbach, D. (2009). *The future of the nursing workforce in the United States: Data, trends, implications*. Boston, MA: Jones & Bartlett.

Burns, J. M. (1978). *Transforming leadership* New York, NY: Grove Press.

Center for American Nurses. (2008). The nursing workforce ecosystem: Creating healthier work environments. Retrieved from http://centerforamericannurses.org/displaycommon.cfm?an=1&subarticlenbr=144

Centers for Medicare and Medicaid Services. (2011). CMS Programs and information. Retrieved from http://www.cms.gov/

Christensen, C. (2009). *The innovator's prescription: A disruptive solution for health care.* New York, NY: McGraw-Hill.

Clancy, C. M., Farquhar, M. B., & Sharp, B. A. (2005). Patient safety in nursing practice. *Journal of Nursing Care and Quality, 20*(3), 193–197.

Council on Graduate Education in the Administration of Nursing. (2010). CGEAN definitions. Retrieved from http://www.cgean.org/cgean-documents.php

Cronenwett, L., Sherwood, G., Barnsteiner, J., Johnson, J., & Mitchell, P. (2007). Quality and safety education for nurses. *Nursing Outlook, 55*(3), 122–131.

Curran, C. R., & Totten, M. K. (2010). Expanding the role of nursing in healthcare governance. *Nursing Economics, 28*(5), 44–46.

Devers, K., & Berenson, R. (2009). Can accountable care organizations improve the value of health care by solving the cost and quality quandaries? Retrieved from http://www.urban.org/uploadedpdf/411975_acountable_care_orgs.pdf

Disch, J. (2002). Creating healthy work environments. *Creative Nursing, 8*(2), 3–4.

Douglas, K., & Kerfoot, K. (2008). Applying a systems thinking model for effective staffing. *Nurse Leader, 6*(5), 52–55.

Friedman, T. (2005). *The world is flat: A brief history of the twentieth-first century.* New York, NY: Farrar, Straus & Giroux.

Fritz, C., & Sonnentag, S. (2006). Recovery, well being and performance-related outcomes: The role of workload and vacation experiences. *Journal of Applied Psychology, 91,* 936–945.

George, B., Sims, P., & Gergen, D. (2010). *Truth north: Discover your authentic leadership.* San Francisco, CA: J Wiley & Sons.

Gorzeman, J. (2008). Balancing just culture with regulatory standards. *Nursing Administration Quarterly, 32*(4), 308–311.

Greiner, A., & Knebel, E. (Eds.). (2003). *Health professions education: A bridge to quality.* Committee on the Health Professions Education Summit of the Institute of Medicine. Washington, DC: The National Academies Press.

Hansen-Turton, T., & Ritter, A. (2008). Insurers' contracting policies on nurse practitioners as primary care providers. *Policy, Politics & Nursing Practice, 9*(4), 241–248.

Heath, J., Johanson, W., & Blake, N. (2004). Healthy work environments: A validation of the literature. *Journal of Nursing Administration, 34,* 524–530.

Infectious Diseases Society of America, Society for Healthcare Epidemiology of America, & Association for Professionals in Infection Control and Epidemiology in America. (2006). Comment on CMS Inpatient PPS Proposed Rule 1488P: Healthcare-associated infections. Retrieved from http://www.apic.org/AM/Template.cfm

Institute of Medicine. (1999). *To err is human: Building a safer health system.* Washington, CD: The National Academies Press.

Institute of Medicine. (2001).*Crossing the Quality Chasm: A New Health System for the 21st Century*. Washington, DC: The National Academies Press.

Institute of Medicine. (2004). *Keeping patients safe: Transforming the work environment of nurses*. Washington, DC: National Academy Press.

Institute of Medicine. (2006a). *Preventing medication errors.* Washington, DC: The National Academies Press: Washington, D.C.

Institute of Medicine. (2006b). *Rewarding provider performance: Aligning incentives in Medicare*. Washington, DC: The National Academies Press.

Institute of Medicine. (2010). The future of nursing: Leading change, advancing health. Retrieved from http://www.iom.edu/Reports/2010/The-Future-of-Nursing-Leading-Change-Advancing-Health.aspx

Kerfoot, K. M., & Ivy, S. (2004). Renewing the spirit: Sanctuaries for healing. *Reflections on Nursing Leadership, 30*(3), 20–23.

Kimball, B., Joynt, J., Cherner, D., & O'Neil, E. (2007). The quest for new innovative care delivery models. *Journal of Nursing Administration,* 37(9), 392–398.

Koloroutis, M. (2004). *Relationship based care: A model for transforming practice.* Minneapolis, MN: Creative HealthCare Management.

Kotter, J. (1996). *Leading change*. Boston, MA: Harvard Business School Press.

Kouzes, J. M., & Posner, B. Z. (2010). *The truth about leadership.* San Francisco, CA: Jossey-Bass.

Kramer, M., & Schmalaberg, C. E. (2003). Magnet hospitals describe control over nursing practice. *Western Journal of Nursing Research, 25*(4), 434–452.

Kuhnel, J., Sonnetag, S., & Westman, M. (2009). Does work engagement increase after a short respite? The role of job involvement as double edged sword. *Journal of Occupational and Organizational Psychology, 82,* 575–594.

Kupperschmidt, B. (2006a). Carefronting: Caring enough to confront. A reprint. *The Oklahoma Nurse, 51*(2), 22–23.

Kupperschmidt, B. (2006b). Addressing multigenerational conflict: Mutual respect and carefronting as a strategy. Retrieved from http://www.nursingworld.org/MainMenuCategories/ANAMarketplace/ANAPeriodicals/OJIN/TableofContents/Volume112006/No2May06/tpc30_316075.html

Leape, L. L. (1994). Errors in medicine. *Journal of American Medical Association, 272,* 1851–1867.

Leape, L. L., Bates, D., Cullen, D., & Gallivan, T. (1995). Systems analysis of adverse drug reactions. *Journal of the American Medical Association, 274*(1), 35–43.

Loehr, J., & Schwartz, T. (2003). *The power of full engagement*. New York, NY: Simon & Schuster.

Mackey, T., & McNeil, N. (2002). Quality indicators for academic nursing primary care centers. *Nursing Economics, 20*(2), 62–65.

Manion, J. (2009). *The engaged workforce: Proven strategies to build a positive healthcare workforce*. Chicago, IL: Health Forum.

Manojlovich, M., & Laschingrer, H. (2002). The relationship of empowerment and selected personality characteristics to nursing job satisfaction. *Journal of Nursing Administration, 32*(11), 586–595.

Maslach, C., & Leiter, M. (2008). Early predicators of job burnout and engagement. *Journal of Applied Psychology, 93*, 498–512.

Maslow, A. (1954). *Motivation and personality*. New York, NY: Harper and Row.

Maxfield, D., Grenny, J., McMillan, R., Patterson, K., & Switzler, A. (2005). Silence kills: The seven crucial conversations in healthcare. Retrieved from http://www.aacn.org/WD/Practice/Docs/PublicPolicy/SilenceKillsExecSum.pdf

McClure, M., Poulin, M., Sovie, M., & Wandelt, M. (1983). *Magnet hospitals: Attraction and retention of professional nurses. American Academy of Nursing Task Force on Nursing Practice in Hospitals*. Kansas, MO: American Nurses Association.

Montgomery, K. L., & Porter-O'Grady, T. (2010). Innovation and learning: Creating the DNP nurse leader. *Nurse Leader, 8*(4), 44–47.

National Quality Forum. (2009). National voluntary consensus standards for patient safety. Retrieved from http://www.qualityforum.org/projects/patient_safety_measures.aspx

National Quality Forum. (2010a). Standardizing a patient safety taxonomy. Retrieved from http://www.qualityforum.org/Search.aspx?keyword=standardizing+a+patient+safety+taxonomy

National Quality Forum. (2010b). Safe practices for better health care. Retrieved from http://www.qualityforum.org/News_And_Resources/Press_Kits/Safe_Practices_for_Better_Healthcare.aspx

Nursing Organizations Alliance. (n.d.). Retrieved from http://www.nursing-alliance.org/index.cfm

Porter-O'Grady, T., & Malloch, K. (2011). *Quantum leadership: Advancing innovation and transforming healthcare* (3rd ed.). Sudbury, MA: Jones & Bartlett.

Porter-O'Grady, T., & Malloch, K. (2010). *Innovation leadership*. Sudbury, MA: Jones & Bartlett.

Robert Wood Johnson Foundation. (2008). Transforming care at the bedside. Retrieved from http://www.rwjf.org/qualityequality/product.jsp?id=30051

Robert Wood Johnson Foundation. (2010). Health policy brief on accountable care organizations. *Health Affairs Web Exclusive*. Retrieved from http://www.healthaffairs.org/healthpolicybriefs/brief.php?brief_id=23

Rogers, E. (1995). *Diffusion of innovation*. New York, NY: Free Press.

Schaufeli, W. B., Salanova, M., Gonzalez-Roma, V., & Bakker, A. B. (2002). The measurement of engagement and burnout; a confirmative analytic approach. *Journal of Happiness Studies, 3*, 71–92.

Schaufeli, W., & Bakker, A. (2003). Utrecht work engagement scale: Preliminary manual. http://www.schaufeli.com/downloads/tests/Test%20manual%20UWES.pdf

Schein, E. (1995). Kurt Lewin's change theory in the field and in the classroom: Notes toward a model of managed learning. *Systems Practice*. Retrieved from http://www.solonline.org/res/wp/10006.html

Senge, P. (1990). *The fifth discipline.* New York, NY: Doubleday.

Sherman, R., & Pross, E. (2010). Growing our future nurse leaders to build and sustain healthy work environments at the unit level. *Online Journal of Issues in Nursing, 15*(1), 1.

Shirey, M. (2006). Authentic leaders creating healthy work environments for nursing practice. *American Journal of Critical Care, 15*(3), 256–267.

Shojania, K. G., Duncan, B. W., & McDonald, K. M. (Eds.). (2001). *Making health care safer: A critical analysis of patient safety practices. Evidence Report Technology Assessment Number 43*. San Francisco, CA: University of California at San Francisco Press.

Simpson, M. (2009). Predicators of work engagement among medical-surgical registered nurses. *Western Journal of Nursing Research, 31*, 144–165.

Sisko, A., Truffer, C., Smith, S., Keehan, S., Cylus, J., Poisai, J. A., Clemens, M. K., & Lizonitz, J. (2009). Health spending projections through 2018: Recession effects add uncertainty to the outlook. *Health Affairs, 28*(2), w346–357.

Stanhope, M., & Lancaster, J. (2004).*Community and public health nursing*. St. Louis, MO: Mosby.

Tapscott, D., & Williams, A. D. (2010). *Macrowikinomics: Rebooting business and the world.* New York, NY: Portfolio Hardcover.

Unruh, L. (2005). Employment conditions at the bedside: A cause of and a solution to the RN shortage. *Journal of Nursing Administration, 35*(1), 11–14.

Weberg, D. (2010). Transformational leadership and staff retention: An evidence-based review with implications for healthcare systems. *Nursing Administration Quarterly, 34*(4), 246–258.

Wheatley, M. (1992). *Leadership and the science.* San Francisco, CA: Barrett-Koehler.

Wheatley, M. (2005). *Finding our way: Leadership for an uncertain time.* San Francisco, CA: Barrett-Koehler.

Whitehead, D. (2006). Workplace health promotion: the role and responsibility of healthcare managers. *Journal of Nursing Management, 14*(4), 59–68.

Wolf, G., Triolo, P., & Ponte, P. R. (2008). Magnet recognition program: The next generation. *Journal of Nursing Administration, 38*(4), 200–204.

Savigny, D., & Tagheed, A. (2009). Systems thinking for health systems strengthening. Washington, DC: Alliance for Health Policy and Systems Research.

Zimmerman, B., & Dooley, K. (2001). Mergers versus emergers: Rethinking structural change in health care systems. *Emergence 3*(4), 65–82.

Zimmerman, B., Lindberg, C., & Plsek, P. (1998). *Edgeware: Insights from complexity science for healthcare leaders.* Irving, TX: VHA Publishing.

CHAPTER 6

INFLUENCING HEALTH-CARE PRACTICE AND POLICY THROUGH ADVOCACY

Objectives:

By the end of the chapter, students should be able to:

1. Define and discuss major issues in U.S. health policy and how these issues affect Americans and advanced practice nurses.
2. Discuss the policy process within the United States, including how policy becomes law, communicating with legislators regarding health policy, monitoring legislation, developing relationships with legislators, and nursing involvement in the political process.
3. Describe the role of nursing groups such as the American Nurses Association (ANA) and others involved in health-care policy in the United States.
4. Discuss the history of health-care reform, and appraise how the history of health-care delivery in the United States affects health-care policy today.
5. Discuss the history of payment for health-care services in the United States and how that history affects current health-care payment policy.
6. Discuss the voice of nursing in reshaping health-care policy in the United States, in particular with respect to primary care.
7. Support the use of health promotion as a key public policy issue for the advanced practice nurse.

This chapter discusses health-care policy in the United States and the importance of involvement of advanced practice nurses with a doctor of nursing practice (DNP) degree in educating the public about health-care issues and in influencing health-care policy. The chapter provides information about the history of health policy and the current state of health care in the United States. Health policy issues affect all people in society and include health disparities, cultural sensitivity, ethics, the internationalization of health-care concerns, access to care, quality of care, health-care financing, and issues of equity and social justice in the delivery of health care. The Institute of Medicine (2001) stated that all nurses should be knowledgeable in the areas of health-care design and implementation policies, health-care finance, practice regulation, access, safety, quality, and efficacy.

DNPs bear more responsibility than simply knowing about health policy. The American Association of Colleges of Nursing (2006) essentials for DNP education list understanding of health policy and governmental actions as an important aspect of DNP education. DNP knowledge in the area of health policy includes, but is not limited to, the following:

- Understanding the decision-making process and how the legislative process can either advance the progress of health-care legislation or slow down the development of health policy
- Assessing and accessing health-care legislation to apply it and educate the public by presenting both positive and negative aspects
- Being informed to speak to legislators to gain support for or against a proposed piece of health-care legislation

Because health policy affects every aspect of the health and well-being of patients, the DNP-prepared nurse should be engaged in the process of policy development, implementation, and public education. Through political activism and leadership, the DNP can assist in the development of health policies at the federal, state, and local levels to meet the needs of individuals, communities, and the nation. Table 6-1 lists the essential competencies in DNP education as outlined by the American Association of Colleges of Nursing.

Table 6-1

Essential Competencies in Doctor of Nursing Practice Education

DNP students should be able to:

1. Analyze critically health policy proposals, health policies, and related issues from the perspective of consumers, nurses, other health professionals, and other stakeholders in policy and public forums.
2. Demonstrate leadership in the development and implementation of institutional, local, state, federal, or international health policy.
3. Influence policy makers through active participation on committees, boards, or task forces at the institutional, local, state, regional, national, or international levels to improve health-care delivery and outcomes.
4. Educate others, including policy makers at all levels, regarding nursing, health policy, and patient care outcomes.
5. Advocate for the nursing profession within the policy-making and health-care communities.
6. Develop, evaluate, and provide leadership for health-care policy that shapes health-care financing, regulation, and delivery.
7. Advocate for social justice, equity, and ethical policies within all health care arenas.

Source: American Association of Colleges of Nursing. (2006). The essentials of doctoral education for advanced nursing practice. Retrieved from http://www.aacn.nche.edu/dnp/pdf/essentials.pdf

American Health Policy Defined

For the last several decades, leaders from both political parties, health-care leaders, business leaders, and social activists have acknowledged that the U.S. health-care system is broken (Berry & Miralito, 2010; Davidson, 2010; Garson, 2010; Herzlinger, 2010). Fixing the broken system is not simple because of the diverse interests among recipients, payers, and providers of health care. Not all groups believe that change in the health-care system is in their best interests, and some groups have more power than others. Insurance companies are opposed to a national health insurance plan that would reduce the numbers of customers they can attract; the pharmaceutical companies do not want any interference in their ability to sell high-end medications by institution of formulations of drugs that might reduce competition and decrease cost.

Health care in the United States has been called a "paradox of excess and deprivation" (Enthoven & Kronick, 1998). Although we have the best technology in the world and can create "miracles" for individuals who can afford it, many Americans are without basic access to health care of any sort. One study noted that 87.6 million Americans do not have health insurance or access to health care, and people who have coverage are paying an increasing amount and receiving fewer benefits each year (Pifer-Bixler, 2009). In the midst of this insurance coverage crisis, the United States pays the highest rate for health care per capita in the world and has a slightly lower life expectancy and higher infant mortality than almost all other industrialized countries around the world (Noah, 2007).

Health care is a finite resource, so society must decide how and where to spend limited health care dollars (Mathews, 2006). At some point, either Americans will have to impose governmental rationing of care, or individuals will have to pay more of the cost of their own care (Kling, 2010). As expensive technologies and therapies continue to develop, access to these treatments and payment for expensive therapies will continue to be at the center of the American health-care policy debate. Let's begin by setting the scene in American health policy and looking at the major foundational issues being encountered today.

Financing Health Care

Although much has changed in our scientific understanding of health and disease, not much has changed in health-care delivery and access to health-care benefits from the early 1900s to today. The hospital is still the primary place where most health-care diagnosis and treatment take place. The following revealing factors about the cost and effectiveness of the U.S. health-care system come from the Kaiser Family Foundation (Kaiser, 2009):

- Health care costs more per person in the United States than in any other nation in the world.
- The World Health Organization (WHO) ranked the U.S. health care system as number 1 in cost, 37 in overall performance, and 72 in ability to meet the health-care needs of the population. These rankings compared 191 WHO member nations on standard health indicators.

- Current spending on health care in the United States is 15.2% of the gross domestic product.
- Spending on health care is estimated to reach 20% of the gross domestic product by 2017, which is not sustainable economically. In comparison, health-care spending accounted for 10.9% of the gross domestic product in Switzerland, 10.7% in Germany, 9.7% in Canada, and 9.5% in France, according to the Organization for Economic Cooperation and Development.
- In 2007, the United States spent $2.26 trillion on health care, or $73,439 per person, private and public sources combined.
- In 2009, 16.7% of U.S. citizens did *not* have health insurance—this translates to 50.7 million people.
- In 2007, $69 billion of uncompensated care was delivered in the United States to uninsured persons.
- The Institute of Medicine estimated that 18,000 lives are lost annually as a consequence of gaps in coverage and calculated the annual cost of achieving full coverage at $34 billion to $69 billion, which is less than the loss in economic productivity from existing coverage ($65 billion to $130 billion annually).
- Every 30 seconds in the United States, someone files for bankruptcy in the aftermath of a serious health problem. About 1.5 million families lose their homes to foreclosure every year because of unaffordable medical costs. Many of these families have medical insurance that does not meet the needs of an ever more costly system.
- The United States spends more on health care than other industrialized nations who provide health insurance to all their citizens, such as the Netherlands, France, Italy, and Israel.
- Retiring elderly couples need $250,000 in savings when they retire just to pay for the most basic medical coverage. Many experts believe that this figure is conservative, and that $300,000 may be a more realistic number.
- The United States spends six times more per capita on the administration of the health-care system than its peer Western European nations (Centers for Disease Control and Prevention, 2009).

What does this enormous outlay of funds in the United States buy? Why does health care in the United States cost so much more on a per capita basis than in other countries? The answer to these and other finance questions are very important. They help to provide an understanding of exactly why health-care reform is needed.

Advancing Your Knowledge

Harold and Sue started their own home cleaning service business 6 months ago. They employ themselves and three others, and the business is expanding. They project adding two other workers in the near future. This business gives jobs to individuals who need them and helps working people to keep clean houses. One weekend, Harold feels pain in his abdomen that eventually settles in his lower right quadrant. He and Sue did not purchase health insurance when opening the business because the cost was prohibitive. Harold decides to go to a walk-in clinic to save money and is told that he has appendicitis and needs surgery to remove his appendix before it bursts. He goes to a surgeon who sends him for the surgery that same day. He is in the hospital less than 24 hours and is discharged home. His postoperative course is uneventful. He receives a bill from the hospital for $15,000, another from the surgeon for $8000, and another from the anesthesiologist for $1500. Harold is sure these bills cannot be correct because his neighbor and friend had the same surgery a year ago and said his insurance company paid only $1200 for hospital fees, $800 to the surgeon, and $350 to the anesthesiologist. He calls the hospital to discuss the bill and is told that the hospital has agreements with insurance companies to provide reduced prices for services, but these same agreements do not apply to people without insurance. Eventually, because of this hospital bill, Harold and Sue close their cleaning service, lay off all the workers, and have to find jobs.

1. What are the issues related to policy in this scenario?
2. How is American small business affected by the cost of health-care insurance?
3. Imagine that you decide to open your own independent practice. How would you handle health insurance for yourself and your workers?
4. Discuss the statement, "The United States has the best health care in the world," which has been uttered by many legislators. Is it true? Is it partially true? Analyze the level of health care in the United States in total.

Advancing Your Knowledge

Thomas and Marianne Lehner are covered by Medicare. They currently are unable to afford supplemental (gap) insurance for other health-related expenses. Thomas has diabetes, hypertension, and hyperlipidemia. Marianne has depression, hyperlipidemia, and irritable bowel syndrome. The monthly cost of medications for the pair is $300 more than what is covered by Medicare Part D. When Marianne goes for a mammogram, she is told that Medicare will pay $50 of the $175 cost for the test, so she decides not to have the mammogram. Some months when money is short, both Tom and Marianne do without medications or take their medications every other day to stretch the funds for these drugs.

1. What is the issue here?
2. What could be the hidden cost for not taking appropriate medications or following the guidelines for disease prevention?
3. What, if anything, could be done to make things better?

In 2008, 31% of health-care dollars in the United States was spent on hospital services, 21% on physician services, 10% on medication and drugs, 6% on nursing home care, 7% on administrative costs, and 4% on dental and home care services (Kaiser Health Care Report, 2009). Hospital care is the most expensive care in the system. One of the reasons for the high cost of hospital care is the amount of uncompensated care hospitals must absorb. People who come to hospital emergency departments or who need immediate care legally and ethically cannot be turned away by hospitals because of an inability to pay. They must be stabilized and plans for continued care must be established before the hospital can discharge the patient. This situation leads to high levels of "uncompensated" care incurred by hospitals, which they must balance with payments from people with insurance or who can pay.

Advancing Your Knowledge

Cory is a 60-year-old man who has been out of work for more than a year. He no longer has health insurance, and he is low on funds for living expenses. He wakes up one morning with stomach pain and nausea. He has several episodes of bloody diarrhea. He does not know what to do, but his neighbor tells him he should go to the emergency department. He does, and the work-up there shows diverticulitis. He is given a prescription for an antibiotic and several shots and sent home. The discharge instructions tell him to see his primary care provider on Monday. He cannot afford to see his physician, and he knows that he will be unable to pay the emergency department bill. He lives in a rented apartment and has a 10-year-old car. He has another episode of bloody diarrhea and stomach pain 2 months later and goes to the emergency department again. The diagnosis is the same, and he gets another prescription for an antibiotic. He feels as though this is a revolving door for him and that he is really not getting better. Cory worries that he will have some serious complications from this frequent diverticulitis without getting consistent care. He feels badly that the hospital is not getting paid for services it provides to him.

1. What could be done to make this situation better in the immediate future?
2. How can this situation be improved over the long-term for Cory and others in the same situation?
3. What will happen to Cory if he continues in this pattern and is unable to find a job or get health insurance until he is 65 and can receive Medicare?

Sometimes care provided in hospitals is not the best level of care for the problem at hand. One example is health-care dollars spent on end-of-life care; more expensive care is not always better care (Kaufman, 2006). Patients who spent their last days in hospice programs rather than in hospitals had lower end-of-life costs than patients not in hospice programs. Patients receiving hospice care or dying at home had a higher level of family satisfaction. Families indicated that the hospice care received was excellent and met the physical, spiritual, and emotional needs of the patient and the family. Nevertheless, 67% of patients in the United States under the care of a physician for a life-threatening disease die in the hospital, and only 33% die at home assisted by hospice programs. In some situations, less dramatic (and less expensive) interventions may lead to better care. Unrealistic family expectations and physician and hospital reimbursement methods all create an incentive to admit dying patients to the hospital.

Advancing Your Knowledge

Lisa and Nancy are neighbors. Both of their mothers died within the past 2 months. They are discussing the experience of being with their mothers through this process. Lisa's mother was 84 and had cancer of the bladder. She was receiving chemotherapy and radiation when she fractured her femur. She was rushed to the hospital where they did surgery to put a rod in the femur to stabilize it and found that the cancer from her bladder had progressed to the bone. She was in a lot of pain, and it was difficult for the hospital nurses to keep Lisa's mother pain-free. Lisa came to the hospital as much as she could, but her work schedule meant that she could not be there all the time. On the third hospitalized day, Lisa's mother had a stroke, was comatose, and required ventilator assistance to breathe. Lisa was very concerned about her mother being in pain and not being able to let anyone know. Her mother died 3 weeks later on a ventilator without being able to speak while Lisa was at work. Lisa now must handle her mother's death and hospital and doctor bills that require most of her mother's money. The idea that her mother died in pain and afraid continues to haunt Lisa, even after several months.

Nancy's mother was 88, had end-stage chronic obstructive pulmonary disease, and was on supplemental oxygen. They decided to ask the primary care physician for a hospice referral. The hospice nurse came to the home and evaluated the needs of Nancy's mother. Hospice brought in supplies, including oxygen and a home health aide. A physician, a social worker, nurses, and a minister all came to the home. Nancy's mother did well with this assistance for 8 months. At the end of that time, she also had a stroke. She was unable to get out of bed on her own. Hospice sent in home health aides and nurses around the clock. Nancy was able to be with her mother as much as possible around her work schedule. Other friends from the neighborhood and from the church came to visit Nancy's mother at her home. Nancy's mother developed pneumonia 1 month after the stroke. She became very short of breath. To ease her anxiety, she received small doses of lorazepam (Ativan) and pain medications when needed. Nancy's mother died at home in her own bed, comfortable and peaceful with friends and family around her. Medicare covered all of the hospice services. Nancy asked that

Continued on page 250

Advancing Your Knowledge *Continued from page 249*

in lieu of flowers for her mother's funeral that friends and family send donations to hospice.

1. Evaluate these two stories and determine what you would do in each of these situations to make things better for the patient and family.
2. How could nurses educated as DNPs work to create public understanding of death and dying? In what policy areas could advanced practice nurses make a difference for patients and families in these situations?

Another cause of waste and overspending in the current health-care system is the need for defensive medical practice. According to a Gallup poll, one in four dollars spent on health care in the United States pays for unnecessary tests and treatments that physicians order to keep from being sued (Ledue, 2010). The poll of surveyed physicians nationwide found that 73% practiced some form of defensive medicine in the past 12 months to protect themselves from frivolous lawsuits. Gallup conducted the 6-week survey across all specialties of physicians. They reported that 26% of overall health-care costs could be attributed to the practice of defensive medicine.

Personal liability insurance or malpractice insurance payments have driven many high-quality physicians out of the practice of medicine. Other physicians have adapted to these issues by "going bare," or not buying malpractice insurance. Nurse practitioners are required in many states to obtain malpractice insurance to be licensed. Experts in health-care reform consider tort reform to be essential to effective health-care reform and control of escalating health-care costs. Potential types of tort reform could include placing caps on the type and amount of damages allowed, limiting the need for defensive medical services by reducing the effect of paid expert witnesses, and eliminating frivolous lawsuits through mediation and arbitration.

The Congressional Budget Office (CBO) estimated cost savings associated with tort reform as follows: total national health-care spending could decrease by about 0.5%, or $11 billion (Simmons, 2009). The CBO asserts that tort reform could affect costs for health care both directly (by 0.2%) by reducing premiums for medical liability insurance and indirectly (by 0.3%) by reducing the use of diagnostic tests and other health-care services when providers recommend those services specifically to reduce their potential exposure to lawsuits. Enactment of a tort reform package also could reduce mandatory spending for Medicare, Medicaid, the Children's Health Insurance Program, and the Federal Employees Health Benefits program by an estimated $41 billion between 2010 and 2020.

Advancing Your Knowledge

S.T. is a nurse practitioner working in a primary care practice with two other nurse practitioners and two physicians. At a meeting of the health-care providers, S.T. asks whether the idea of a sliding scale for people without insurance might be used to increase access to care for people who are unable to afford or obtain health insurance. Although the other health-care providers in the practice are interested in the idea, there are many problems that such a practice would present. The most pressing issue would be the cost of testing, treatments, and referrals. A patient must be treated for any presenting problem with the "community standard" of care. For example, if a patient comes to the office with diabetes but cannot afford to see a cardiologist when his electrocardiogram is slightly irregular, the practice could be held responsible legally if the referral is not arranged and completed by the patient. If a patient has no insurance or is unable to afford all of the tests, procedures, and referrals warranted by community standards, the practice is putting itself in jeopardy by taking this patient. Even if the patient signs a statement saying that he or she does not want a test or procedure, such a statement does not protect the practice from legal issues later.

1. How do the millions of Americans without access to health care get help for chronic problems?
2. Is some care better than no care, or should everyone receive the "community standard" of care or nothing?
3. How would you propose tort reform to decrease costs in health care, while holding health practitioners to appropriate standards of law?

Prevention Versus Cure in Health-Care Policy

Some experts are of the belief that health care in the United States has focused on illness care rather than on health promotion and disease prevention. This focus has contributed to the increasingly expensive system in the United States (Lee, 2009). Medicare and Medicaid and many private insurers heavily weight payment toward cure and away from less expensive prevention. Prevention is described as a personal issue rather than one that is the responsibility of the health-care provider (Van Leuven, 2006). Still, promoting health and preventing diseases not only improves the health of the population, but it also lowers the cost of health care overall (Lee, 2009).

Health Policy and the Aging Population

The aging U.S. population poses another challenge to health financing because of the chronic, debilitating, and expensive diseases that accompany aging. Currently, individuals older than 65 represent 12% of the U.S. population, but it is projected that by 2040, 40% of the population will be older than 65 (Kaufman, 2006). This increase in the number of older adults in the United States means increasing incidences of diabetes, heart disease, stroke, dementia, and joint problems. All of these chronic diseases require careful monitoring and provision of care and put major stressors on the health-care system.

Medicare and Health Policy

Medicare, which covers all individuals older than 65 and younger persons with disabilities, is the largest insurance program in the United States, paying out more than $500 billion annually (Kaiser Foundation, 2010). The CBO estimated that if health costs continue to increase at a pace consistent with past trends, Medicare alone will constitute 17% of the U.S. gross domestic product by 2082 (Congressional Budget Office, 2010). In other words, 17% of what is "produced" in the United States will be health care, which represents a nearly sixfold increase from 2006 (Medicare.gov, 2010).

Although the idea of a national health insurance plan such as Medicare to help senior citizens is very popular, the Department of Justice found that billions of dollars are spent on fraudulent claims (Siskel, 2010). The Department of Justice is sponsoring the HEAT initiative to recognize and prosecute fraudulent Medicare claims. An important aspect of this initiative is to educate the public regarding the need to identify and report suspicious Medicare billing practices.

Many other policy issues plague the U.S. health-care system, including increasing out-of-pocket expenses, lack of physical access to health care, overuse of emergency departments, uncoordinated medical records, and a declining number of primary care providers (Berry & Miralito, 2010). U.S. health care overall has problems with efficiency, effectiveness, and equity (Blankenhorn, 2010). All of these issues are influenced by and rely on health policy and legislation.

Critical Thinking Questions

1. What do you think are the biggest health policy issues facing the United States today, and why are they more critical than the other issues that exist?
2. Who should decide how health-care dollars are spent, and how should they decide this?
3. What could nurses, especially DNP-prepared advanced practice nurses, do to educate Americans about health-care policy? How can DNP-prepared advanced practice nurses present issues fairly and overcome all of the misconceptions people have about health-care policy?
4. How could wasteful spending in Medicare be reduced? Give examples of some of the difficult choices to be made when it comes to determining what to fund.
5. We know that 85% of Medicare dollars are spent on expensive treatments and care near the end of an elderly adult's life (Fisher, 2008). What changes could be made to continue to meet the needs of individuals who are at the end of life and reduce spending on treatments that may not prolong life? What better options might the DNP propose to policy makers?

Policy Process

Before delving deeper into the substance of health-care policy, it is important to understand the policy-making and policy-changing processes. The health policy process is subject to a complex array of considerations and influences. Scientists believe that in an ideal world, health policy would be formulated in a rational, linear process, moving from data collection, to interpretation, to scientific consensus. Translating science to policy is far messier and convoluted because it involves societal priorities, resource allocation, changing cultural values, special interests, politics, and other competing motivations that may or may not serve the public good. In other words, health policies are affected by and have an effect on a host of issues outside of simple science.

Public policy is an attempt by the government to address a public issue. The government, whether at the city, state, or federal level, develops public policy through laws, regulations, decisions, and actions. There are four parts to public policy making: problems, players, stakeholders, and the policy. The *problem* is the issue that needs to be addressed. The *player* is the individual or group that is influential in forming a plan to address the problem in question. Players may have agendas that are not in the best interests of the public but further their own best interests instead. *Stakeholders* are individuals who are directly affected by the policy developed. *Policy* is the finalized course of action decided on by the government. In most cases, policies are open to interpretation by nongovernmental players, including people in the private sector. When the federal government creates a policy that is unfunded and requires states to meet requirements that cost the state money, the state often interprets the policy differently than the federal government intended. For example, the Patient Protection and Affordability Act of 2010 requires states to spend more dollars in the area of Medicare and provide services to an expanded number of persons. How this requirement is met is up to each state, and the interpretation of the law or policy also is in the hands of the state.

Who decides how medical care is distributed among society? Does social justice play a role in the decision, or do individuals who have adequate resources receive adequate care, while the poor receive less than adequate care? Nurses who become actively involved in the health-care policy debate can play a role in the decisions about health-care cost containment and distribution.

How Does Federal Policy Become Law?

Policy becomes law through the legislative process. Five steps are required for a proposed bill to become a law. Table 6-2 provides an overview of this process.

The legislative process begins before Congress drafts a bill and ends after legislation is signed. Other governmental institutions are involved, including various executive branch agencies, such as the Environmental Protection Agency (EPA). Within Congress, there are many different committees. These committees are charged with promulgating specific types of legislation. Certain committees are more relevant to health-care policy making. See Table 6-3 for a list of committees that involve themselves with health policy.

Once a bill is passed by both houses of Congress and signed by the president, it goes to an executive agency where another part of the process begins. The agency creates a way to implement the law, often by writing rules and regulations. Rule writing is based on implementation guidelines established in the Administrative Procedures Act, which includes holding public hearings for citizen

Table 6-2

How a Bill Becomes a Law

Step	Process
1. Draft of proposed law	The draft is called a bill, is sponsored by a member of Congress, and is recommended for consideration. Each bill is assigned to a standing or permanent committee for consideration.
2. Standing committee	The bill goes to a subcommittee to study and modify. The bill is debated and edited line by line and sometimes word by word.
3. Back to full House or Senate	There is more debate and a vote on the bill. The bill is then sent to the other legislative house for its debate and approval. Often changes are made to reconcile the bill for both the House and the Senate.
4. Sent to President for signature	If approved by both the House and the Senate, the bill is sent to the President for signature. If the President does not sign the bill (a presidential veto), it goes back to the House and Senate.
5. Supermajority vote	If after a veto, a supermajority (two-thirds of all members) of the House and Senate votes for the bill, Congress successfully overrides the President's veto.

Table 6-3

Key Congressional Committees in the Senate and House That Speak to Nursing and Health Care Issues

Senate	House of Representatives
Appropriations Committee: Committee that controls the federal purse strings and determines federal funding for all government functions, from defense to biomedical research	Appropriations Committee: Committee that controls the federal purse strings and determines federal funding for all government functions, from defense to biomedical research
Labor, Health and Human Services-Education (LHHS) Appropriations Subcommittee: Specialized subcommittee that determines federal funding for federal agencies, including HHS, NIH, CDC, and HRSA, and administers the nursing workforce development programs	Labor, Health and Human Services-Education (LHHS) Appropriations Subcommittee: Specialized subcommittee that determines federal funding for federal agencies, including the HHS, NIH, CDC, and HRSA, and administers the nursing workforce development programs
Health, Education, Labor and Pensions: Authorizing committee with jurisdiction over all non-Medicare and non-Medicaid health-care policy issues	Energy and Commerce Committee and Health Subcommittee: Authorizing committee with policy jurisdiction over the Medicaid program, Part B of the Medicare program, and all non-Medicare and non-Medicaid health-care issues

Continued from page 254 Table 6-3

Key Congressional Committees in the Senate and House That Speak to Nursing and Health Care Issues

Senate	House of Representatives
Finance Committee and Health Subcommittee: Authorizing committee with policy jurisdiction over Medicare and Medicaid	Ways and Means Committee and Health Subcommittee: Authorizing committee with policy jurisdiction over Medicare Part A (shares jurisdiction over certain parts of Medicare with the House Energy and Commerce Committee).

feedback. The legislative process ends here with an implemented and enforceable law and accompanying regulations.

State laws follow similar processes. However, state law can be superseded by federal law. For example, a state can set its own different minimum wage law only as long as that minimum wage is higher than the federally mandated level. Although states may pass laws allowing marijuana to be used for medical purposes, the federal government says that all use and sale of marijuana is illegal. Federal officials can prosecute persons who are using and selling medical marijuana despite any state law allowing it.

Outside government, additional parties, such as the media, grassroots groups, organizations, political action committees, lobbyists, and other interested groups and individuals are also involved in lawmaking. These external, unofficial players help to mediate the political dialogue about what government should do.

Influence of Lobbyists

Lobbyists are hired by groups to represent issues important to that group. They spend time with legislators to explain the goals of the organizations that they represent and press for favorable legislation regarding those goals. In 2009, there were more than 17,000 federal lobbyists based in Washington, DC (Reuters Press, 2009). Lobbying activities are also performed at the state level, and lobbyists try to influence legislation in the state legislatures in each of the 50 states. In many states, the state medical association, a local arm of the American Medical Association, sends a physician to each day of the legislative session. They call this program "Doctor of the Day" and say that this person is there to attend to any health needs of legislators. The real purpose of the Doctor of the Day is to spend time discussing health-care issues with legislators and promoting the agenda of the medical association. At the local municipal level, some lobbying activities occur with city councils and county commissions, especially in large cities and more populous counties.

Not only do lobbyists share their constituents' opinions and provide information to lawmakers, but they also use money supplied by their employers to influence lawmakers. There are laws that require lobbyists to be registered and that restrict or prohibit the use of lobbyist funds for the purpose of persuading legislators, but these laws can be difficult to enforce because there is no "watch-dog" agency monitoring lobbyist activity.

There are many powerful lobbies for health-care legislation at the federal and state government levels, including those hired by pharmaceutical companies, insurance companies, the American Medical Association, the American Nurses Association, and the American Association of Retired Persons (AARP). All of these groups persuade legislators to enact and support legislation that benefits them. If an issue and opinion on it are compelling enough, one or more legislators will introduce a bill in one of the houses of the legislature, and lawmaking begins. Coalitions are formed among these groups to achieve sufficient leverage and votes for passage of legislation that serves their joint purposes.

Personal Interaction With Legislators

Members of Congress, state representatives, and local commissioners or other political figures pay attention to mail from constituents because each citizen's vote counts. Drafting a concise, well-thought-out personal letter is one of the most effective ways Americans have of influencing lawmakers. However, members of Congress get hundreds of letters and e-mails every day. Following are some tips that can help a letter have greater impact. It is usually best to send letters to the representatives from your local congressional district or to the senators from your state.

- Be clear and to the point
- Be considerate and polite; show respect for the legislator
- Address a single issue in each communication
- Use your credentials so that the legislator understands your area of expertise
- Thank the legislator for his or her history of supporting a policy agenda
- Provide personal contact information
- Keep communication limited to one page (three paragraphs) with a (1) bold statement of your reason for writing, (2) specific information about the topic, and (3) request for desired action by the legislator.

E-mail is an effective way to connect with a legislator and provide information for the legislator regarding health-care issues. E-mail is a good approach because it provides immediate correspondence in most cases and flexibility for the staff as to when they read and reply. Using e-mail attachments is an efficient way to send important documentation to support a position on health-care policy. E-mail is so easy to use, however, that legislators are often bombarded by unmitigated volumes during campaigns from organizations, which may lessen the impact of individual e-mails. Most legislators do keep tabs and tally the opinions of constituents that arrive via e-mail.

Personal meetings with legislators at the national, state, or local level are an even more effective way to get your point across and have your ideas heard. The meetings are usually set up by the aides to the legislator. Provide the staff member

Table 6-4

Meeting With Your Legislators

- Do your homework. Know as much as you can about the subject you would like to discuss, be aware of recent legislation in this area, and be knowledgeable about the legislator's record on the issue you wish to discuss.
- If the legislator is unavailable, be willing to meet with a staff member. Staff members are often responsible for outlining issues for legislators and may have a better ability to get your message heard than you would if you spoke to the legislator in person.
- Be sure to have hard facts and statistics that can provide empirical data regarding the outcomes of legislation.
- It is often a positive step to develop a facts sheet and send it to the legislator in advance of the meeting and bring the facts sheet to the meeting to help the discussion stay focused.
- If the legislative person with whom you meet has a question for which you do not have an answer, respond with an answer after the meeting when you have had time to find a solid answer.
- Be polite; discuss but never argue with a legislator. It is important to get your immediate message across, but it is also important to develop a long-term relationship with this legislator for when other issues arise. It is important to acknowledge that the legislator represents a large group of people with divergent ideas on policy issues and that sometimes the legislator must conform to the majority even if that majority does not have the same ideas about an issue as you do.
- It is a good idea to ask the legislator or his or her staff member how the legislator plans to vote on the issue you are discussing. If the vote is in favor of your ideas, thank the legislator for his or her support and ask the legislator what you could do to build support among other legislators. If the legislator or staff member opposes your position, let him or her know that you will continue to provide information to support your position and hope that the legislator will review the information and revise his or her position on the issue. If the legislator is unsure how he or she will vote on an issue, ask what information you could provide to help him or her decide in your favor.
- Send a thank you note to the legislator or staff member or both.

with the best time for scheduling a visit and the purpose of the visit. Provide information about a particular topic or appeal for specific action on an upcoming piece of legislation. Table 6-4 provides information on how to conduct a meeting with your legislator.

Critical Thinking Questions

Pick a topic in health care or an issue you feel passionate about related to health promotion and disease prevention. Develop a plan for getting your ideas heard by legislators and making an impact within the community, state, or nation.

1. What is your idea? How can you back up what you want with facts and figures?
2. Write a letter or e-mail to a legislator, using the steps outlined in this chapter.

Continued on page 258

Critical Thinking Questions *Continued from page 257*

3. Call a legislator to make your ideas known.
4. How will you become politically active? In what areas will you become active?
5. How does being educated as a DNP change your professional outlook on legislative issues? How does it change your professional responsibility?
6. Name five things you would like to advocate for in the area of health care over the next several years. What plan can you develop to make this happen?
7. How does the quote "think globally, act locally" apply to health care?

Political Action for Nurses

Traditionally, nursing as a professional group has been active in health policy discussions. In a survey to determine the level and type of nurse practitioner public policy involvement, 59.6% were involved in three or fewer public policy activities (Oden, Price, Alteneder, Broadley, & Ubokudom, 2004). The most frequently indicated activities included voting (87%) and giving money to a campaign (57%). Lack of time was the most frequently cited barrier, whereas improving the health of the public was cited most often as a benefit. Overall, nurse practitioners felt they had limited knowledge on how to go about changing public policy, were somewhat interested in public policy issues, believed the actions of public policy makers were very important, and believed these actions influenced the public's health. Most (79%) had received some information or education on public policy change. The nurse practitioners most active in public policy had high public policy efficacy expectations and perceived a high number of benefits to public policy involvement.

If nurses are involved in health policy discussion and formation, nursing values become a consideration. There are multiple avenues for nurses to become involved in changing health policy; belonging to a professional organization is a first step, but where to go from there? Nurses usually learn to be politically active in several steps, as follows:

- The first stage is to decide that nurses have a responsibility to become involved in groups that are active in health-care policy. This step requires nurses to understand that they have valuable knowledge and information about health-care policy and that they have a voice to make this information known to people in power.
- The second stage is learning about the political process at the local, state, and national levels and becoming educated as to what the current issues are in each of these venues and where nursing stands in the debate. Volunteering to be on committees within the workplace or the community is an excellent way in which to learn and grow in political and policy awareness.
- The third stage is to become politically aware and involved. This stage includes contacting local and state nursing or legislative groups that are involved in policy development and becoming active in these committees as a nurse and health-care expert.

The opportunities within professional nursing organizations and community, state, and national policy organizations and boards for nurses to become involved are virtually unlimited. As nurses become involved, they can affect and set the agenda for policy development within groups. Involvement begins with recognition of the connection between policy and practice. Interest in policy is often ignited when passion for practice coincides with need for policy change. If every professional nurse set aside some time each week to learn about policy in the newspaper or on local or national television, write letters to officials involved in policy setting, make phone calls, or go to local or state meetings where policy is discussed, nursing values and the voice of nurses would be more significantly present in policy debates and decision making.

Leavitt, Chaffee, and Vance (2007) differentiated between the nurse citizen, nurse-activist, and nurse-politician. The *nurse citizen* registers to vote; votes in elections; keeps informed about health-care issues; speaks out when services are inadequate; participates in public forums; interacts with local, state, and federal elected officials; and joins politically active nursing organizations. The *nurse-activist* writes letters, e-mails or telephones public officials, registers others to vote, contributes money to political campaigns, volunteers to work on political campaigns, lobbies decision makers and provides statistical and anecdotal information, forms or joins coalitions that support an issue of concern, and writes letters to the editor of a local paper. The *nurse-politician* runs for elected office, seeks appointments to agencies that regulate public health and welfare, seeks appointments to government boards in the public and private sector, and uses nursing knowledge and expertise to create or change policy in the public and private sectors. All nurses have the ability to become involved in health-care policy. Becoming active in this area is a responsibility of all professional nurses.

One of the first questions asked by nurses when encouraged to participate in the policy debate is, "how do I get involved?" Mason, Leavitt, and Chaffee (2007) proposed four spheres of political action in which nurses should consider becoming involved. Table 6-5 lists and describes the four spheres and gives examples of each.

All four of the spheres of policy influence described are intertwined and may compete with each other for allocation of resources. Nurses, as responsible professionals, must be active in these four spheres to ensure that health care meets the needs of the public. Although this involvement in policy may seem like a burden for the already overburdened nurse, it is an essential component of the nurse's responsibility to patients and to community.

The American Association of Colleges of Nursing essentials for DNP practice in the area of health-care policy and advocacy identify health-care policy as a framework for health-care delivery. The current system does not meet the needs of the population, and the new health-care reform legislation bills do not completely overhaul the system (Ledue, 2010). Health-care reform will be an ongoing debate and struggle for decades and beyond. Because of the extensive knowledge that advanced practice nurses have in the area of health-care delivery

Table 6-5

Spheres of Political Action

Sphere of Political Action	Where	Examples
1	Workplace	No-smoking areas in hospitals, requirements for overtime, authority to intervene on a patient's behalf, decisions concerning unlicensed personnel substitutes for RNs and allowing loved ones to be with the patient during an emergency, shared governance, committee membership. *Advanced practice nursing examples:* Office protocol, after-hours call, hospital rounds, use of drug samples, peer review, patient scheduling, and reimbursement for services.
2	Government	*Local:* Laws regarding collection of garbage, use of pesticides and other chemicals in the community, availability of school nurses, home care, creation of health centers and clinics for underserved people. *State government:* Alcohol use, smoking, public health centers, food safety, the environment and responses to emergencies such as hurricanes, floods, and epidemics. Medicaid spending priorities, end-of-life decision making, and use of state health-care dollars all are ways each state makes health-care decisions. *Federal:* Voting age, military service, drug safety through the U.S. Food and Drug Administration (FDA), entitlement programs such as Social Security and Medicare. Federal research in the areas of health from the National Institutes of Health. Groups that work to support the health of Americans, such as the U.S. Surgeon General, the U.S. Public Health Service Commissioned Corps, Centers for Disease Control and Prevention (CDC), Health Resources and Services Administration (HRSA), Institute of Medicine (IOM), Congress, and the President, all of whom create and pass health-care legislation. The Supreme Court, which hears arguments on the legality of legislation, such as *Roe v. Wade,* which legalized abortion.
3	Professional organizations	Republican and Democratic parties; for nurses, the American Nurses Association, state nurse associations, other political action groups. In the area of health policy, these organizations have a responsibility to represent the policy goals of members, keep members apprised of health-care issues, legislation, and shifts in governmental policy.

Continued from page 260 Table 6-5

Spheres of Political Action

Sphere of Political Action	Where	Examples
4	Community: Local or global	Nurses have a duty to promote health and well-being through policy development and legislation within communities of all sizes, and the community provides the resources for health maintenance, civic organizations, planning boards, business groups, and community councils, food banks, and local charity organizations.

and social justice, political activism in the area of health-care policy and reform is an essential part of the DNP's role. The DNP degree prepares nurse leaders in advanced practice who can engage with their professional colleagues to share in policy reform by providing vision, innovation, and evaluation skills to reform health care. As a foundation, the DNP-prepared nurse should be knowledgeable about influencing health-care policy, understanding the foundations of health-care financing, knowing how new health-care policies are formulated and how these policies become law, and creating ways to address issues such as social justice and equity in health care.

To become involved in the legislative process, access federal health care legislation through the Library of Congress at http://thomas.loc.gov/. This Web site provides information about bills, resolutions, presidential nominations, the Congressional Record, treaties, and committee reports. The site has an instruction page that guides users to help them find what they are looking for. In the area of legislation, it provides a summary of bills before Congress, a full version of the entire bill, and the status of the bill as it passes through the legislative process. States likewise have Web sites that provide a list of statutes and bills before the state legislature. Local community legislation can be accessed through county or local government sites. These sites also supply a list of federal, state, and local government officials with e-mail addresses and telephone numbers.

Critical Thinking Questions

To develop a sense of how to read and understand health-care legislation and how to discuss these legislative issues with patients and others in a knowledgeable way, go to http://thomas.loc.gov/ and click on one of the federal health care legislative bills listed. First, determine who has sponsored the bill and what committee is reviewing and discussing the bill. Then click on the icon for "bill

Continued on page 262

Critical Thinking Questions *Continued from page 261*

text" and read the bill. Locate a section of the bill entitled "Resolved," which is usually where the issues contained within the bill can be found.

As you look at the bill, think about the following:

1. Who is the bill meant to help? Does the bill have a substantive plan for action?
2. How will the implementation of this bill be financed—new taxes, fines, or current restructure of spending?
3. Are there unintended consequences from implementation of the bill that you can discern?
4. Who is sponsoring the bill, and are there cosponsors? Why might these individuals have espoused this bill?
5. Are there stated amendments to the legislation?
6. How would you influence the sponsors of this bill, the cosponsors, the committee considering the bill, and Congress as a whole on the issues concerned in the bill?

Because DNP graduates are experts in clinical practice, their expertise should help shape health policy. Advanced practice nurses are aware of the problems created by lack of health insurance. They understand that although individuals without health insurance often can afford to see a primary care provider, specialist care is beyond their means. This situation creates a scenario where simple prevention of diseases such as diabetes, heart disease, and stroke are outside the reach of people without insurance until they have a major complication such as renal failure or myocardial infarction. When such a complication occurs, the emergency medical system, the most expensive type of care, is activated, and these patients are now beyond prevention and in tertiary care, which is the most expensive aspect of care. DNP-prepared nurses possess a higher level of health policy knowledge and are able to engage with legislators and the public to educate and introduce ideas for improving the care of the population while decreasing cost. As the United States strives to meet standards set by the Institute of Medicine (2001) to redesign health care financing, practice regulations, safety, quality, and efficiency, nurses who are prepared with the DNP degree can contribute greatly to meeting these aims and standards.

Critical Thinking Questions

1. Name the congressional representatives from the district where you reside. What are their party affiliations? What congressional committees are they on? Visit the Thomas Web site of the Library of Congress and Web sites of the congressional representatives to find health-related bills they have sponsored or cosponsored. Where do they stand on health-care issues?
2. Name the two senators who represent your state in Washington, DC. What are their party affiliations? What Senate committees are they on? Visit the

Thomas Web site of the Library of Congress and the Web site of each senator to find health-related bills they have sponsored or cosponsored. Where do they stand on health-care issues?
3. Name the state legislators who represent the area where you reside. What are their party affiliations? What state legislation have they sponsored or cosponsored? What health-related accomplishments are they responsible for either funding or starting in the town or area where you reside?
4. Who are your local councilmen or town leaders (mayors, other elected officials)? What health-related issues are these leaders involved in?
5. What other groups in your state or community are active in health-related issues? What do they stand for?

Nursing Groups Reshaping Health-Care Policy

Voicing support for policy change sometimes requires a network or coalition that advises nurses regarding issues of interest and provides leadership to drive a strategic, timely response. Nurses often form strategic alliances within the nursing community and with other organizations with similar interests in health-care issues. These alliances or coalitions give nurses a stronger voice and provide a coordinated and united approach that can have more impact than each organization acting individually. Coalitions simplify the work of legislators and their staff members by providing policy input from a large group of people that is succinct and well stated, rather than many different communications from individuals. Legislators are able to understand the political weight of a policy stance based on the size and membership of the coalition.

Nurses are a powerful group politically in the United States by virtue of their numbers. Nurses as a group are also well educated and feel strongly about ethical and social justice issues. National and international nursing organizations represent nursing views in political advocacy. As coalitions, nursing organizations are powerful and have the ability to create and change health-care policy.

International Council of Nurses

The International Council of Nurses is a federation of more than 130 national nurses associations. Its mission is to ensure quality nursing care for all people and sound health policies globally. This group has created a policy statement stipulating that nurses should accept responsibility for health policy and decision making in all countries around the world (International Council of Nurses, 2000). The International Council of Nurses promotes and supports efforts to prepare nurses in the areas of leadership and policy development, including how to engage in the political process, how to form coalitions, and how to work with the media to exert influence within the public debate over health-care issues.

Sigma Theta Tau International Honor Society of Nursing

Another international nursing organization that supports policy debate and development in nursing is Sigma Theta Tau International Honor Society of Nursing. The policy position statement of this group notes that Florence Nightingale was involved in policy development and that many visionary nurse leaders since that time have been involved in policy discussions and development (Sigma Theta Tau International, 2005). The policy position statement of Sigma Theta Tau International asserts, "Sigma Theta Tau International is committed to providing opportunities and forums for nurses and others around the world to be informed, share knowledge, openly discuss health care, nursing and social concerns, and speak to public, health and nursing policy issues." In regard to this commitment, Sigma Theta Tau International disseminates articles on various health and social issues relevant to health policy.

American Nurses Association

The American Nurses Association (ANA) represents American nurses in the areas of health policy development and legislation. The ANA has stated that practicing nurses have hands-on experience of the outcomes of health-care laws and regulations. Because nurses work with these laws at a practical level, they have a unique perspective on health-care policy. The ANA uses the insights of nurses to craft position statements regarding health-care policy legislation and the need for health-care policy. These statements explain, justify, or recommend a course of action that is reflective of positions of the ANA. Nurse members can view and comment on these positions at http://www.nursingworld.org/positionstatements. An example of an ANA position statement is presented in Box 6-1.

The ANA also endorses certain legislation. An example of a letter not only endorsing legislation but also requesting changes be made to represent the needs of nurses is presented in Box 6-2.

American Organization of Nurse Executives

Nurse executives and administrators are represented in policy advocacy by the American Organization of Nurse Executives (AONE) founded in 1967 as a subsidiary of the ANA. The mission of this group is to shape health care through innovative and expert nursing leadership. Through membership in AONE, nurse leaders can participate in professional development, advocacy, and research to advance nursing leadership, promote excellence in nursing practice, and work toward shaping health-care policy. AONE supports its members through the following (AONE, 2010):

- Providing vision and actions for nursing leadership to meet the health-care needs of society
- Influencing legislation and public policy related to nursing and patient care issues

Box 6-1

American Nurses Association Position Paper on Adult Immunization

Adult Immunization—12/12/02

The American Nurses Association supports:

1. Vaccine delivery strategies that remove barriers to access for all persons, regardless of ethnicity, socioeconomic status, immigration status, or geography.
2. Public policy that removes barriers to access to immunization for all adults.
3. Research to evaluate consumer and professional attitudes and behaviors in regard to immunization delivery and to guide the design of evidence-based programs to improve vaccine acceptance and immunization levels.
4. Clinical practices linking assessment of vaccination status and administration of vaccines to other recommended preventive measures and strongly recognizing nursling's role in this process.
5. Forums for health-care professionals to develop, share, disseminate, and become educated about current information regarding indications, efficacy, safety, and delivery of adult immunization and consumer educational materials that reflect current research in these areas.
6. Collaborative and cooperative agreements and partnerships with private and public sector organizations to promote adult immunizations in a variety of settings and to advance ongoing vaccine research.

Source: ANA, 2002. From http://www.mendeley.com/research/american-nurses-association-position-statement-adult-immunization/

Box 6-2

Example of Letter of Endorsement of Health-Care Policy Legislation

January 6, 2010

The Honorable John Boehner
H-232, US Capitol
Washington, DC 20515
The Honorable Harry Reid
522 Hart Senate Office Bldg
Washington, DC 20510

Dear Speaker Boehner and Majority Leader Reid:

The 43 undersigned nursing organizations commend the work of the House and Senate to reform America's health-care system. This legislative effort represents a movement toward comprehensive and meaningful change that will improve access to quality care. On pages 1–6 of this letter, we have outlined specific provisions contained in either the House or the Senate bills that are critical to the nursing profession and respectfully request that they be included in the final health-care reform bill. Additionally, on pages 6 and 7, we have highlighted provisions that were incorporated in

Continued on page 266

Box 6-2

Example of Letter of Endorsement of Health-Care Policy Legislation

Continued from page 265

both bills, and we seek your continued support of these important issues. Finally, we would like to raise your attention to page 7, where we address provisions contained in either the House or the Senate bills that require vital modifications. As you negotiate the differences between the House's *Affordable Health Care for America Act of 2009* (H.R. 3962) and the Senate's *Patient Protection and Affordable Care Act* (H.R. 3590), please consider our nursing requests cited below.

Health-Care Provisions Needing Modifications

As stated earlier, the Nursing Community supports the Medicare Graduate Nurse Education demonstration program, Section 5509 of the Senate bill. While the Nursing Community supports this provision, the current legislative language dramatically limits the scope to only five hospitals, and we request that this arbitrary limitation be removed. Additionally, we also have serious concerns about Section 5509 (a)(2)(A) relying on 1861 (v) of the Social Security Act (SSA) and its related interpretation in the Code of Federal Regulations for the determination of reasonable costs of the demonstration. This could tie reasonable costs to those of the existing Nursing and Allied Health pass-through funding, which would run directly counter to the intent of this Graduate Nurse Education demonstration.

The Accountable Care Organization (ACO) Pilot Program, which is included in the House bill (Sec. 1301) and Senate bill (Sec. 2706), will provide improved incentives for performance-based care. The Senate bill includes Nurse Practitioners and Clinical Nurse Specialists as participants, but not CNMs and CRNAs. The Nursing Community requests that this Senate provision include CNMs and CRNAs. In addition, the Nursing Community could support the House provision only if it clarifies that APRNs are full participants.

Additionally, we support the development of a National Health Care Workforce Commission under section 5101 of the Senate's bill. Quality data on the national health-care workforce is critical to ensure that care is comprehensive and coordinated and all providers are used to their full scope of practice. This can occur only with the collaboration from all health-care providers in the planning and development of national standards for data collection and analysis. We recommend that the membership of this commission has an equal representation among health professionals.

Comparative effectiveness research based on the collection of standardized, evidence-based performance information that will accurately measure quality and enable transition to a value-based payment system is a critical area of inquiry at a time when health-care consumers and reformers are seeking quality care focused on prevention that is affordable and accessible by all. While the Nursing Community supports these provisions, we recommend report language that specifically identifies that nurse-sensitive quality and performance measures are a critical data component of the research.

Both the House and the Senate versions of the bill offer numerous programs that would augment the nursing workforce for the benefit of the nation's health. We would like to reiterate our appreciation to both the House and the Senate committees for the significant efforts to meet the nursing needs of not only our underserved populations, but the entire nation. The nursing community appreciates the consideration of our above requests.

- Offering member services that support and enhance the management, leadership, educational, and professional development of nursing leaders
- Facilitating and supporting research and development efforts that advance nursing administration practice and quality patient care

AONE has a political action committee that advocates for policies supporting nursing education and leadership. The AONE political action committee supports coalition efforts to work collaboratively with the greater nursing community and other partners to address issues crucial to health care, health reform, and advancement of the nursing profession. The current priorities of this group include expanding the nursing workforce, promoting the role of the nurse in primary care, supporting the role of nursing to improve patient outcomes, increasing care coordination and decreasing health-care costs, supporting data gathering and research activities to articulate the economic value of nursing, and supporting the rights of nurses internationally.

History of Health-Care Delivery, Payment, and Reform in the United States

Throughout history, most health care has been provided in the home. This care was sometimes referred to as "domestic medicine" because it was delivered by the female head of the household or a servant at her discretion. Further assistance came from outside of the home from people who were believed to have special healing gifts. Receiving care from strangers became more common throughout the early part of the 19th century, and people began to travel long distances to see healers. As travelers journeyed to see healers, Christian women opened their homes to serve as refuges for travelers who were ill.

History of Health-Care Delivery in the United States

The U.S. health-care delivery system, spurred by scientific discovery, developed in a similar way. Care was provided initially through domestic medicine; then by persons known to have special skills; and then, as cities grew, through congregate care in alms houses, asylums, and hospitals. Even surgery was performed in the home until well into the 20th century. After World War I, hospitals began to thrive because they were convenient locations for efficient physician practice and training. Bellevue in New York City became one of the most famous public hospitals in the United States. In the late 1800s and early 1900s, modern nursing and the foundations of the current health-care system in the United States developed.

Early Nurse Leaders as Role Models for DNP-Prepared Nurses

Advances in health-care delivery in the United States have always been tied to the nursing profession (Cherry & Jacob, 2005). During the late 19th century, several very strong women in nursing were practicing at an advanced practice level. These nurses were expert clinicians and clinical scholars. Florence Nightingale (1820–1910) was the founder of modern nursing. She advocated infection control and a clean environment to improve health outcomes and used statistics to uncover and monitor trends and outcomes in care to create the profession of nursing. Her influence was most strongly felt in the education nurses received and in the establishment of fundamental principles within the discipline (Bostridge, 2008).

Lillian Wald (1867–1940) made home visits to people living in an impoverished community in New York City at the turn of the 20th century. Wald developed and implemented the role of the public health nurse, and she cofounded the Visiting Nurses Association—which still exists today. She worked to improve the health of the community by working with the political and business community to create playgrounds for children and to clean up the water. Wald and her nurses established the Henry Street Settlement House, which was built to help families in poverty to achieve better lives for themselves and their children.

Isabelle Hampton Robb (1860–1910) was the first superintendent of nurses at Johns Hopkins School of Nursing and the first president of the Society of Superintendents for Training Schools for Nurses, which later became the National League for Nursing. She was also very politically active in health-care legislative issues and was the first president of the Nurses' Associated Alumnae of the United States and Canada, which later became the ANA and the Canadian Nurse Association. She wrote the first books on nursing ethics (1901). Other leaders in the cause of nursing and health care that may have been the models for the DNP include Clara Barton, who established the American Red Cross; Margaret Sanger, who created Planned Parenthood; and Mary Breckenridge, who began the Frontier Nursing Service and midwifery practice. These nursing leaders not only provided care to their patients but also opened the eyes of the public and legislators to the need for adequate health care for all members of society.

History of Payment for Health-Care Services

Throughout the history of health care in the United States, there has been a policy debate regarding the right to health care. Some people see health care as a privilege that should be allocated according to ability to pay. Other people perceive health care as a right to be distributed according to need. In the United States at the present time, health care is not a right but a privilege. In the United States, citizens have never been entitled to health care. Health care for the most part has been perceived as a purchased benefit for persons who can afford the services. Health care in the United States has an associated cost, so people pay or have insurance (private, from their employer, or government provided) that pays, or they do without needed services. Most Americans who have health insurance receive it as a benefit of employment, have it provided as an entitlement by a governmental agency, or purchase it privately from an insurance company.

In 1929, when physicians and hospitals began charging more than most individuals could easily pay, the first modern group health insurance plan was formed. A group of teachers in Dallas, Texas, contracted with Baylor Hospital for room, board, and medical services in exchange for a monthly fee. Several large life insurance companies entered the health insurance field in the 1930s and 1940s as the popularity of health insurance increased. In 1932, nonprofit organizations called Blue Cross and Blue Shield first offered group health plans. Blue Cross and Blue Shield plans were successful because they involved discounted contracts negotiated with physicians and hospitals. In return for promises of increased volume and prompt payment, providers gave discounts to the Blue Cross and Blue Shield plans.

Employee benefit plans proliferated in the 1940s and 1950s. Strong unions bargained for better benefit packages, including tax-free, employer-sponsored health insurance. Wartime (1939–1945) wage freezes imposed by the government accelerated the spread of group health care. Unable by law to attract workers by paying more, employers instead improved their benefit packages, adding health care. Insurance was provided for working people, but nonworking people were left out of the system, which offered a favorable risk pool to insurers of young and mostly healthy (i.e., employed) people, and people who were too sick or too old to work were not covered.

Government programs to cover health-care costs began to expand during the 1950s and 1960s. When the government created Medicare and Medicaid programs in 1965, private sources such as Blue Cross Blue Shield still paid 75% of all health-care costs. However, by 1995, individuals and companies paid for only about half of health care, and the government paid the other half.

During the 1980s and 1990s, the cost of health care increased rapidly, driven both by improving medical technology and by the growing inefficiencies of the health-care system. At that point, most employer-sponsored group insurance plans switched from fee-for-service plans to the less expensive managed care plans. As a result, most Americans with health insurance were enrolled in managed care plans by the mid-1990s.

In 1993, President Clinton presented to the U.S. Congress a health-care reform plan that would have guaranteed health insurance for all Americans. Congressional leaders opposed the plan because it was too expensive and excessively regulated. In 1994, members of Congress introduced a series of alternative proposals, but they never reached a compromise. In 1996, Congress did pass the Mental Health Parity Act, which required some employers to offer health plans with psychiatric benefits. Congress also passed the Health Insurance Portability and Accountability Act in 1996. This act protected individuals from losing their health insurance when they moved from one job to another or became self-employed. However, the act did not ensure the overall quality or comprehensiveness of insurance offered by employers.

Managed care kept cost increases in check for a while during the 1990s, but eventually costs started creeping up again, creating the current crisis.

The managed care model, where physicians were paid per patient per month regardless of the amount of care provided, created a public perception that physicians were reimbursed for not providing needed care. This perception caused employers and individuals to opt out of managed care as a health insurance option (Greene et al., 2008). The ideal for managed care is to provide the most effective care at the time it is required; however, this does not take into account the wish of most people to have extensive testing and treatment that may or may not be effective for themselves and their loved ones (Elkin et al., 2008). As patients demanded more treatments and tests, costs, even in managed care, began to increase. Today, employers are reducing or eliminating outright health-care benefits for employees; employers are allowing employees to choose to receive higher wages and forego health benefits (Mitka, 2008); hospitals are consolidating and becoming less accommodating to low-income patients as they seek to push back against insurers (Thompson & Lee, 2007); and a growing portion of the population has no health insurance at all (U.S. Department of Health and Human Services, 2009).

History of Health-Care Reform in the United States

Fundamental health-care reform has not occurred in the United States since the 1960s when Medicare and Medicaid legislation created national and state health insurance programs for older adults and low-income families. Health-care reform is such a hot button issue because there are so many differing views of what should be changed and how. Health-care costs seem uncontrollable, and 46 million Americans remain uninsured. This situation is troubling, as is the waste in health-care spending. How have we gotten here, and what reforms have been discussed in other administrations? The Kaiser Family Foundation created *Focus on Health Reform Brief* (Hoffman, 2009), which reviews health care reform from 1900 to the present.

In the early 1900s, Theodore Roosevelt campaigned on a platform calling for health insurance for all workers. Opposition to this idea of "socialized medicine" was strong. In 1912, when the English Parliament passed the National Insurance Act, the American Association for Labor Legislation called for social insurance for the American worker. The editor of the *Journal of the American Medical Association* stated that this type of insurance would benefit the public as no other health legislation had. World War I soon began, and the idea of health insurance took a backseat. However, during the war, California proposed a law to provide universal health insurance to all residents of the state. When insurance companies took out advertisements in the *San Francisco Chronicle* stating that universal insurance would "spell the social ruin" of the state of California, they killed the ballot referendum.

Polls of Americans since the 1930s have shown support for guaranteed access to health care and health insurance for all and a role for government in regulating insurance and health-care payments (Kleefeld, 2009). Support lessens when money comes into play, however. Historians have found that many national health insurance proposals have failed because of the complexity of a national health insurance program, ideological differences, and the lobbying strength of special interest groups.

The next effort to institute a national health insurance plan came in the era of the "Fair Deal" from 1945–1950. After World War II, workers were in scarce supply, and employers offered health insurance to attract workers. President Truman proposed a national health insurance program but was unable to pass legislation because of a Republican Congress in his first term and because of Southern Democrats (fearing interference with segregation) in his second term. During this time, the American Medical Association (AMA) continued to oppose a national health insurance plan as "socialized medicine." The AMA and other opponents of national health insurance were successful in eroding public support using fear of socialism at a time when communism was growing in Russia and China.

During the "Great Society" from 1960–1965, a well-educated middle class became a powerful force in society. Because of the increased productivity within the United States, health insurance provided by employers was deemed to be a safe and effective method for bargaining by trade and labor unions. However, employers were less willing or able to afford the rising cost to ensure the sick and elderly. The health-care reform focus turned to the elderly population. Generally, elderly adults were among the most medically needy in society, given their fixed incomes and poorer health, and were in greater need of medical care. Congress passed a single bill with three layers, called Medicare:

- Medicare Part A pays for hospital care and limited skilled nursing and home health care.
- Medicare Part B (paid for in part by premiums) is optional and helps pay for physician care.
- Medicaid, a totally separate program, not only assists states in covering long-term care for poor people but also provides health insurance coverage for certain classes of poor and disabled persons.

The final bill proposed by President Johnson left elderly adults in need of private coverage for some services, such as prescription drugs, long-term care, and eyeglasses. No governmental cost controls were enacted, and the government distanced itself from the financial aspects of the program by selecting *fiscal intermediaries* (usually private insurance organizations such as Blue Cross) to apply their standards of "reasonableness" for physician fees.

Labor unions, civil rights organizations, the American Hospital Association, and the health-care industry all supported these programs as necessary to care for elderly, sick, and poor individuals in the United States. Despite the AMA opposition to Medicare as socialized medicine, the legislature incorporated it into the Social Security Act and signed it into law in July 1965.

As the economy of the United States continued to grow, high levels of inflation began to increase health-care costs. Medicare and Medicaid grew rapidly from 4% of the national budget in 1965 to 11% in 1973. In addition, millions of Americans younger than 65 still had no access to health insurance. During this time, Congress passed regulations in an attempt to stem the increases in health-care costs. These regulations led to certificate-of-need programs for hospitals, rate setting, health maintenance organizations, and health planning. Senator Ted Kennedy proposed a universal single payer national health insurance plan to be financed through payroll taxes. President Nixon countered the Kennedy plan with his Comprehensive Health Insurance Plan, which called for universal coverage, voluntary employer participation, and a separate program for the working poor and unemployed. By 1974, Congress reached a compromise between these two plans and enjoyed bipartisan support for health-care reform.

From 1976–1979, the economy was stagnant, and inflation continued. President Carter focused on cost containment and hospital cost control. In 1983, Congress passed legislation to change the payment method for hospital care. The Medicare Prospective Payment System changed hospital payments from a charge-based system to a predetermined, set rate based on the patient's diagnosis.

During the Reagan administration, because of the effect of substantial tax cuts and large increases in defense spending, the federal debt reached record levels. Health-care costs continued to increase, representing 12% the nation's gross domestic product in 1990. During the Presidency of George H.W. Bush, many plans for health-care reform began to surface, such as health-care tax credits, purchasing pools, single-payer plans, and employer mandates (play-or-pay) plans.

President Clinton campaigned on the promise to have a health-care reform plan to Congress within 100 days of taking office. Clinton's plan, the Health Security Act, called for universal coverage, employer and individual mandates, competition between private insurers, and regulation by government to keep costs down. Under this plan, private insurers and providers would compete for business or groups of businesses and individuals in *health-purchasing alliances*. President Clinton wanted every American to have a "health security card" similar to a Social Security card.

To accomplish his goals, President Clinton created a Health Care Task Force, chaired by his wife Hillary Clinton. This group accepted and processed input from 34 closed working groups with 600 experts. While this complex health-care plan was being developed, others in Congress proposed their own health-care plans, which began to splinter support of the majority Democrats in Congress. In the end, a divided Congress did not pass the bill. Some reform did occur during the Clinton presidency, however, including the Children's Health Insurance Program, which expands the Medicaid program to provide health coverage to more low-income children.

The first term of George W. Bush was riddled with national crises and a focus on the "war on terror." Although President Bush was opposed to a national health insurance plan, he did support tax incentives and reductions for employers who provided health-care insurance to employees and medical savings accounts for individuals and families. In his second term, President Bush signed into law a Medicare drug benefit program. This act provided prescription drug coverage for Americans older than 65 as a part of their Medicare benefit (Medicare Part D). Senior citizens must choose a Medicare Part D plan from private insurers that includes the medications they are taking. Similar to Medicare Part B, there is a monthly fee for Medicare Part D.

As greater numbers of Americans found themselves without health care or with health care that was too expensive to meet their needs, the call for greater reform became stronger. One legislative priority for the Obama administration was to initiate comprehensive health-care reform and pass laws that improved health care for all Americans. The three major goals of health-care reform were (1) to increase access to health care, (2) to reduce health care costs, and (3) to increase the quality of health care in the United States. In 2010, Congress narrowly passed the Patient Protection and Affordable Care Act, Public Law No. 111-148, and President Obama signed it into law.

Patient Protection and Affordable Care Act of 2010

The Patient Protection and Affordable Care Act expands access to medical care and primary health-care services to approximately 32 million more Americans. The new law has a tremendous impact on the provision of health care for all Americans. Following are some of the changes made by the Patient Protection and Affordable Care Act:

- The bill creates a mandatory prevention and public health fund to support established programs that focus on prevention and public health, and it increases funding for the National Health Service Corp. These two measures indicate a shift to more government support for health promotion and disease prevention.
- Children cannot be denied insurance because of pre-existing conditions, and children can remain insured on their parents' health insurance until age 26.
- Adults with a pre-existing condition can join an insurance "high-risk" pool to purchase insurance coverage. Currently, the largest groups of uninsured Americans are unmarried young adults and individuals with pre-existing conditions. Offering insurance coverage for individuals with pre-existing conditions allows them to continue receiving care. For example, a diabetic patient who was not covered by his employer's benefits plan can now continue to receive medical care and medications. Without insurance coverage, long-term hyperglycemia would likely result in a heart attack, renal failure, or any of the other long-term effects of untreated diabetes. Continuing health care for these individuals can prevent heart attack or renal failure and can result in significant cost savings.

- Senior citizens who fall into the "Medicare doughnut hole"—a coverage gap that requires Medicare patients to pay for the full cost of medications when their medication spending ranges from $2700 to $6154—will get a 50% discount on some drugs.
- In 2011, a new fee on drug manufacturers will be implemented to help pay for the upcoming changes.
- The fine on withdrawing funds from a Health Savings Account for non-medical expenses will increase by 5% to 10%.
- Employers will need to start including the cost of health care on their employee W-2 forms.
- In 2011, the bill mandates that chain restaurants and vending machines disclose the nutritional content in foods sold.
- Medicare will pay a 10% bonus to primary care providers to increase interest among physicians and advanced practice nurses to work in primary care, health promotion, and disease prevention.
- Medicaid will be able to offer more home-based and community-based services to disabled individuals.
- In 2012, the Center for Medicare and Medicaid Services (CMS) will implement plans to decrease readmissions to the hospital through a "pay for performance" incentive program. This program serves to motivate hospitals to reduce unnecessary readmissions by ensuring that patients are discharged with appropriate home and community care, medications, and education.
- Beginning in 2014, employers with more than 50 workers must provide a health insurance benefit or face a fine from the federal government. Small businesses will receive a subsidy from the federal government to help defray the cost of this insurance benefit for employees. Unemployed individuals will be required to purchase health insurance, but the federal government will subsidize the payments for this insurance. Individuals at higher income levels will be able to purchase reasonably priced health insurance through insurance exchanges where risk for the insurer is pooled among a large group. This portion of the act is the most controversial. Many states have undertaken lawsuits to prevent this aspect of the bill from being enacted. The belief is that persons should not be required to purchase health insurance.
- In 2014, the law will institute a ban on lifetime caps on the amount of payout from insurance companies on any individual illness a plan member experiences.
- Between 2015 and 2018, a new health-care provider payment schedule will be implemented, based on quality rather than volume as it is now. New plans must cover checkups and other preventive care without copays. All plans will be affected by 2018.
- Insurance companies can no longer drop someone's coverage because of illness. Insurers must now reveal how much money is spent on overhead.

Any new plan must now implement an appeals process for coverage determinations and claims. New screening procedures will be implemented to help eliminate health insurance fraud and waste. The Secretary of Health and Human Services will set up a new Web site to make it easy for Americans in any state to seek out affordable health insurance options. The site will also include helpful information for small businesses.

The Congressional Budget Office (2010) estimated that the new health-care bill will cost $940 billion over the next 10 years. At the same time, the bill will reduce the U.S. budget deficit by $143 billion over the next 10 years. The CBO predicted that over the second 10 years, the health-care reform bill will reduce the deficit by $1.2 trillion. The report from the CBO also stated that the bill will extend Medicare's solvency by at least 9 years and reduce the rate of its growth by 1.4%.

Immediately after the Patient Protection and Affordable Care Act was passed, states and individuals challenged it. The provision of the legislation that mandates that all citizens obtain health insurance has been challenged by 19 states on the grounds that the requirement infringes on state sovereignty. Legal experts believe that the final decision on this aspect of the health-care plan may have to be decided by the Supreme Court (Mears, 2010).

Some states already require all citizens to have health insurance. In 2006, former Governor Mitt Romney signed a Massachusetts law that is considered a landmark of political compromise and shared responsibility. Since enacting an individual mandate, the state has reduced its number of uninsured citizens by about 300,000. One of the lessons learned in the 4 years since Massachusetts passed its health-care bill is that a shortage of primary care physicians reduces the efficacy of the bill because although individuals now have access, they have nowhere to go to get basic health care (Schratz, 2010). This situation presents an opportunity for advanced practice nurses to fill that gap and provide needed patient-centered primary health care.

Public Response to Health-Care Reform

The response of Americans to this health-care reform initiative has been mixed. In a study completed by the Kaiser Family Foundation (2010), 55% of people questioned stated that they were confused about the reform laws, did not have enough information about the reform laws, and were unsure how these laws would affect health care. The same poll asked participants to rate the impact of these new laws on the U.S. economy. Of participants, 45% responded that they thought the laws would increase the U.S. budget deficit, 25% stated it would decrease the budget deficit, 16% said it would not have much of an impact, and 13% were unsure what financial impact the laws would have.

Among all respondents to a poll from the Kaiser Family Foundation in June 2010, regardless of political affiliation, 41% felt very favorable toward the new legislation, 23% were somewhat favorable, 10% were somewhat unfavorable,

12% were very unfavorable, and 14% did not know or refused to answer. When the survey asked questions about the effect of the new law on families, 41% felt their family would be better off under the new laws, 20% felt there would be no difference for their family, and 32% felt they would be worse off when the new laws became effective.

Critical Thinking Questions

1. How does the Patient Protection and Affordable Care Act of 2010 improve health care in the United States? What does it do to reduce cost? What does it do to increase access to care and quality?
2. What are the drawbacks of this plan? Why are some people opposed to the plan?
3. What are the "unknowns" in this law that trouble some Americans?
4. What are some of the misconceptions in the public view of this plan?
5. Why do you think there is strong opposition to requiring people to obtain health insurance?
6. How will advanced practice nurses be able to increase their visibility as health-care providers as the various components of this bill become law?
7. Go to the Library of Congress Web site and read the full summary of the plan. What do you think of the plan overall? Are there parts you would change? Why?
8. What are the next steps in legislation that would improve access and quality in health care in the United States? What are the benefits or challenges in providing the best health care at the lowest cost to the most people?

Regardless of public opinion, the new health-care legislation does place a great deal of emphasis on primary care, health promotion, and disease prevention as essential elements of care and cost reduction.

Nurses Reshaping Primary Care

One of the challenges in meeting the new expansion in coverage predicated by recent health-care reform is the current shortage of primary care health-care providers and the likelihood that this shortage will remain for the foreseeable future. One way to combat the shortage is through the use of nurse practitioners as independent primary care providers. At the present time, two-thirds of advanced practice nurses are working in primary care, with 20% working in rural areas where the shortage of primary care providers is even more critical. Each year, an estimated 8000 nurse practitioners graduate, with 7000 prepared to work in primary care (Stokowski, 2010). Graduates of medical programs are avoiding primary care as a specialty because of lower reimbursement and increased time commitment. Only 7% of fourth-year medical students plan careers in adult primary care (Bodenheimer, 2010). It seems that advanced practice nurses may be the keystone to the provision of primary care. Nonetheless, several public policy barriers block nurse practitioners from practicing to their full potential in the area of primary care.

A coalition of advanced practice nurses, including the National Organization of Nurse Practitioner Faculty, American Association of Nurse Practitioners, American College of Nurse Practitioners, Gerontological Advanced Practice Nurses Association, National Association of Pediatric Nurse Practitioners, and National Association of Nurse Practitioners in Women's Health, has provided a list of key issues necessary to promote advanced practice nurses in the area of primary care. These issues include the following:

- Full recognition and use of nurse practitioners as primary care providers in all health-care systems and models: This calls for removing barriers to practice, such as policies regarding collaboration or supervision of nurse practitioners, and allowing nurse practitioners to sign death certificates and create do not resuscitate (DNR) orders.
- Full recognition of nurse practitioner practices in coordinated care models, such as medical homes: Current medical home policies do not allow nurse practitioners to be the director of this type of care model. This creates further barriers to nurse practitioner practice, especially in the area of whole person primary care.
- Full participation of nurse practitioners and nurse practitioner practices in accountable care organizations: This would allow nurse practitioners to be listed on insurance panels so that patients can choose a nurse practitioner as their primary care provider.
- Full participation of nurse practitioners and nurse practitioner practices in long-term care and transitional care models included in the legislation: This would allow nurse practitioners to be full partners in initiatives to improve care coordination and the management of patients with long-term chronic diseases.
- Maintenance of the nondiscrimination language contained in the Senate Finance Bill: This would give equal status in Medicare to primary care physicians and primary care nurse practitioners.
- Maintenance of the funding stream for nurse-managed clinics in the HELP (Health Education, Legislation and Policy) bill: This would continue funding nurse managed clinics where nurse practitioner students are often educated in the area of primary care.
- Maintenance of the Graduate Nurse Education Funding Stream as proposed in the Senate Finance Bill: This could continue the federal traineeship for nurse practitioners.
- Authorization of nurse practitioners to certify patients eligible for home health care services: This would remove a barrier to independent practice for nurse practitioners and allow them to certify patients and order home health for patients who require this service.

Public Policy Barriers to Primary Care

The barriers faced by nurse practitioners in fulfilling the critical need for primary care providers can be found in the individual state practice acts, which govern oversight and autonomy in practice and prescriptive authority. The regulation of nurse practitioner practice is uneven among states. In 28 states, the state board of nursing is the sole regulator of nurse practitioner practice, whereas in 22 other states, boards of medicine or pharmacy have regulatory authority over nurse practitioners, along with the state boards of nursing. Changes in state and federal policies regarding nurse practitioner practice are essential to improving access to primary care providers.

Prescriptive authority for nurse practitioners is an important aspect of providing primary care. All states now have prescriptive authority for nurse practitioners although some states limit the type of drugs that can be prescribed by advanced practice nurses. Other states allow nurses to prescribe expanded levels of medications but require re-education each year for prescribers. All but two states, Alabama and Florida, allow nurse practitioners to obtain Drug Enforcement Administration (DEA) numbers from the federal government. These numbers are important because pharmacies use these numbers to bill insurance companies for medications (American Academy of Nurse Practitioners, 2010).

Another serious health policy barrier to nurse practitioner practice in primary care is payer policies. There are discrepancies between nurse practitioner and physician reimbursement from Medicare and most private insurance companies for the same level of care. In the new health care bill, nurse midwives for the first time will receive the same reimbursement as physicians. However, nurse practitioners working in other areas including primary care will continue to receive less per patient than the physician. Continued reimbursement discrepancy is a disincentive for advanced practice nurses. The lower rates of reimbursement make it more difficult for nurse practitioners to open their own practices, meet expenses, and provide themselves with a salary. This reimbursement plan seems contrary to research that shows that nurse practitioners are able to provide quality primary care and do a better job at health education, health promotion, and disease prevention than their physician colleagues (Laurant, 2005; Pohl, Hanson, Newland, & Cronenwet, 2010). The new legislation funds nurse-managed health centers, but these centers may not be financially viable without payment policy changes.

Because of these policy barriers, many nurse practitioners have been reluctant to open their own practices to meet the community needs for primary care. With greater opportunities accompanying health-care reform, more nurse entrepreneurs will take on these challenges.

What do these new laws do, with regard to nursing, to improve health care in the United States? These new laws stimulate growth in nursing education via loan forgiveness, increased scholarships, and increased funding for bridge programs to help nurses complete their baccalaureate or graduate degrees. The laws establish grants to provide traineeships for nurses through federally qualified health centers. They also establish funding to pay for the clinical training of advanced practice nurses so that community health-care settings and hospitals where nurse practitioner students complete clinical hours can receive reimbursement.

Health Promotion as Public Policy

Health promotion is an important aspect of primary care (Flocke, Crabtree, & Strange, 2007) and of public policy orientation. To promote health, the clinician must have a working knowledge of behavior change mechanisms, must set behavior change goals with the patient and family, must continue to monitor the ability of the patient to reach those goals (Aittasalo, Miilunpalo, Kukkonen-Harjula, & Pasanen, 2006), and must have the backing of public policy that supports reimbursement for health promotion activities. There are health consequences to many decisions made by policy makers, and these should be recognized and accepted as such. For instance, why are visits to a primary care physician (who tells a patient to lose weight) covered, whereas membership to Weight Watchers is not?

Health promotion has been defined by the WHO as "the process of enabling people to increase control over their health and its determinants, and thereby improve their health" (World Health Organization, 2008). Another definition of health promotion comes from *The American Journal of Health Promotion,* where health promotion is described as "the science and art of helping people change their lifestyle to move toward a state of optimal health" (Minkler, 1989, p. 112). Health promotion is taking action to be healthy before (and to avoid) becoming sick. Payers of health care have begun to recognize that health costs are best contained through health promotion and disease prevention, rather than rescuing individuals with catastrophic health crises that could have been prevented through healthier lifestyles. It is important in the United States from a cost perspective as well as from a health perspective. Behaviors with a negative health impact, such as overconsumption of food, lack of exercise, smoking, and stress, contribute heavily to approximately 40% to 50% of morbidity and mortality in the United States (McGinnis & Foege, 1993; Woltz, 2000). Modifiable risk factors account for almost half of premature deaths among Americans (Danaei, Ding, Mozaffarian, Taylor, Rehm, Murray, & Ezzat, 2009). If citizens could be encouraged to change health behaviors—lose weight, stop smoking, and reduce stress—health-care costs could be substantially reduced.

Many health-care providers believe that health promotion is a straightforward process that simply requires the provision of information and instructions to decrease certain behaviors and increase others. For example, people are advised to stop smoking, lose weight, exercise, and eat more fruits and vegetables. However, it has become evident that simply providing information is insufficient to change behaviors (Harrison, 2010). Sometimes behaviors persist because of long habit, family values, or lack of funds. Sometimes the limited choices available in the community environment inhibit the ability to make healthy changes. The longer a person smokes, the more difficult it is to stop smoking; a family may value children who are overweight as a sign of health or wealth; and poor people usually have diets rich in simple carbohydrates and sugars because these foods are less expensive than proteins and vegetables. If a person wants to exercise by walking and the neighborhood is unsafe, it may be difficult to walk routinely. In short, changing health behaviors is a complex process.

Motivating people to make healthy lifestyle choices and changes is a difficult part of health-care practice (Berry & Miralito, 2010), and individuals who struggle with unhealthy behaviors require sustained support to overcome these problems. Several studies show the benefits of a team approach, including nurses, psychologists, educators, and coaches, in making meaningful and lasting behavior change (Noar, Benac, & Harris, 2007). Health promotion awareness and activities begin with public policy that addresses the known prerequisites of health, such as income, housing, food, security, literacy, employment, and quality working conditions. New population-based initiatives need to be developed and implemented at local community levels that promote health via the teaching of positive life practices and the provision of environmental supports to sustain them (Kelly, Melnyk, Jacobson, & O'Haver, 2010). Health policy should meet the needs of community members and provide opportunities to promote and improve health.

Advancing Your Knowledge

T.M., an advanced practice nurse with a DNP, has developed an after school program for children 12 to 15 years old to reduce obesity. The program incorporates education for both parents and children, an exercise program for the children with goals and prizes for reaching the goals, and a celebrity cooking class as part of the program. T.M. gets permission to test her program at a boys and girls club in a nearby neighborhood. She recruits 20 children and receives permission from parents to work with them. Not all of the children are obese, but all are overweight. The program proves to be successful in helping these children and families understand better the problems associated with childhood obesity, including adult obesity, heart disease, and diabetes. The program discusses the need for diet and exercise and how to get both without exorbitant cost. The celebrity chef program, as part of the overall program, is a great success, with local civic leaders coming to cook with the children once a week during the 12-week program. Overall, the children reach many of their exercise goals and are able to identify healthy snacks that they like and what foods to avoid or eat sparingly for good health. Of the 20 children in the program, 17 lose weight, and 10 have lower blood pressure than when the program started, and all of the families are invested in continuing the work begun during this program.

1. What are the health policy implications that could come from this program? How could health policy and advanced practice intersect around the issue of childhood obesity?

2. What is it about nursing, and advanced practice nursing in particular, that makes it incumbent on advanced practice nurses to be invested in health promotion?
3. Why should the United States as a whole be invested in health promotion?
4. What forms of health promotion could be paid for by the government or insurance that in the long run would save money and improve the quality of life of individuals?
5. Create your own community health initiative that would be advantageous for health promotion.

History of Health Promotion

The ideas of health promotion and disease prevention are not new to the 20th and 21st centuries. Consider the following health promotion time line:

- Hippocrates, a Greek physician born in 460 BCE, wrote that the body was influenced by outside forces. He felt that these forces could influence the health of a person. He believed that prescribing clean water, a healthy diet, and good hygiene for patients was the basis for medical care (National Center for Health Promotion and Disease Prevention, Veterans Health Administration, 2011).
- In the 19th century, Far and Snow, two English scientists, examined patterns of death in communities in London and found that people got sick depending on which part of the River Thames supplied their drinking water. Some parts of the river transmitted cholera, and the people whose drinking water came from that part of the river got sick and died at higher rates than others (Hennekens & Buring, 1987).
- The yearly checkup began in the United States in the 1920s as medical science advanced to treat medical conditions more successfully if they were diagnosed in the early stages.
- In the 1960s, health researchers began to look to the community to determine how health promotion and disease prevention could be moved outside of the clinical setting into the community.
- In 1978, WHO and the United Children's Fund (UNICEF) held a conference in the Soviet Union attended by 134 nations. In this summit, attendees recognized that health was more than the absence of disease and that health was influenced and affected by social, economic, and natural environment issues. At the end of this conference, both WHO and UNICEF adopted this philosophy for health promotion around the world (Green & Kreuter, 1990).
- In the United States, the Surgeon General called for preventive health in the 1979 report *Healthy People*. This report became the foundation for a prevention agenda and set objectives for communities to use to improve health. This report is reissued every 10 years to update the country on

the advances made in health promotion and disease prevention in priority areas. The most current report is *Healthy People 2010*, which provides health promotion goals for this decade.

- The Ottawa Charter of 1986 was the first international document to outline the need for and goals of health promotion. To reach a state of complete physical, mental, and social well-being, an individual or group must be able to identify and realize aspirations, to satisfy needs, and to change or cope with the environment. Health is seen as a resource for everyday life, not the objective of living.

WHO has since described fundamental conditions that must be present for health: peace, shelter, education, food, income, a stable ecosystem, sustainable resources, and social justice and equality. These conditions constitute a much expanded view of what is required for health and one that supports a holistic framework of determinants of health that could affect well-being and decrease the cost of medical services. Nursing has a worldview that persons are whole and complete at any moment, and advanced practice nurses take this nursing concept into the area of primary care and advanced practice.

Health Policy for Health Promotion

One way to stimulate interest in changing health behaviors is to initiate health policy that regulates the cost of health insurance based on health habits. This policy would be the same as having a good driver discount on automobile insurance. One such system is called *accountability-based wellness*; employees receive discounts on health insurance premiums based on attendance at wellness programs. These programs have shown measurable improvements in health indicators (Harrison, 2010). In these types of programs, participation saves the employee money and helps to create positive health habits. What if health-care insurers, including the government, charged more for health-care visits for "noncompliant" patients? For example, if a person refused to attend a smoking cessation class that was offered to him, insurance rates would increase. Consider how legislation would look if it were designed this way. Would it be unfair to anyone?

Thorpe & Ogden (2010) created a menu of potential legislative and government-driven reforms that could improve health. First on the menu are federal financial incentives for workplace health promotion programs. These types of programs would provide incentives for employers to adopt comprehensive worksite health promotion programs that could attract workers and sustain their commitment to behavior change. The motivation to employers could be in the forms of tax incentives, reduced employer insurance costs, or grant funding.

The second item Thorpe proposed is school-based interventions. Schools are held accountable for maintaining academic standards; they could also be held responsible for creating and achieving certain health standards for students.

These health standards could be accomplished through initiatives to improve school lunches, selections of healthy foods in vending machines, and promoting physical education. In addition, parents could be given reports on their child's health. Teacher-parent conferences about student progress not only could discuss academic achievement but also how the child rates on physical and health matters.

The final item on the menu includes community health centers where health promotion activities would take place. These health centers could be funded through local taxes, grants from health-care institutions, or federal grants. Classes in nutrition, exercise, managing chronic health problems, and stress reduction could be provided for the community at little or no cost. Incentives for community members to attend could be provided by local grocery store coupons for healthy food or local events.

Advancing Your Knowledge

J.F. is an advanced practice nurse with a DNP who is the manager of a community health clinic. Primary care services are provided in the clinic as well as educational classes, psychological services, physical therapy, occupational therapy, nutrition counseling, exercise classes of different levels, yoga classes, stress reduction classes, nutrition and cooking classes, and child care and childbirth classes. Self-help sessions such as Alcoholics Anonymous and Narcotics Anonymous are held at the community center. There are teen dances that are carefully chaperoned and discussion groups for adolescents about drug and alcohol use and sexuality. All members of the community are able to use the center and attend classes for free. The center is sponsored by the local government using a federal grant. Over the past 5 years, data from the center have shown a decrease in obesity and smoking, fewer teen pregnancies, successful self-efficacy, and reduced use of alcohol and drugs among community members. People who use the community center for primary care or physical services pay on a sliding scale based on income; however, they pay an extra $5 per visit if they smoke, abuse alcohol, or have a body mass index greater than 40. They pay an extra dollar if they have uncontrolled hypertension or blood sugar levels.

1. What do you think of this type of community center from an ethical perspective?
2. What do you see as barriers to starting something like this?
3. How could advanced practice nurses advocate for community centers similar to this one?
4. What services would you add to this clinic?
5. If the center could show considerable cost savings to the health-care system based on the health promotion and disease prevention activities provided there, who would be happy? Who would not?

The DNP as a Leader in Health Promotion

The DNP is well positioned to be a leader in health promotion initiatives. WHO (2008) proposed three important roles for health-care providers in the area of health promotion: advocate, enabler, and mediator. The first role is that of *advocate* for health promotion and disease prevention initiatives. An advocate is a person who pleads for a cause or propounds an idea; the DNP nurse with advanced education in health, population-based care, and leadership is well positioned to be an advocate for health promotion initiatives within the community and the nation.

The second role is that of *enabler*, or one who helps something to happen or supports another to achieve an end. In the area of health promotion, an enabler is a person who supports opportunities for individuals to take charge of their health to make healthy choices. DNP-prepared advanced practice nurses can use their skills in leadership and their knowledge of population-based health to create interventions to assist patients and families to live healthier lives. Examples of interventions are the development of after-school exercise programs for children, creating links for teens to discuss sexual practices and sexually transmitted infections, and assisting older adults in care coordination so that they can be independent for as long as possible. As an enabler, the DNP establishes an environment within the community that provides information on healthy choices and teaches life skills.

The final role is that of the *mediator*. A mediator acts as a link between parties who disagree. In the area of health promotion, the mediator coordinates actions between governmental agencies, industry, local authorities, the economic sector, social service and volunteer organizations, and the media to meet health promotion needs of citizens. The DNP-prepared nurse is educated to be a leader who can mediate between different societal segments within a community or in other areas to promote health and wellness. For example, the DNP could create appropriate access to care for cultural groups in the community and work with the state and local legislature to create policies that improve health and reduce the risk for disease.

The rapidly changing environments in technology, work, energy production, and urbanization are elements that affect health promotion. Systematic assessments of societal and environmental elements within the community related to health and health promotion and actions to ensure positive health policy are needed. To accomplish this assessment and action, health-care providers who are educated in population-based health issues and actions should assist communities to set priorities, make decisions, plan strategies, and implement them to achieve better health. Any health-care strategy must also address the conservation of natural resources and creation of healthy environments.

Advancing Your Knowledge

The year is 2025. The Toney family includes a grandmother, mother, father, and two children. Mother works as an accountant for a firm making advanced technology computers. Father works as an air traffic controller. Both children are in school. Grandmother lives with the family. Mother has a work program that allows her to attend an exercise program twice a week for the last hour of her work day. She also receives stress management time 2 other days a week when she can get a massage, participate in a mindfulness mediation class, or simply spend time in the corporate garden area where soft music is played. These additions to her day are completed within the 8 hours of work so that she can get home to be with her family. The cafeteria at work provides healthy meals that are low in fat and sugar and high in fiber. Her employer has noted fewer sick days and higher productivity since these services have been provided for employees.

Father has a high-stress job and receives stress management time during the workday each day, including exercise, massage, and other services. He has lunch in a garden dining area where healthy foods are provided. He also has access to the health club at work where there are exercise and fitness classes. Both children have 1-hour periods of exercise during school hours and find these energizing and fun. All foods served at school are low in fat, high in fiber, low in sugar, and very tasty. Each child has classes in school regarding sustainable environmental issues that promote health and preserve the earth's resources. Grandmother attends a community center senior program where dancing, exercise, and tai chi classes are provided each week. She also participates in a cooking class to learn about nutrition and how to keep herself and her family healthy.

The family often has "fast food" for dinner, which mother picks up on the way home. Fast food consists of salads (vegetables and fruit), whole grain sandwiches with low-fat meats, and whole wheat pasta. In the evening, the whole family takes a walk after dinner, and then there is time for entertainment.

1. What do you like or not like about this scenario? What changes would you make?
2. How could we achieve these types of changes in our society? Who would be the advocate for healthy workplaces, healthy schools, a healthy environment, and healthy aging?
3. How can health-care providers convince the public to adopt healthy behaviors and discontinue unhealthy habits?
4. Why is the DNP well positioned to advocate and enable such changes to take place?

DNP-educated advanced practice nurses with knowledge of leadership, health policy, and advocacy are positioned to become champions of health promotion policy in their communities and at state and national levels. Community groups, individuals, health professionals, health service institutions, and governments must work together to create a system where an environment conducive to health promotion is at the center of policy making. The health sector and health-care providers must foster a health promotion direction, moving beyond the responsibility for providing clinical and curative services. Health services should expand to include health promotion mandates that are sensitive to cultural and community needs and differences. DNPs should cultivate a change in attitudes of policy makers and a reorganization of health delivery systems to refocus on the total needs of the community. Table 6-6 lists Web sites useful for the DNP who is invested in health-care policy and advocacy.

Table 6-6

Web Sites for Policy and Legislation

Name of Web Site	URL
American Academy of Nurse Practitioners	*http://www.aanp.org/AANPCMS2*
American Association of Nurse Executives	*http://www.aone.org/*
American Nurses Association	*http://www.nursingworld.org/*
Centers for Disease Control and Prevention	*http://www.cdc.gov/*
Gerontological Advanced Practice Nurses Association (GAPNA)	*https://www.gapna.org/cgi-bin/WebObjects/GAPNA*
Global Policy Forum	*http://www.globalpolicy.org/*
Information on U.S. senators	*http://www.senate.gov/general/contact_information/senators_cfm (Find your senator in the upper search boxi)*
International Council of Nurses	*http://www.icn.ch/*
National Association of Clinical Nurse Specialists (NACNS)	*http://www.nacns.org/*
National Association of Pediatric Nurse Practitioners	*http://www.napnap.org/index.aspx*
National Organization of Nurse Practitioner Faculty (NONPF)	*http://www.nonpf.org/displaycommon.cfm?an=1&subarticlenbr=25*
Nurse Practitioners in Women's Health (NPWH)	*http://www.npwh.org/i4a/pages/index.cfm?pageid=1*
Safe Patient Project—lists all patient safety bills before state legislatures	*http://www.safepatientproject.org/2010/02/2010_state_patient_safety_legi_1.html*
Sigma Theta Tau International Honor Society of Nursing	*http://www.nursingsociety.org/default.aspx*
USA.gov—contacting elected officials at the federal and state levels	*http://www.usa.gov/Contact/Elected.shtml*
U.S. Department of Health and Human Services	*http://www.hhs.gov/*
Write Your Representative—information on U.S. congressmen and congresswomen	*https://writerep.house.gov/writerep/welcome.shtml*

Conclusion

Involvement in the health-care policy debate is an important aspect of practice for professional nurses. Health-care policy decisions determine the present and future objectives of the health-care system. Nurses, as members of a profession, are interested in healthy populations and advocate for social justice, health, and all its determinants. Advocacy for policy and resources that are needed to implement health-care programs is an important role for advanced practice nurses.

Health care within the United States is not a right but a privilege that must be paid for personally or through health insurance. Although the United States may have the most advanced health-care technology in the world, many Americans are without access to basic health care. How the nation chooses to distribute the finite resources within health care becomes a policy debate. This debate has gone on for many years with little change in the way health care is accessed. The United States spends more per capita on health care than any country in the world, but it does not rank among the best countries for providing health-care services or achieving positive health outcomes.

A health-care reform bill, the Patient Protection and Affordable Care Act of 2010, was passed in March 2010. This bill is the first real recent change in the way health care in the United States is distributed. As with most new legislation, what the bill does and how it works to improve the health of all Americans are still to be seen. Changes to the bill are being contemplated and will be suggested by legislators at both the federal and the state levels. DNPs must be part of the debate about where health-care dollars are spent and how health care is provided in the United States. To be successful contributors to this process, DNPs must be knowledgeable in all aspects of health care legislation and the policy process.

References

Aittasalo, M., Miilunpalo, S., Kukkonen-Harjula, K., & Pasanen, M. (2006). A randomized intervention of physical activity promotion and patient self-monitoring in primary care. *Preventative Medicine, 42*(1), 40–46.

American Academy of Nurse Practitioners. (2010). Nurse practitioner prescriptive authority. Retrieved from http://www.aanp.org/NR/rdonlyres/8A2583FC-981F-45FD-BB6D-094BDF4AEE7A/0/AuthoritytoPrescribeMap72710Color.pdf

American Association of Colleges of Nursing. (2006). The essentials of doctoral education for advanced nursing practice. Retrieved from http://www.aacn.nche.edu/dnp/pdf/essentials.pdf

American Organization of Nurse Executives. (2010). Organizational information. Retrieved from http://www.aone.org/membership/about/press_releases/press_releases.shtml

Berry, L., & Miralito, A. (2010). Innovative health care delivery. *Business Horizons, 53*(2), 157–169.

Blankenhorn, D. (2010). U.S. still lags in health care value for money. Retrieved from http://www.smartplanet.com/blog/rethinking-healthcare/us-still-lags-in-health-care-value-for-money/1331

Bodenheimer, T. (2010). Primary care: Current problems and proposed solutions. *Health Affairs, 29,* 799–805.

Bostridge, M. (2008). *Florence Nightingale: The woman and her legend.* New York, NY: Viking Press.

Centers for Disease Control and Prevention. (2009). National Center for Health Statistics. Retrieved from http://www.cdc.gov/nchs/

Cherry, B., & Jacob, S. (2005). *Contemporary issues in nursing: Issues, trends and management* (3rd ed.). St. Louis, MO: Mosby.

Congressional Budget Office. (2010). Cost estimates for health care legislation. Retrieved from http://www.cbo.gov/publications/collections/health.cfm

Danaei, G., Ding, E. L., Mozaffarian, D., Taylor, B., Rehm, J., Murray, C. J., & Ezzati, M. (2009). The preventable causes of death in the United States: Comparative risk assessment of dietary, lifestyle, and metabolic risk factors. PLoS Med 6(4): e1000058. doi:10.1371/journal.pmed.1000058

Davidson, S. (2010). *Still broken: Understanding the U.S. health care system.* Stanford, CA: Stanford University Press.

Elkin, E., Ishill, N., Riley, G., Bach, P., Gonen, M., Begg, C., & Schrag, D. (2008). Disenrollment from Medicare managed care among beneficiaries with and without a cancer diagnosis. *Journal of the National Cancer Institute, 100*(14), 1013–1021.

Enthoven, A., Kronick, R. (1989). A consumer-choice health plan for the 1990s. Universal health insurance in a system designed to promote quality and economy. *New England Journal of Medicine. 320*(1):29–37.

Fisher, E. (2008). Dartmouth study on end of life Medicare spending. Kaiser Daily Health Policy Report. Retrieved from http://www.kaisernetwork.org/daily_reports/rep_index.cfm?DR_ID=51385

Flocke, S., Crabtree, B.J., & Strange, K.C. (2007). Clinician reflections on promotion of healthy behaviors in primary care practice. *Health Policy, 84*(2–3), 277–283.

Garson, A. (2010). The U.S. health care system, 2010: Problems, principals and potential solutions. *Circulation, 101,* 2015.

Green, L., & Kreuter, M. (1990). Health promotion as a public health strategy for 1990s. *Annual Review of Public Health,* 11, 311–334.

Greene, S., Reiter, K., Kilpatrick, K., Leatherman, S., Someres, S., & Hamlin, A. (2008). Searching for a business case for quality in Medicaid managed care. *Health Care Management Review, 33*(4), 350–360.

Harrison, J. (2010). Health behavior initiatives. Retrieved from http://www.marketwire.com/press-release/Accountability-Based-Wellness-Saves-Money-Improves-Health-1322578.htm

Hennekens, C.H., & Buring, J.E. (1987). *Epidemiology in medicine.* Boston, MA: Little, Brown.

Herzlinger, R. (2010). Health care reform and its implications for the US economy. *Business Horizons, 53*(2), 105–117.

Hoffman, C. (2009). Focus on Health Reform. Publication # 7871. Kaiser Family Foundation. Retrieved from http://www.kff.org/healthreform/upload/7871.pdf

Institute of Medicine. (2001). Crossing the quality chasm: A new healthcare system for the 21st century. Retrieved from http://www.iom.edu/~/media/Files/Report%20Files/2001/Crossing-the-Quality-Chasm/Quality%20Chasm%202001%20%20report%20brief.pdf

International Council of Nurses. (2000). Participation of nurses in health services decision making and policy development. Retrieved from http://www.icn.ch/publications/position-statements/

Kaiser Family Foundation. (2009). Health care report. Retrieved from http://www.kaiseredu.org/topics_im.asp?imID=1&parentID=61&id=358

Kaiser Family Foundation. (2010). Health tracking poll, conducted April 9-14, 2010. Retrieved from http://www.kff.org/kaiserpolls/upload/8067-C.pdf

Kaufman, S. (2006). *And a time to die: How American hospitals shape the end of life.* Chicago, IL: The Chicago University Press.

Kelly, S., Melnyk, B., Jacobson, D., & O'Haver, J. (2011). Correlates among healthy lifestyle cognitive beliefs, healthy lifestyle choices, social support and healthy behaviors in adolescents: Implications for behavioral change strategies and future research. *Journal of Pediatric Health Care, 25*(4), 216–223. Retrieved from http://www.sciencedirect.com/science?_ob=ArticleURL&_udi=B6WKK-4YX65M7-2&_user=10&_coverDate=04%2F22%2F2010&_rdoc=1&_fmt=high&_orig=search&_origin=search&_sort=d&_docanchor=&view=c&_searchStrId=1521119587&_rerunOrigin=google&_acct=C000050221&_version=1&_urlVersion=0&_userid=10&md5=b60458c17b7b3416f691041e182c4f29&searchtype=a - vitae

Kleefeld, E. (2009) Poll: Americans overwhelmingly favor universal health care: Until taxes are mentioned. Retrieved from http://tpmdc.talkingpointsmemo.com/2009/05/poll-americans-overwhelmingly-favor-universal-health-care----until-taxes-are-mentioned.php

Kling, A. (2010). American health care policy issues. Retrieved from http://econlog.econlib.org/archives/2010/08/american_health.html

Laurant, M. (2005). Substituting nurses for doctors results in high quality care, few savings. *Medical News Today.* Retrieved from http://www.medicalnewstoday.com/articles/23495.php

Leavitt, L., Chaffee, M., & Vance, C. (2007). Learning the ropes of policy, politics and advocacy. In D. Mason, J. Leavitt, & M. Chaffee (Eds.), *Policy and politics in nursing and health care* (5th ed., pp. 239–241). St. Louis, MO: Saunders.

Ledue, C. (2010). Poll: One in four health care dollars spent unnecessarily. *Health Care Finance News*. Retrieved from http://www.health carefinancenews.com/news/poll-one-four-healthcare-dollars-spent-unnecessarily

Lee, K. (2009). Health care affordable quality coverage for all. *Otolaryngology, 140*(6), 775–781.

Mason, D., Leavitt, J., & Chaffee, M. (Eds.). (2007). *Policy and politics in nursing and health care* (5th ed.). St. Louis, MO: Saunders.

Mathews, J. R. (2006). Social justice versus market incentive: Allocating finite health care resources. Retrieved from http://www.suite101.com/content/social-justice-v--market-incentive-a9312

Mears, B. (2010). Judge rejects motion to dismiss 20 states' lawsuits against health care law. *CNN US*. Retrieved from http://www.cnn.com/2010/US/10/14/health.care.challenge/index.html

McGinnis, J. M., & Foege, W. H. (1993). Actual causes of death in the United States. *Journal of the American Medical Association, 270*(18), 2207–2212.

Medicare.gov. (2010). How big is Medicare? What does the future hold. Retrieved from http://www.medicare.gov/

Minkler, M. (1989). Health education, health promotion and the open society, an historical perspective. *Health Education Quarterly, 16*(1), 17–30.

Mitka, M. (2008). Health insurance costs remain a burden for employers and working families. *Journal of the American Medical Association, 300*(16), 1863–1968.

National Center for Health Promotion and Disease Prevention, Veterans Health Administration. (2011). The VA history in health promotion and disease prevention. Retrieved from http://www.prevention.va.gov/index.asp

Noah, T. (2007). A short history of health care. *Slate*. Retrieved from http://www.slate.com/id/2161736

Noar, S., Benac, C., & Harris, M. (2007). Does tailoring matter? A meta-analysis of tailored health behavior change interventions. *Psychological Bulletin, 133*(4), 673–683.

Oden, L., Price, J., Alteneder, R., Broadley, D., & Ubokudom, S. (2004). Public policy involvement by nurse practitioners. *Journal of Community Health,* 25(2), 139–155.

Pifer-Bixler, P. (2009). 87.6 million Americans uninsured over last two years. *Health Report CNN*. Retrieved from http://articles.cnn.com/2009-03-04/health/uninsured.epidemic.obama_1_families-usa-health-insurance-health-coverage?_s=PM:HEALTH

Pohl, J.M., Hanson, C., Newland, J.A., & Cronenwet, L. (2010). Unleashing nurse practitioners' potential to deliver primary care and lead teams. *Health Affairs, 29,* 900–905.

Reuters Press. (2009, September 13). How many lobbyists are there in Washington. Retrieved from http://www.reuters.com/article/2009/09/13/obama-lobbying-idUSN1348032520090913

Schratz, L. (2010). Evidence based health care reform: Lessons learned from Massachusetts. *Breitbart Health Report*. Retrieved from http://biggovernment.com/lschratz/2010/01/19/evidence-based-health-care-reform-lessons-from-massachusetts/

Sigma Theta Tau International. (2005). Policy position statement. Retrieved from http://www.nursingsociety.org/aboutus/PositionPapers/Pages/policy.aspx

Simmons, J. (October 12, 2009). Adding tort reform to healthcare reform could lower costs. *HealthLeaders Media.*

Siskel, E. (2010). Reducing fraud, waste, and abuse in Medicare spending. A report to the Congressional Subcommittee on Health and Subcommittee on Oversight,

Committee on Ways and Means, United States House of Representatives. Retrieved from http://www.mainjustice.com/2010/06/15/doj-eliminating-medicare-fraud-waste-a-priority/

Stokowski, L. (2010). The nurse practitioner will see you now. *Medscape Nursing.* Retrieved from http://www.medscape.com/viewarticle/723986

Thompson, J., & Lee, V. (2007). The effect of health insurance disparities on the health care system. *AORN Journal, 86*(5), 745–748.

Thorpe, K., & Ogden, L., (2010). Foundation that health care reform lays for improved paymen, care coordination and prevention. *Health Affairs 29*(6), 1183–1187.

U.S. Department of Health and Human Services. (2009). Overview of the uninsured in the United States. Retrieved from http://aspe.hhs.gov/health/reports/05/uninsured-cps/index.htm

Van Leuven, K. (2006). The reality of health promotion. *California Journal of Health Promotion, 4*(4), 36–40.

Woltz, M. (2000). Statement from the National High Blood Pressure Education Program: Prevalence of hypertension, *American Journal of Hypertension, 13*(1), 103–104.

World Health Organization. (2008). Workplace health promotion: The workplace a priority setting. Retrieved from http://www.who.int/occupational_health/topics/workplace/en/

CHAPTER 7

Ruth McCaffrey
Todd Swinderman

INFORMATION SYSTEMS/TECHNOLOGY AND PATIENT CARE TECHNOLOGY FOR THE IMPROVEMENT AND TRANSFORMATION OF HEALTH CARE

Objectives:

By the end of the chapter, students should be able to:

1. Describe the current uses of informatics in health care today, in particular, the benefits of informatics for advanced practice nurses.
2. Describe the history of health-care documentation and how information has increased and changed to improve patient outcomes.
3. Classify the way in which information technology has been effective in health-care delivery systems:
   a. Explain the basic elements of data and data storage.
   b. Recognize computer terminology and definitions.
   c. Construct a method and define the selection criteria for choosing a computer system for documentation and billing.
4. Describe the ways in which advanced practice nurses can and should use information systems and technology in practice to improve outcomes, reduce health-care costs, and improve overall health quality:
   a. Describe and appraise the role of the informatics nurse in supporting advanced nursing practice.

   b. List Web sites that are useful for advanced practice nurses in the area of technology and informatics.
   c. Analyze the effectiveness of telemedicine, and formulate a plan for using telemedicine in advanced practice.
5. Describe privacy issues related to health-care informatics and technology. Discuss methods for maintaining patient privacy and the ethical treatment of patient information.
6. Describe patients' use of information on the worldwide Web. Evaluate the pros and cons associated with this information, including accuracy of information.
7. Appraise the use of a Web site for a practice. Describe the components needed to develop a Web site.
8. Analyze methods for learning about and increasing the use of informatics to improve patient outcomes and safety at all levels of nursing education.

As the health-care system in the United States becomes more focused on disease prevention, health promotion, and population-based health, knowledge of and the ability to use medical informatics will become essential for leaders. The doctor of nursing practice (DNP) graduate will be challanged to be familiar with uses of informatics and appropriate methods to evaluate and implement informatics technology in health-care settings.

In 1984, the Panel on the General Professional Education of the Physician and College Preparation for Medicine prepared a report on the need for informatics knowledge among all persons providing health care. The objectives recommended by the panel include that all health-care providers should be able to do the following (Jordon, 2002, p. 35):

- Manage information bases for use in treating patients
- Treat patients more efficiently and cost-effectively by using national databases as references
- Rely on technology to free up provider time to be used on personal aspects of patient care
- Improve the education process through the incorporation of information technology, decision-making science, and computer-assisted instruction.

This chapter provides information relevant to the need for and uses of information systems in health care, the use of advanced technologies in advanced practice nursing, and transforming health care through the use of information systems. Specifically, this chapter discusses (1) the need for increased use of informatics in health-care settings, (2) methods for evaluation and implementation of informatics systems, and (3) general ways in which informatics can increase knowledge and improve population-based care.

Current Uses of Informatics in Health Care Today

Health-care informatics is the intersection of three distinct disciplines: information science, computer science, and health care. Regardless of the practice setting—clinical practice, administration, research, or education—technology can be used to support nursing in direct and indirect care practice. Knowledge required for competence in the area of health-care informatics includes understanding available resources, devices, and methods required to optimize the acquisition, storage, retrieval, and use of information in health, biomedicine, and nursing. Tools for health-care informatics include not only computers but also clinical guidelines, formal medical terminologies, and information and communication systems. Over the last decade, health-care organizations embraced the Internet as a medium for publishing general health information and allowing patients to gain more knowledge about medical conditions, treatment plans, and options for care. In 2009, more than 90% of the approximately 5000 member institutions of the American Hospital Association reported having Web sites, with most having descriptive information about their facilities and services (American Hospital Association, 2009).

Electronic Health Records

In addition to Web sites, another major use of informatics is the electronic health record (EHR). The term *electronic health record* is used interchangeably with the term *electronic medical record.* "Gradually, the informatics community has been adopting 'electronic health record' as a name more in keeping with modern perspectives on comprehensive health care, health maintenance, and multidisciplinary practice" (Hunter, 2001, p. 186). "Besides providing complete, accurate patient data, regardless of location of the patient, the system will provide decision support, contain clinical reminders and alerts, and provide links to related knowledge bases" (Thede, 2003, p. 320). The Institute of Medicine (IOM) at the National Institutes of Health recognized the important role that the EHR could play in the health of Americans. To establish standards for EHRs, the IOM has provided a list of eight standards that all computerized medical records should offer, as follows (Association for Healthcare Research and Quality, 2010):

- Physician access to patient information, such as diagnoses, allergies, laboratory results, and medications
- Access to new and past test results among providers in multiple care settings
- Computerized provider order entry
- Computerized decision-support systems to prevent drug interactions and improve compliance with best practices
- Secure electronic communication among providers and patients

- Patient access to health records, disease management tools, and health information resources
- Computerized administration processes, such as scheduling systems
- Standards-based electronic data storage and reporting for patient safety and disease surveillance efforts

The EHR automates and streamlines the clinician's work flow, while increasing the accuracy and consistency of information provided about the patient and treatment plan. In this way, the EHR is able to generate a complete record of a clinical encounter and support other care-related activities, such as office intiative treatments, referrals, and medications. The EHR can also support care and patient treatment by including evidence-based decision support, quality management, and outcomes reporting.

The American Recovery and Reinvestment Act (ARRA) of 2009 was created to assist health-care business and practice in increasing its use of information technology. This act contains the Health Information Technology for Economic and Clinical Health (HITECH) Act and created the Office of the National Coordinator for Health Information Technology (ONC), which reports to the Secretary of Health and Human Services. The goals of this act are to provide incentives for standardization of terminology and data and to facilitate electronic exchange of data by 2014. Establishing an EHR is included in the HITECH Act, with incentives for nurse practitioners practicing in federally qualified health centers or rural health clinics.

In 2004, the U.S. Department of Health and Human Services formed the Office of the National Coordinator for Health Information Technology (ONCHIT). The mission of this office was to oversee the widespread adoption of EHRs in the United States within 10 years. Health-care technology has lagged behind other industries, which are transforming the delivery of health care in the United States, necessitating the government-proposed EHR initiative (Laramee, Bosek, Kasprisin, & Powers-Phaneuf, 2010). To encourage the use of EHRs throughout the United States, Medicare will reduce payments by 1% each year to health-care facilities that do not reach the benchmark of using an EHR system by 2015. Physicians, dentists, podiatrists, optometrists, and chiropractors are eligible for $44,000 in Medicare incentives for adopting qualified EHRs (Abraham, 2010).

The Regional Health Information Organizations (RHIO), in cooperation with the U.S. National Health Information Network, is working toward a health information exchange (HIE) with the ultimate goal of establishing a standard EHR for most Americans by 2014. The RHIOs and HIE would enable clinical and biomedical data sharing; this is similar to having a savings account at one bank and using an automated teller machine (ATM) at any other bank around the country to withdraw cash. As applied to health care, it means that all health-care providers could access just one universal medical record per individual. That record would contain an individual's history, allergies, medications, test results, and any other care received from any and all health practitioners. Such consistency in the records not only would eliminate waste but also would reduce medical errors. HIE requires standardization and interoperability of multiple systems. For interoperability to occur, there must be consistent standards, and all systems must be willing to share and communicate in a standard format.

Computerized Patient Records

A computerized patient record (CPR) is a system where care providers "... directly enter patient data, findings, and notes into a computer system that may be linked to a hospital-wide database and decision support system. The difference between CPR and an EHR is that the CPR is usually limited to one facility (acute care, ambulatory clinic, etc) and, at times, to one episode of occurrence" (Patel, Kushniruk, Yang, & Yale, 2000, p. 570).

Computerized provider (physician) order entry entails care providers placing orders directly into the computer. The system sends orders directly to the performing departments, expediting treatment and eliminating the problem of illegible orders. Clinical decision support (CDS) is available at the time of order entry.

Institute of Medicine Report on the Need for Informatics in Health Care

A report from the IOM entitled, "Crossing the Quality Chasm: A New Healthcare System for the 21st Century" (IOM, 2001), emphasized the use of information technology to produce care that is safe, effective, efficient, patient-centered, timely, and equitable. This report documented the need for increased use of information technology in health care. Areas that could be improved based on the information in the IOM report include patient safety, increased compliance with guidelines and improved diagnostic ability, patient-centered care through education based on the use of Web sites and information pages, customized disease management, cost reduction by eliminating redundant laboratory tests, and timeliness of information dissemination to both clinicians and patients. The IOM listed informatics as a core competency for all health-care professionals and stated that informatics knowledge is essential to patient-centered care, working in interdisciplinary teams, evidence-based practice, and quality improvement.

Despite the IOM report, the use of health-care informatics among health-care providers continues to lag significantly behind advances in informatics science and is being challenged to "catch up" so that information can be used to improve the lives of Americans (Jordan, 2002). The U.S. government economic stimulus package targeted financial assistance to health-care practices of all sizes for the purchase and use of information systems. When practices are purchased by hospitals or other health-care systems, information technology is often provided to the practice. These services are usually supported by information systems departments at the main health-care institution, but adequate education and customization of these technologies require input from health-care providers within the practice setting. As health care moves toward an information-based system of care delivery, advanced practice nurses prepared with a DNP must provide leadership in the field to encourage the use of appropriate information technologies to promote health and manage the health-care needs of large groups.

Medical and nursing science has created an explosion of knowledge in the areas of health promotion, disease treatment, and well-being. Although this information has benefits, it also creates problems when attempting to keep pace with an escalating body of knowledge. Persons who are unfamiliar with informatics and are unable to critique information presented in the ever-expanding literature that appears on the worldwide Web and medical databases will be left to ponder conflicting information and become more uncertain. Information does not always equal knowledge or truth. Being a wise and educated consumer of information is another essential factor for the advanced practice nurse.

Use of Informatics in Critical Thinking and Decision Making

Decision making is a critical component of nursing education and is an important competency for advanced practice nurses. Emphasis among health-care leaders has been placed on using critical thinking in the area of patient safety. Advanced practice nurses make critical decisions about patient care based on judgment, intuition, diagnostic reasoning, and knowledge obtained from the evidence of research. Patel and Currie (2005) theorized that the most effective methods employed by nurses in problem solving include pattern recognition, focused problem solving, and deliberate problem solving. In a study, these authors found that although advanced practice nurses usually make appropriate decisions, they are not always able to articulate the evidence-based reasons for the decisions made. Errors in decision making were found to be due to incorrect or incomplete knowledge, biases, or information overload. These authors discussed the use of technology to support decision making and human performance in the clinical area. They posited that using effective health-care information systems could assist clinicians in gathering data more systematically and efficiently. Informatics systems could reduce the information overload by creating a systematic analysis of practice and population data and allow advanced practice nurses to focus on higher-order thinking skills. Electronic documentation has the potential to benefit the patient and the entire multidisciplinary health-care team by rapid communication, results, assessments, alerts for laboratory values and allergies, and CDS for maximal clinical decision making. EHRs that are available to authorized care providers through secure Internet or intranet access allow care providers to obtain information and intervene quickly based on real-time nursing assessments.

Patel and Currie (2005) found that when health-care providers did not use an EHR, they focused their documentation on exploration and discovery. After beginning to use an electronic documentation system, however, their documentation was aimed in the direction of problem solving, problem detection, and hypothesis-driven reasoning. Technology can reduce the amount of time and effort used to retrieve basic information and can assist in accessing population-based data and knowledge derived from research. Information technology will change the way advanced practice nurses think and reason and support decision making that is evidence-based and consistent with nursing values.

Clinical decision support "... is software that [is] designed to be a direct aid to clinical decision-making, in which the characteristics of an individual patient are matched to a computerized clinical knowledge base and patient specific assessments or recommendations are then presented to the clinician or the patient for a decision" (Sim et al., 2001, p. 528). CDS can help providers in checking relevant laboratory results and allergies and in other decision making. Some computer software simply flags laboratory values that are high or low, with a special flag for values that are potentially dangerous. Other CDS software provides the clinican with a decision tree or a standardized plan of care for the elements entered into the computer. For example, if a patient has a blood sugar value of 350 mg/dL, the laboratory value will be flagged as dangerously high, and the clinican will be provided with a plan that includes obtaining further laboratory work and initiating treatment, medication, and follow-up and a list of other signs and symptoms that may indicate diabetic ketoacidosis and require hospitalization. If a clinician orders trimethoprim-sulfamethoxazole (Bactrim) for a patient who is allergic to sulfa drugs, the computer will flag this prescription to remind the clinician of the patient's allergy and ask for a different drug to be prescribed.

History of Information Technology in Health Care

In 1966, the U.S. government began to use computer systems to process the standardized forms required for reimbursement of health-care services provided to elderly patients through Medicare (Saba, 2001b, p. 180). During that time, Saba explained that billing studies were conducted to determine how computer technology could be effective in the health-care industry and what areas of nursing might be automated. The initial attempts to create electronic medical records began based on the findings from these investigations.

In the 1970s, nursing began to contribute actively to the design of information systems by consulting with health-care agencies about selecting and using information technology and helping install and use information systems in hospitals (Ball, Hannah, & Douglas, 2000). In 1971, two events were pivotal in advancing information technology. First, health maintenance organizations came into being and were caring for large numbers of clients using systems of primary care providers and referrals for specialist care. Second, a computerized medical information system was introduced to the health-care industry. This system revolutionized the way adopting hospitals maintained patient records and has a continuing impact on nursing documentation as the CPR is honed and implemented in increasing numbers of health-care institutions (Staggers, Thompson, & Snyder-Halpern, 2001).

For information systems to assist in classification and aggregation of patient data, standarized terminology must be developed so that data are consistently identified and evaluated. In the 1980s, diagnostic-related groups (DRGs) were established as a standard data tool within Medicare as a system of prospective payment for health-care services. This plan changed the way hospitals were reimbursed for services and required additional nursing documentation to describe services provided. Although DRGs created standard terminology for medical care, there was no such terminology created for nursing care. In 1982, the ANA formed the Steering Committee of Classification of Nursing Practice. This group was charged with developing strategies to name, identify, and classify the phenomena of nursing practice, whether at the bedside or in advanced practice nursing (Saba, 2001a).

In 1994, the American Nurses Association (ANA) recognized nursing informatics as a speciality and created a certification for eligible individuals. *Nursing informatics* now is a collaborative effort that includes registered nurses, educators, systems analysts, Web analysts, security coordinators, and system administrators; the focus is to enhance nursing practice through the creative use of technology, maximizing nursing productivity, improving the work environment infrastructure, and further supporting the excellence in patient care.

In his State of the Union Address on January 20, 2004, President George W. Bush became the first president to call for the use of technology in health care. He called for the use of information technology to capture health records to avoid dangerous medical mistakes, reduce costs, and improve care.

Nuts and Bolts of Informatics in Health-Care Delivery

Using informatics technology in practice requires an understanding of the different uses of this technology and the effect this technology can have on nursing practice and on patient care. There is much to know about informatics, but several areas are of particular importance to advanced practice nurses. Understanding computer technology creates a mechanism whereby an advanced practice nurse can comprehend and gain insight into the way computers and informatics software work and how they can improve health care. One of the roles of advanced practice nurses is to educate patients. With so much information on the Internet, it is challenging to guide patients to good sources of quality information. Evaluating consumer health information services is an important role for the advanced practice nurse to help patients receive information that is useful and not harmful. When educating patients, the development of Web sites could be a useful tool. Being able to use the Internet to distribute quality information to patients can increase patient satisfaction and improve the health of patients. When patient data are collected using informatics technology, it must be appropriately stored so that it can be used and so that patients are protected. Advanced practice nurses must understand the definition of informatics data, where it comes from, and how it is stored and retrieved for use.

Computer Terminology

The first step in understanding information technology and computers is to understand the terminology that is used in the field. As in health care, nursing, and other professions, taxonomy provides insight into what and how things work. Table 7-1 defines common computer terms that may be useful to advanced practice nurses (Rohan Academic Computing, 2010). Although the list is not exhaustive, Table 7-1 provides definitions of many of the most commonly used terms when either buying or using a computer information system.

Table 7-1

Common Computer Terminology

Access provider—company that provides Internet access and, in some cases, an online account on its computer system

Bandwidth—transmission capacity of the lines that carry the electronic traffic of the Internet. In many cases of health-care records, the bandwidth may be too small to transmit desired information (audio/video). This has imposed severe limitations on the ability of the Internet to deliver everything that is demanded from it. However, fiberoptic cables will ensure that bandwidth will soon be essentially limitless and free

Baud—unit of measurement that denotes the number of bits (the basic piece of information for computer storage) that can be transmitted per second. For example, if a modem is rated at 9600 baud, it is capable of transmitting data at a rate of 9600 bits per second

Browser—software interface to the worldwide Web; it interprets hypertext links and lets you view sites and navigate from one Internet node to another. Companies that produce browsers include Internet Explorer, Mozilla Firefox, America Online (AOL), and Flock

Bug (or glitch)—mistake, or unexpected occurrence, in a piece of software or in a piece of hardware. A bug usually causes the program to shut down, stop working, or work improperly until the bug has been removed

Cache—browser cache plays an important role in providing a smooth and speedy surfing experience. Cache is a temporary holding area for images, sounds, videos, and other items that may appear on a Web page that you visit. The browser cache works by eliminating the need to re-download an image or Web page if the content has not changed since your last visit. Size of the disc cache varies depending on the size of your hard drive and if you have manually altered the size of your browser (e.g., Microsoft Internet Explorer, Netscape). Typical cache size is 10% of your hard-drive space. In some cases, it is necessary to "refresh" the cache to obtain materials that are being downloaded

Central processing unit (CPU)—"brain" of the computer. Sometimes referred to simply as the processor or central processor, the CPU is where most calculations take place. In terms of computing power, the CPU is the most important element of a computer system

Clipboard—area used to store cut or copied information. The clipboard can store text, graphics, objects, and other data. The clipboard contents are erased when new information is placed on the clipboard or when the computer is shut down

Continued on page 302

Continued from page 301 Table 7-1

Common Computer Terminology

Configuration—(1) components that make up a computer system (which model and what peripherals); (2) physical arrangement of those components (what is placed and where); (3) software settings that enable two computer components to talk to each other (as in configuring communications software to work with a modem)

Coaxial cable—type of cable that contains two conductors and is required for data transmission on the Internet. The center conductor is surrounded by a layer of insulation, which is wrapped by a braided-metal conductor and an outer layer

Cookies—most commonly refers to a piece of information sent by a Web server to a Web browser that the browser software is expected to save and send back to the server whenever the browser makes additional requests from the server. Depending on the type of cookie used and the browser's settings, the browser may accept or not accept the cookie and may save the cookie for either a short time or a long time. Cookies might contain information such as login or registration information, online "shopping cart" information, or user preferences. When a server receives a request from an Internet browser that includes a cookie, the server is able to use the information stored in the cookie. For example, the server might customize what is sent back to the user or keep a log of particular users' requests. Cookies are usually set to expire after a predetermined amount of time and are usually saved in memory until the browser software is closed down, at which time they may be saved to disc if their "expire time" has not been reached. Cookies do not read your hard drive and send your life story to the CIA, but they can be used to gather more information about a user than would be possible without them

Dedicated line—telephone or data line that is always available. A leased telephone line can be dedicated for computer data communications. This line is not used by other computers or individuals, is available 24 hours a day, and is never disconnected

Digital signature—means of proving that a file or e-mail message belongs to a specific person, similar to a driver's license being used to prove identity in real life. Digital signatures have the added benefit of verifying that your message has not been tampered with. When you sign a message, a hash function—a computation that leaves a specific code, or "digital fingerprint"—is applied to it. If the fingerprint on the recipient's message does not match the original fingerprint, the message has been altered. Digital signatures are often used in combination with strong encryption software to create a secure channel of communication, in which both privacy and identity are protected.

Domain name—located to the right of the "@" sign in an e-mail address, or about 10 characters into a URL. U-Wipe's domain name is *u-wipe.com*. The domain name of info@nrlab.com is *nrlab.com*. Domain names are issued by the National Science Foundation, and they come with different extensions based on whether the domain belongs to a commerical enterprise (*.com*), an educational establishment (*.edu*), a government body (*.gov*), the military (*.mil*), a network (*.net*), or a nonprofit organization (*.org*). Some domains also use a geographical notation (e.g., the United Kigdom, www.amazon.co.uk)

Firewall—mechanism that isolates a network from the rest of the Internet, permitting only specific traffic to pass in and out

Freeware—programming that is offered at no cost. However, it is copyrighted so that you cannot incorporate its programming into anything you may be developing

Continued from page 302 Table 7-1

Common Computer Terminology

Home page—document that is displayed when you first open a Web site

Host—main computer system to which users are connected

HTML (hypertext markup language)—system for tagging various parts of a Web document that tells the Web client programs how to display the document's text, links, graphics, and attached media

IP (Internet Protocol)—unique string of numbers that identifies a computer on the Internet. These numbers are usually shown in groups separated by periods: 124.198.76.1. All resources on the Internet must have an IP address

OS (operating system)—a computer by itself is essentially bits of wire and silicon. An operating system knows how to talk to this hardware and can manage a computer's functions, such as allocating memory, scheduling tasks, accessing disk drives, and supplying a user interface. Without an operating system, software developers would have to write programs that directly accessed hardware—essentially reinventing the wheel with every new program. With an operating system, developers can write to a common set of programming interfaces called APIs and let the operating system do the dirty work of talking to the hardware

PDF (portable document format)—electronic facsimile of a printed document

Pixel (picture element)—digital images are composed of touching pixels, each having a specific color or tone. The eye merges differently colored pixels into continuous tones

Pop-up—graphic user interface display area, usually a small window, that suddenly appears in the foreground of the visual interface. Pop-ups can be initiated by a single or double mouse click or rollover (sometimes called a *mouseover*), can be initiated by voice command, or can be timed to occur

RAM (Random Access Memory)—most common type of computer memory and where the computer stores system software, programs, and data currently in use. It was formerly called *dynamic RAM (DRAM)* because it is volatile—that is, the contents are lost when you turn off the computer (or crash). RAM is measured in megabytes. Some computer programs can back up data while you are working on it, and the files can be recovered when you turn the computer back on. However, this is not automatic, and the computer program must be set to do this task

ROM (read-only memory)—similar to software that is hardwired into your computer—basic, permanent information that tells the computer things such as how to load up the operating system when you turn it on

Router—special purpose computer that attaches to two or more networks and routes packets from one network to the other. A packet is information that has been incapsulated with a "to" and a "from" address and other pertinent, decriptive information for processing. A router uses network layer addresses (e.g., IP addresses) to determine if packets should be sent from one network to another. Routers send packets to other routers until they arrive at their final destination

Server—usually a computer that provides the information, files, Web pages, and other services to the client who logs on to it. The client/server setup is analogous to a restaurant with waiters and customers. The waiter takes the information and serves it to the customers who are at the right place in their computer

Continued on page 304

Continued from page 303 **Table 7-1**

Common Computer Terminology

Spyware—software that transmits information back to a third party without notifying the user. Some privacy advocates also call legitimate access control, filtering, Internet monitoring, password recovery, security, and surveillance software "spyware" because they all can be used without notifying the users

UPS (uninterruptible power supply)—unit that switches to battery power whenever the power cuts out

URL (Universal Resource Locator or Uniform Resource Locator)—Internet equivalent of addresses. Similar to other types of addresses, they move from the general to the specific. For example, first, *www* in an address is the worldwide Web, then an address within this web is given, and finally the aspect of the worldwide Web is provided (*.gov* for government,*.com* for commercial, or *.edu* for education)

Virus—piece of programming code usually disguised as something else that causes some unexpected and usually undesirable event. A virus is often designed so that it is automatically spread to other computer users. Viruses can be transmitted as attachments to an e-mail, can be transmitted as downloads, or can be present on a disc or CD

Worldwide Web (WWW)—usually known simply as the *Web,* a client/server hypertext system for retrieving information across the Internet that was originally developed by CERN laboratories in Geneva, Switzerland. Continuing development of the Web is overseen by the World Wide Web Consortium

Zipped—compressed version of a program or document

Evaluating Consumer Health Information Sources

In the IOM (2001) report, "Crossing the Quality Chasm: A New Health System for the 21st Century," the authors found that the information technology landscape had changed dramatically. The share of households with Internet access grew from 26.2% in December 1998 to 41.5% in August 2000, an increase of 58% in 20 months (U.S. Census Bureau, 2000). The 2010 U.S. census found that 80% of American households had a computer with Internet access (U.S. Census Bureau, 2010). The explosive growth of the Internet opened up many new applications that have implications for consumers of health-care services. Consumers use the Internet to search for health information, to obtain information useful in selecting a health plan or provider, and to participate in formal and informal support groups. Comparative performance data are available on the Internet for many health plans and, depending on the geographic area of interest, for hospitals and providers.

It is important for advanced practice nurses to be aware of the nature of information patients review on the worldwide Web and to have the capacity to evaluate patient information. At the present time, there are no standards for Web postings, and not all information on the Web is accurate or in any way substantiated. Many Web sites are designed to sell a product and can claim results that do not stand up to scientific inquiry. It is important to discuss issues of accuracy with patients and to become a resource for any questions they may have. Web sites with accurate and adequate information usually include the source of information on the Web posting providing links to evidence and information posted and have a documented mechanism for reviewing and updating material on the Web site.

The popularity of the Internet has made it easier and faster for practitioners, patients, and families to retrieve health information. Most of the information presented on the Web is valuable; however, the Internet also allows rapid and widespread distribution of false and misleading information. It is important for health-care providers to consider carefully the source of information and to be knowledgeable about Web sites when speaking to patients and families about the information presented there. Following are specific questions to ask when evaluating the usefulness and accuracy of information presented on a Web site:

- Who runs the Web site?
- What is the purpose of the Web site?
- Is the information presented on the Web site reviewed for accuracy?

The first question to ask is who runs the Web site? Reputable Web sites make it clear who is responsible for the information presented on the site. The National Cancer Institute clearly labels its Web site with "NCI" on every major page, along with a link to the site's home page. A second question is who pays for the Web site? The source of funding should be readily apparent on the site. Federal government sites are labled *.gov,* educational institutions are labeled *.edu,* nonprofit organizations are labeled *.org,* and commercial sites are labeled *.com.* The source of funding can affect what content is presented, how the content is presented, and the purposes for posting the content.

A logical follow-up question is what is the purpose of the Web site? Often, there is an icon on the site labeled "about this site," which should state the site's purpose and help users evaluate the trustworthiness of the information presented there. It is important to determine the original source of information on the Web site. Many Web sites use information from other Web sites, but it is important to identify clearly the original source to gauge the accuracy of information. The site should also identify the evidence on which the material presented there is based. Medical facts and figures should have references and citations from journals. Opinions and advice should be clearly labeled as such to avoid confusion between opinion and evidence-based knowledge.

Another important job in determining information accuracy is figuring out how and if the information was reviewed before it was posted on the Web site. The NCI Web site contains summaries from the Phyicians Data Query (PDQ) database that are peer-reviewed and updated by six cancer specialists. This Web site also provides an 800 telephone number where users can request fact sheets.

There should be evidence that the Web site itself is regularly updated and reviewed for content; this is very important because medical information and knowledge changes so rapidly. Does the Web site collect data about users? Is there a cost to retrieve information, or does the site solicit funds for an organization?

These are both signs of Web information with an agenda, and materials should be carefully verified before using. Reputable Web sites should always provide a way for users to contact the Web site owners with problems, feedback, and questions.

Many health-care companies send e-mails to advertise products or attract people to their services. Such e-mails should also be viewed with a critical eye. The accuracy of health information may be influenced by the desire to promote a product or service. The best way to minimize the dissemination of false or misleading information in e-mails is to identify respected sources of sound health information and use them as primary references to confirm the claims in the e-mails. The Federal Trade Commission (FTC) enforces consumer protection laws to reduce the amount of misleading or false health-care claims on the Internet. The FTC provides a Web page that can help people understand what questions to ask and how to spot scams and misleading information on Web sites (http://www.ftc.gov/curious). The U.S. Food and Drug Administration (FDA) also has a Web page that helps people find out more information about medicines and medical products (www.fda.gov/Drugs/DrugSafety/PostmarketDrugSafetyInformationforPatientsandProviders/).

Advancing Your Knowledge

F.A. is an advanced practice nurse in a rural clinic. One of his patients, a 56-year-old farm worker, comes to the office with a copy of an e-mail he received about lowering cholesterol. The patient is receiving a statin drug to reduce cholesterol, but he always complains about how much it costs. The e-mail provides information about a wonderful new product that is guaranteed to lower cholesterol and decrease bad cholesterol. It states that the first month will be free just for calling a specific number. When reviewing the product through the FDA Web site, F.A. finds that this is an unregulated herbal product that is not controlled for the quality of the drug, amount supplied, and efficacy. F.A. talks to his patient and acknowledges the frustration of having to pay for the statin and shows the patient the information obtained from the FDA about the product advertised in the e-mail. He also tells the patient that because the drug is not regulated for quality, it may have an increased side-effect profile that could ultimately cost more money to fix. The patient is surprised to know that supplements are not regulated by the FDA and agrees to continue taking the statin because he does not want to take what he calls a "mystery drug" that is not regulated.

1. How could the advanced practice nurse use information on the Internet to benefit patients?
2. List ways that you could improve patient care by providing patients with approved Web sites for their use to gather health-care information.
3. How can assisting patients to evaluate information obtained on the Internet benefit your work as a health-care provider?

Using the Internet to Distribute Quality Information

One method of distributing quality educational material to patients and populations is to develop a Web site and be conscientious about the material placed on the site. Developing a Web site is a specialization among computer programmers and requires not only computer skills but also design skills. A Web site is placed on a server so that it can be accessed from other computers. Most individuals or groups have access to free server space, but these spaces are limited in size, so it may prove beneficial to pay for server space.

The Internet can also be used to post customized health education messages to suit the needs of groups of individuals. Individual practice Web sites or group Web sites for diseases such as diabetes, hypertension, or heart disease are launched to allow patients to learn about their disease, treatment options, and methods for reducing complications. For example, you may design a Web site to provide information to diabetic patients about diet, medication, and exercise and to serve as a place to keep track of their home glucose testing results The same Web site could be used as a way for patients to ask general questions that could be posted on a "blog" and answered by the health-care provider. Health information is an important aspect of care that can be facilitated by using the Internet and informatics. Documentation and billing are other areas within a health-care practice that can benefit from the use of informatics, but choosing the correct system is essential.

Choosing a System for Documentation and Billing

Electronic documentation and billing can save time, increase practice revenue by using appropriate codes and levels for billing, and perfect the level of documentation to improve care and create a more complete record for use in the future. It is estimated that normal chart upkeep in an office (ensuring all pertinent laboratory reports and other paperwork make it into the appropriate place in the paper chart) costs $8 per year per patient. In an electronic record system, this cost is reduced to $2 per year per patient (Freeman, 2010).

Purchasing an EHR system is probably one of the most important decisions a small medical practice will make. These systems require major investments of time and money, and they bring fundamental change to the practice's clinical and business processes. Automation has a significant impact on all aspects of a health-care practice and dramatically alters the way health-care services are delivered. The average implementation for a small practice (one or two providers) can take 12 to 18 months, including planning, design, implementation, and training. For practices with three to five providers, the implementation time can be longer. Larger group practices with multiple specialties require even more time partly because of the greater number and variety of templates to be designed, the additional staff requiring training, and the greater number of system interfaces to be developed. The first step in the process of choosing a documentation and billing system is to evaluate the practice, plan what you want the system to do, and have a vision for what a successful implementation and use of the system will look like.

Questions to ask before choosing a system for documentation and billing include the following:

- What are the goals for documentation and billing? Does the system automatically update codes as they change? How do providers want to input their documentation? How might computers affect the work flow in the office? How will the system be seen by patients?
- What types of hardware are required?
- What are the goals and functions needed from the system in terms of hardware (computers, information storage, and other devices) and software?
- What is the price?
- How will you choose a vendor for buying the system?

Questions to ask potential vendors include the following (Miller, West, & Brown, 2005):

- Does the vendor have service level agreements that define how quickly it responds to service calls?
- Does the vendor provide support 24 hours a day, 7 days a week? Is there an extra charge?
- Are upgrades included in the maintenance fees?
- How frequent are the system updates?
- Does the vendor have a training plan and a project plan you can review?
- How many installations does the vendor have in your area?
- Does the vendor have a testing plan? (Testing the system is necessary to ensure integrity of the data and increase the success of implementation.)
- Can the system be implemented modularly? (This allows some budgeting flexibility.)

It is important for all persons who will use the system to be involved in choosing the system that best meets their needs. One of the most critical aspects of choosing a system is the support given to users by the company where the system is purchased.

Basic Elements of Data and Data Storage

The 2008 ANA publication, *Nursing Informatics: Scope and Standards of Practice,* charged nursing informatics "... to manage and communicate data, information, knowledge and wisdom in nursing practice" (ANA, 2008, p. 1). Data are simple numbers, such as a pulse measured in beats per minute, respirations per minute, or an oral temperature. The three together become information, and when combined and interpreted by the nurse, they become knowledge. A change in one data element may affect the other elements.

A database is a collection of information or data that is arranged in individual records and is searchable. A database is usually arranged for ease and speed of retrieval. Many software tools are used to search databases. The aim of many analyses of large databases is to draw causal inferences about the outcomes of actions, treatments, or interventions. One example of a large database that might be useful in advanced practice is the Minimum Data Set (MDS) (http://www.resdac.org/MDS/data_available.asp). The MDS is a federal database that stores information on any resident of an extended care nursing facility who is covered by Medicare or Medicaid. The MDS identifies health problems, functional status, medication use, and care plans for each patient. The database is searchable and could be used to determine the incidence and prevalence of certain diseases in an extended care nursing facility or to determine medication use by older adults in extended care. It could be used by advanced practice nurses to determine who seeks extended nursing facility care by researching the common reasons for admission to a facility.

Another large national database that is available to all providers is the National Quality Forum data set (http://www.hcpro.com/QPS-242258-873/National-Quality-Forum-creates-standardized-set-of-data-for-electronic-health-records.html). It provides data to measure performance and accelerate improvements in patient quality of care. This database is useful in all health-care settings. The Department of Veterans Affairs has launched a trial of a "lifetime electronic record," which would allow health-care providers to exchange patient information over a nationwide health information network database (Healthcare IT News, 2010). Accessing these databases can provide valuable information about health management and disease treatment.

A database can be useful for a single practice. It could keep track of each patient's annual preventive testing requirements or medications so that at any given time the nurse could print out a list of patients who need tests or medication refills. A database monthly report could show that one patient has run out of blood pressure medication and has not yet called for a refill. This type of data-based information allows for improved patient care and follow-up. Patient follow-up is essential not only to improve patient care, but also because insurers monitor provider follow-up. Without the aid of informatics, providers could not adequately provide follow-up to large numbers of patients.

Data-based reports regarding payment and reimbursement can be included in an office-based database. From this information, the provider can determine whether accurate coding is being used to bring in the appropriate reimbursement for services. A database can be set up by a computer professional, the office staff can enter data, and the provider can easily run reports and access data. In some cases, hospitals and other treatment centers can upload data directly to a practice database. This allows for the provider to see laboratory and radiology results from the office when a patient is in the hospital.

Technology is also useful in population-based health initiatives. For example, if we know that a specific region of the United States has a higher incidence of breast cancer, we can use information systems to determine what environmental or regional exposures are within the region that could cause this problem and encourage removal of these enviornmental toxins and increase the surveillance for women in the area. Another example is using information systems to correlate levels of obesity. When we are able to see patterns in the community, programs can be developed to make changes to reduce the medical burden of obesity. Without informatics, it would be too time-consuming and almost impossible to gather the data necessary to make these determinations. Without information systems to gather, store, and manage this type of data, the knowledge could be cumbersome or difficult to acquire.

Advancing Your Knowledge

T.M., a nurse practitioner who is working in a clinic in the South, notices three patients in a 2-week period who present with high fever, flu-like symptoms, extreme lethargy, and myalgias. T.M. notes that this is not a typical flu, and the flu vaccine administered this year does not seem to have a preventive effect. T.M. searches a statewide infectious disease database from the Department of Health using the patients' age, gender, and symptoms as parameters. T.M. discovers that there has been a recent outbreak of five cases of dengue fever in the state. T.M. reads the list of presenting symptoms and the length of illness, which both coincide with the findings from the patients in her practice. T.M. calls the health department, which confirms that dengue fever is a likely diagnosis and registers the patients from the practice in the database. A notice is sent out to other primary health-care providers in the area describing the presentation of dengue fever and the information about the cases in the area.

1. How has the use of health-care databases and information assisted T.M. and her patients?
2. How will the information from this one practice be useful to others in the area?
3. Without informatics, how would this information be passed on? How long would it take? What might be the result of others in the community not being informed about the outbreak of dengue fever?

Data storage is the ability to retain data in an accessible repository for use at a later date. The primary method for storage of data uses the random access memory (RAM) on the hard drive of the computer. Secondary data storage is on hard disk, tapes, or other external devices, such as external memories or Universal Serial Bus (USB) devices. The importance of data storage cannot be stressed enough.

Loss of medical data can cause reduced reimbursement for services or reduced ability to report quality indicators to the appropriate source. Saving data in secure files and frequently "backing up" data are important aspects of information storage. Data can be saved on USB ports, tapes, or external drives to ensure that a second file exists that can be used in the event something happens to the RAM space. Having a backup file can mean the difference between a slight computer setback and losing important data that is irretrievable.

Data can be stored or transmitted using barcode technology. Barcode technology is used for tracking patients, supplies, and equipment or for medication and blood administration. The barcoding of supplies used in surgical suites helps avoid unintentionally leaving items inside of patients during surgery. Care providers placing medication orders directly using computerized physician order entry software, pharmacists reviewing and profiling medications, and registered nurses verifying and administering medication using barcode technology have reduced medication errors. Radiofrequency identification (RFID) technology has been adopted to track patients, staff, and equipment. RFID can be used in medication administration in place of barcodes. RFID armbands are encoded with information and exchange information with receivers. RFID tags can quickly track patients; this tracking is especially valuable during triaging and during mass casualty events, such as hurricanes.

Communication Between Databases

Communication between databases requires standardization of language, interoperability, and cooperation among all systems. Systematized Nomenclature of Medicine Clinical Terminology (SNOMED CT) "is the universal health care terminology that makes health care knowledge usable and accessible wherever and whenever it is needed. This strong foundation is leading the health care industry in building a seamless infrastructure of worldwide care while integrating an overwhelming amount of clinical data" (International Health Terminology Standards Development Organisation, 2004).

Health Level Seven (HL7) is one of several standards organizations (International Organization for Standardization), and its mission is "[to] provide standards for the exchange, management and integration of data that support clinical patient care and the management, delivery and evaluation of healthcare services. Specifically, to create flexible, cost effective approaches, standards, guidelines, methodologies, and related services for interoperability between healthcare information systems" (Health Level Seven International, 2004). Communication includes connecting device to device, such as individual nurse computers to the database server. Communication can be in the form of a local area network (LAN) or wireless area network (WAN). Wireless networks have greatly improved the mobility of devices. The Internet has facilitated advanced communication between health-care providers and patients.

Changes are occurring rapidly. As the DNP-prepared nurse participates in monitoring and reporting quality indicators, understanding information systems and technology, and understanding complexity science, he or she will be needed increasingly for leadership in transforming health care. DNP-prepared nurse informaticians have the challenge of designing and building technology and information systems, and DNP-prepared caregivers and leaders have the challenge of implementing technology and information systems into practice.

Advancing Your Knowledge

C.D. is a clinical nurse specialist in a large urban health-care organization. She is part of a group of clinical nurse specialists that is developing an electronic documentation system for nurse sensitive indicators that must be reported to the management group on a quarterly basis. Information from all of the hospital departments must be collected, integrated, and compared with benchmarks.

1. How could the clinical nurse specialist group be instrumental in creating a plan for such a system?
2. In what ways could the system provide higher levels of data that would be useful to the health-care organization?
3. How might nursing work flow be affected by such a system?
4. How could such a system be designed, and who should design it?
5. Describe your level of computer knowledge and proficiency. List the ways you have used computer technology and informatics in the area of patient care.

Role of Informatics in Supporting Advanced Nursing Practice

Informatics is one of the seven essential areas of core content for DNP education identified by the DNP taskforce created within the American Association of Colleges of Nursing (2004). Essential knowledge in this area includes the understanding and use of technology and information for the improvement and transformation of health care. Because DNP education prepares nurses in one of three practice categories—direct nursing care, nursing care of community, or nursing practice supporting care—technology and information management becomes content within the specialty.

DNPs are challenged to be leaders in the use of technology and information management technology to promote advances in patient data management, improve patient care, and increase patient safety. To accomplish this, the DNP student must learn to use informatics technology to manage individual and aggregate health care and financial data and educate others in the use of technology. As leaders in the practice of nursing, DNPs will be called on to assist in the design of effective and efficient information management systems that may be used to assess productivity, make decisions, create Web-based learning tools, and support and improve patient care (American Association of Colleges of Nursing, 2004). Table 7-2 lists objectives for DNP students regarding information technology.

Clinical informatics is the effective use of information in patient care, clinical research, and education. The ultimate goal of clinical informatics is the streamlining of the processes involved in patient care: providing clinicians with accurate data in a timely manner, improving the quality of care, and reducing costs. Nursing informatics has been defined by the ANA as an advanced practice nursing role that uses computer and information science integrated with nursing science to facilitate the use of data information and knowledge to support patient care. The

Table 7-2

Objectives for DNP Education Regarding Information Technology According to the American Association of Colleges of Nursing

1. Design, select, use, and evaluate programs that evaluate and monitor outcomes of care, care systems, and quality improvement including consumer use of health-care information systems.
2. Analyze and communicate critical elements necessary to the selection, use, and evaluation of health-care information systems and patient care technology.
3. Demonstrate the conceptual ability and technical skills to develop and execute an evaluation plan involving data extraction from practice information systems and databases.
4. Provide leadership in the evaluation and resolution of ethical and legal issues within health-care systems relating to the use of information, information technology, communication networks, and patient care technology.
5. Evaluate consumer health information sources for accuracy, timeliness, and appropriateness.

informatics nurse supports patients, nurses, and other practitioners in decision making and in the development of evidence-based practice.

Using informatics in practice can improve collaboration between health-care professionals and provide opportunities for education, research, and program development. Informatics allows advanced practice nurses to manage the care of populations of patients to improve outcomes, measure performance, and benchmark treatments and protocols (American Association of Colleges of Nursing, 2004). Many insurers request aggregate data from health-care providers in regard to patient profiles and specific indicators such as patient satisfaction, patient volume, diagnostic tests and medications ordered, and number of referrals to specialists. These data allow the insurance company to benchmark practice patterns and determine the need for changes in reimbursement patterns. In the future, health insurers and the government will be asking providers for more data related to "pay for performance" measures, compliance with national guidelines, and patient satisfaction with services. Without access to this information via a database, it could take hours or weeks of staff time that would increase costs for the practice.

Informatics Competencies for Advanced Practice Nurses

To gain support for the use of information technology in health care, Curran & Abbot (2003) created competencies for advanced practice nurses that included the objectives from the IOM and some others. These authors believed that advanced practice nurses should have the ability to generate and manage individual and aggregate level information (Curran & Abbot, 2003). Table 7-3 lists informatics competencies for advanced practice nurses.

Table 7-3

Informatics Competencies for Advanced Practice Nurses

Computer Skills

1. Access shared data sets.
2. Extract data from clinical data sets.
3. Extract selected literature resources and integrate them with a personally usable file.
4. Use applications to aggregate and analyze data for forecasting accreditation, clinical value, nurse sensitive outcomes, evidence-based practice, and quality improvement.
5. Use applications to format and present data.
6. Use decision support systems, expert systems, and aids for differential diagnosis.
7. Use interactive communication devices with patients and other health-care providers.

Informatics

1. Support efforts toward development and use of structured languages.
2. Promote the integrity of nursing information and access necessary for patient care with an integrated computer-based patient record.
3. Evaluate computer-assisted instruction as a teaching tool.
4. Provide for efficient data collection.
5. Discuss the impact of computerized information management on the role of the nurse.
6. Describe ways to protect data.
7. Describe general application systems to support clinical care.
8. Describe general applications available for research.
9. Understand the principles of data display to facilitate analysis.
10. Use optimal search strategies to locate clinically sound and useful studies from information resources.
11. Critically analyze data, information, and knowledge for use in site-specific evidence-based practice.
12. Identify, evaluate, and apply the most relevant information.
13. Synthesize best evidence.

Informatics Skills

1. Convert information needs into answerable questions.
2. Use data and statistical analyses to describe and evaluate practice.
3. Evaluate health information on the Internet using a structured critique format.
4. Assist patients to use databases to make informed decisions.
5. Act as an advocate of system users including patients and colleagues.
6. Perform basic troubleshooting in applications.
7. Incorporate structured languages into practice.
8. Apply the principles of data integrity, professional ethics, and legal requirements for patient confidentiality and data security.
9. Design and use database reports.
10. Demonstrate knowledge and clinical decision-making processes within site-specific practice.
11. Evaluate the appropriateness of the monitoring system for the type of data needed.
12. Convert data into information and then knowledge.

Source: Curran, C. R. (2003). Informatics competencies for nurse practitioners. *AACN Clinical Issues, 14*(3), 320–330.

Using the Web as a method to provide health information and education to patients and families is an advanced nursing informatics competency. Web design requires specialized knowledge, but some programs provide a self-directed approach to putting information on the Web. One Internet-based program that teaches how to design your own Web site can be found at http://www.thesitewizard.com/gettingstarted/startwebsite.shtml. Spending some time creating a Web site for a practice or clinic can save time in the long run by providing easy-to-access information on the Web. It could also save the practice money by allowing patients to send messages, refill prescriptions, and schedule appointments without going through an office person. Interactive Web sites could be used to speed communication between patients and health-care providers. For example, if all of the diabetics in a practice had a Web site on which to post their daily or weekly blood sugar values, the provider could see at a glance which patients needed to come in for assessment of blood sugar elevations.

Advancing Your Knowledge

In one large practice, there are more than 1000 postmenopausal women who are at risk for or who have osteoporosis. The advanced practice nurse thinks that many of these women have not had a bone density test and do not understand the risks for untreated bone loss. The advanced practice nurse creates an osteoporosis page on the practice Web site and e-mails all female patients asking them to review the page. The Web page contains a simple explanation of why osteoporosis occurs and displays pictures of good bones versus osteoporotic bones. The Web site lists risk factors and signs and symptoms of osteoporosis but also tells patients that this type of problem can exist without symptoms until a fracture occurs. The site provides national incidence and prevalence data on the disease and links to national osteoporosis information sites. Within 1 month of this page being published, 100 women made appointments to come in to the practice to set up a dual-energy x-ray absorptiometry scan to determine whether they had osteoporosis. Of the 100 patients tested, 47 had osteoporosis, and 19 had osteopenia. All of these women were provided with proper treatment and scheduled follow-up examinations.

1. How long would it take an office to contact 1000 or even 100 women with this information using traditional telephone or letter communication?
2. What other diseases and syndromes could be positively affected using Web education? Who would design these Web sites? What knowledge would they require?
3. How could awareness of other health problems be increased using this method?

Continued on page 316

Advancing Your Knowledge *Continued from page 315*

4. What are the positive and negative aspects of patients' reading about health information online? As an advanced practice nurse, how do you approach patients when they ask questions about or present information obtained online?
5. How could you use a Web site in your practice to improve health promotion behaviors?

Another advanced nursing competency that can be aided by informatics is synthesizing the latest knowledge about diagnosis and treatment of diseases. Several electronic information sites provide daily e-mails to update advanced practice nurses on the latest findings from research. The ANA has a "smart brief" that can be accessed by members of the ANA or members of the American Association of Nurse Practitioners. Box 7-1 provides a sample smart brief. The e-mail address to subscribe to ANA smart brief is ANA@smartbrief.com.

Another daily e-mail update on research findings for health-care providers is Physician's First Watch (http://firstwatch.jwatch.org/). This site reviews

Box 7-1

American Nurses Association Smart Brief Examples

Meditation May Benefit Patients With Multiple Sclerosis

Swiss researchers found that patients with multiple sclerosis who engaged in an 8-week mindfulness meditation program showed better results in measures of depression, anxiety, and fatigue compared with patients who received the standard care.

Obese People Who Have Surgery Have Higher Suicide Rates

A U.S. study found that severely obese adults who undergo bariatric surgery have a higher suicide rate in the years after the procedure compared with the general population. The reason for the higher suicide rate is unclear, but researchers say pre-existing depression or other mental health conditions might play a role. The surgery itself is not thought to be a contributing factor.

Few Patients Choose At-home Dialysis Despite Its Advantages

A study of patients with end-stage kidney disease found that patients who received peritoneal dialysis had about the same survival rate as patients who underwent hemodialysis at hospitals or other health facilities. However, a separate study found that only 11% of patients opted to have dialysis at home despite its benefits. "We need to do a better job of educating people of the advantages of peritoneal," a kidney expert said.

Exercise Cuts Risk for Fractures in Women, Study Finds

Women with osteopenia who engaged in 20 minutes of exercise at home daily, interspersed with 6 months of supervised weekly training every year, for 60 months during a study were 32% less likely to sustain fractures during a follow-up, research showed. Women who subscribed to lifetime moderate exercise had a 78% reduced risk of fracture during the 7-year follow-up study, researchers reported.

Source: ANA Smartbrief. (2010). Retrieved from http://www.smartbrief.com/ana/

numerous medical journals from the United States and Europe and summarizes recent research findings, providing the full citation for further investigation. Box 7-2 lists some of the current information from Physician's First Watch. Both of these daily e-mail sites are convenient and can help to keep nurses up-to-date on important issues in patient care.

Telehealth Advanced Practice Nursing

Another innovation in information technology is telemedicine or telehealth. *Telehealth* is the practice of health-care delivery, diagnosis, consultation, and treatment and the transfer of medical data through interactive audio, video, or data communications that occur in the physical presence of the patient. Different methods of technology and delivery are used in this expanding area of

Box 7-2

Examples of Research From First Watch

Fear of Falling Makes Falls More Likely

Among elderly adults, perceived risk and physiological risk are factors in falls. Some elderly adults with no obvious physiological predispositions to falling nonetheless fear falling—and actually do fall. In this prospective study, investigators assessed the prevalence of perceived risk and physiological risk for falls and falling among 494 community-dwelling elderly adults (mean age 78; 54% women) in Sydney, Australia. During the year before enrollment, 149 elderly adults (30%) fell at least once, and 214 (43%) fell during 1-year follow-up. In a multivariate analysis, perceived risk and physiological risk for falls (measured with validated instruments) were independent risk factors for falls. Although most participants (69%) correctly perceived their risk, 11% had low physiological but high perceived risk, and 20% had high physiological but low perceived risk. Among elderly adults with low physiological risk, individuals with high perceived risk experienced significantly more injurious falls than individuals with low perceived risk. Similar results were found for elderly adults with high physiological risk.

Breastfeeding Protects Newborns Against Common Infections

Infants exclusively breastfed for 6 months have fewer and less severe infections their first year of life, according to a study in the *Archives of Disease in Childhood*. Researchers interviewed roughly 900 new mothers in Crete throughout the infants' first year to assess breastfeeding habits and the infants' health. Overall, infants exclusively breastfed had 0.7 fewer infections in their first year than infants with partial or no breastfeeding. Mothers who exclusively breastfed their infants for at least 6 months reported fewer physician visits for acute otitis media, acute respiratory infection, and thrush. In addition, hospital admissions for infection were lower in breastfed infants. Asked to comment, Dr. F. Bruder Stapleton of *Journal Watch Pediatrics and Adolescent Medicine* said, "These data confirm once again the value of exclusive breastfeeding on the health of infants in the first 6 months of life."

Source: *Archives of Disease in Childhood* article (free abstract) http://adc.bmj.com/.

health care. One method transfers digital images from one location to another. A digital image is taken using a digital camera ("stored") and then sent ("forwarded") by computer to another location. This method is typically used for nonemergent situations, when a diagnosis or consultation may be made within 24 hours and sent back. Telepathology is a common use of this technology in telehealth. Images of pathology slides may be sent from one location to another for diagnostic consultation. Dermatology is a natural specialty for store and forward technology. Digital images may be taken of skin conditions and sent to a dermatologist for diagnosis. Radiologic images can also be saved at a central location and sent to numerous clinicians for interpretation and diagnosis.

Providing health-care services via telemedicine offers many advantages. It can make specialty care more accessible to underserved rural and urban populations. Video consultations from a rural clinic to a specialist can alleviate prohibitive travel and associated costs for patients. Videoconferencing also opens up new possibilities for continuing education or training for health-care practitioners in isolated or rural areas, who may be unable to leave a rural practice or may not have the funds to take part in professional meetings or educational opportunities.

Another widely used technology by telehealth providers is a two-way interactive television when a "face-to-face" consultation is necessary. The patient and possibly the provider are at the originating site. The specialist is at the referral site, most often at an urban medical center. Videoconferencing equipment at both locations allows a real-time consultation to take place. The technology has decreased in price and complexity over the past 5 years, and many programs now use desktop videoconferencing systems.

There are many configurations of an interactive consultation, but most typically it is from an urban-to-rural location. The patient does not have to travel to an urban area to see a specialist, and, in many cases, access to specialty care is provided where none has been available previously. This kind of telehealth has been found to be effective with almost all specialties of medicine, including psychiatry, internal medicine, rehabilitation, cardiology, pediatrics, obstetrics and gynecology, and neurology. Also, many peripheral devices can be attached to computers and can aid in an interactive examination. An attached otoscope allows a physician to see inside a patient's ear; a stethoscope allows the consulting physician to hear a patient's heartbeat.

Here is a simple example of telemedicine: Imagine a scenario where a patient is on a camping vacation and develops a rash that is itchy, red, and spreading. Using a camera mounted on the top of his laptop, this patient e-mails his nurse practitioner and sends her a picture of the rash and a description of the rash. The nurse practitioner, after diagnosing the rash, could find a nearby pharmacy and call in the appropriate medication for this rash, and the patient could continue to enjoy his camping vacation.

Home health care is another booming area of telemedicine, popular in Japan, the United Kingdom, and the United States. The Department of Veterans Affairs initiated home telehealth as part of its telehealth program. Using cameras with voice technology in the homes of older adults, clinicans can observe and talk to these elderly patients to ensure they are safe and have what they need. Telehealth does not have to be a high-cost proposition. Many telehealth projects provide valuable services to people with no access to health care using low-end technology. The Memorial University of Newfoundland Telemedicine Project has been using low-cost store-and-forward technology to provide quality care to rural areas in underdeveloped countries for many years (Elford, 1998).

The military and some university research centers are involved in developing robotics equipment for telesurgery applications. A surgeon in one location can remotely control a robotics arm for surgery in another location. The military has developed this technology particularly for battlefield use, and some U.S. academic medical centers and research organizations are also testing and using the technology (Francis, 2006).

Telehealth Barriers

Several barriers to the practice of telehealth exist. Many states do not allow out-of-state physicians to practice unless licensed in their state. The Centers for Medicare and Medicaid still has several restrictions for Medicare telehealth reimbursement. Many private insurers also do not reimburse, although some states, such as California and Kentucky, have legislated that insurers must reimburse the same as for face-to-face consultations. Fear of malpractice suits (Hatch, 2010) is another consideration for health-care providers, as is acceptance of the technology and lack of "hands-on" interaction with patients; most patient satisfaction studies to date have found patients to be satisfied with long-distance care (Ekeland, Bowes, & Flottorp, 2010).

Many potential telehealth projects have been hampered by the lack of appropriate telecommunications technology. Regular telephone lines do not supply adequate bandwidth for most telehealth applications. Many rural areas still do not have cable wiring or other kinds of high-bandwidth telecommunications access required for more sophisticated uses, so the people who could most benefit from telehealth may not have access to it. See Box 7-3 for an example of a DNP project in telehealth.

Box 7-3

DNP Project in Telehealth

Treatment Fidelity Evaluation of Telehealth Stage-Based Motivational Interviewing Interventions

Susan L. Benson, DNP, APRN

Combat veterans with post-traumatic stress disorder (PTSD) smoke more than other veterans, are less likely to quit, and do not seek out or participate in smoking cessation treatment. These individuals are underserved and understudied. A promising approach to behavioral change is motivational interviewing (MI). MI is a client-centered, directive

Continued on page 320

Box 7-3

DNP Project in Telehealth *Continued from page 319*

therapeutic style that enhances readiness for change. This nonconfrontational intervention is particularly suited for PTSD patients who are easily angered. MI interventions can be delivered via telehealth in a "health buddy" device with weekly telephone counseling sessions. It is critical that these interventions stay "true" to their theoretical stage-based roots in all phases in order to know that significant results were due to the MI method.

- *Purpose:* The parent study tested the feasibility of telehealth care management and tobacco cessation for veterans with PTSD.
- *Methodology:* This nonexperimental study used stage-based MI interventions via a smoking library of text, weekly counseling fidelity tools, and patient satisfaction surveys. The counseling was tailored to the veteran's stage of change to quit smoking. Patient receipt of the interventions and the cognitive and behavioral changes enacted by the veteran were measured descriptively, as were the patient satisfaction surveys with the health buddy and MI counseling.
- *Results and Discussion:* Ten subjects were recruited. Delivery doses of MI were analyzed and found to be adequate. Fidelity checklist frequency of use was true to MI-consistent behaviors.
- *Implications for Nursing:* Only 3.5% of studies with a psychosocial intervention report their treatment fidelity measures, meaning that the participants were able to participate and did so at the recommended levels to support smoking cessation. This makes it very critical that researchers earning DNPs become aware of the value of treatment fidelity.

Completed spring 2009
University of Colorado-Denver College of Nursing

Source: Downloaded from Doctors of Nursing Practice LLC http://www.doctorsofnursingpractice.org/

Advancing Your Knowledge

In a rural federally funded primary care practice outside of Gainesville, Florida, three nurse practitioners work together to care for a population of underserved and often uninsured persons in several small communities. They have a mobile office in which they travel to different communities each day. To be as efficient and effective as possible, the mobile van has a video connection to a large academic medical center in Gainesville. The nurse practitioners have the ability to send e-mails to a physician for quick response and consultation and a digital x-ray machine. They have the ability to send Doppler readings of pregnant patients to the hospital for evaluation and to set up appointments for follow-up care if required. The nurse practitioners have a monthly 1-hour meeting with physicians and other practitioners at the academic medical center to discuss cases and receive updates on new treatment guidelines. These advanced practice nurses also have the ability to participate in online continuing education unit programs and learn about new advances in health care. They are also connected to social workers and insurance personnel to assist patients to get the financial help they need to obtain medications and other health-care–related items.

1. How does this telehealth program help patients? How does it save money? How does it provide for improved patient outcomes?
2. Develop a telehealth practice. How would it be structured? Who would pay? How could monetary savings be evaluated? How would it benefit patients?
3. What areas of leadership could a DNP-prepared nurse use to support this type of information technology in other areas?
4. How could the barriers of state licensure be overcome?

Barriers to the Use of Informatics in Health Care

The following discussion addresses barriers to the implementation of health information systems, including:

- Cost
- Inexperienced users
- Lack of standardization within computer systems
- Changes in work flow
- Technology issues when systems fail
- Confidentiality

Cost is the first barrier. Information systems are costly not only to purchase but also to maintain, and often choosing the best system for the needs of the institution or group is confusing. In a survey completed by the American Academy of Family Practice, more than 60% of 5000 respondents listed cost as the biggest barrier to implementation of information technology in practice (Miller & Sim, 2004). These physicians felt that the upfront cost was high, not to mention the additional cost for implementing and maintaining the systems over time. The survey also revealed that physicians believed that more time per patient after implementing an EHR would be needed, increasing the cost per patient visit. Another concern is that after investing in the expense of information technology for office use, it quickly becomes obsolete and requires further expense for updates.

Cost is not the only issue. Resistance and inexperience by users also create complications when implementing new technology into practice. Providers and office staff must learn to use information technology tools in practice and adapt methods of documentation to fit the parameters of the technology. Many providers resist learning how to use computer-based technologies in practice. In a survey of 685 nurses, approximately 20.3% did not want EHRs to be introduced into their work environments, 45.1% found the EHR useful, and 34.6% found it necessary for EHRs to be implemented into their work environments (de Veer & Francke, 2009).

Other barriers noted by primary care providers to adaptation of computer technology in primary care include a lack of standardization for computerized medical records and lack of support for implementation and ongoing use. Health-care providers have stated that they are frustrated by the change in work flow created by informatics and the lack of a consensus on what information should be included. Some health-care providers have expressed concern that information technology and equipment come between patients and providers (Miller & Sim, 2004).

When technology fails or stops working, it can significantly slow the office flow. Workaround systems have to be initiated, and they tend to be slower and cumbersome. Technology repair can be costly and can take time. When connecting systems such as Medicare billing "go down" or stop working, this can be frustrating for office personnel and can slow reimbursement.

Confidentiality is likewise an issue with technology. The development of passwords and the implementation of levels of information disclosure based on the role of the user must be maintained, and information use must be monitored.

The major factor that limits the use of health information technology is lack of knowledge about what types of health information technology and implementation methods improve care and manage costs for specific health organizations. A lack of understanding among advanced practice nurses in the areas of informatics technology, specific information technology health functions used in the workplace, and perceived benefits of using information technology still exists (Gaumer, Koeniger-Donohue, Friel, & Sudbay, 2007).

Overcoming the Barriers to Health-Care Technology Use

Overcoming the barriers to the use of information technology is important to promoting the success of information systems and EHRs. Information technology will become increasingly important and will be required as a tool for billing, reporting, and compliance with federal and state health care standards (Shortliffe, 2006). The DNP-prepared nurse with more education and understanding of information technology and the benefits that can be achieved from the use of informatics can serve as a change agent and foster better understanding to overcome perceived barriers.

DNPs must be able to articulate the need for these types of data when informatics products are being acquired or designed for a health-care facility. DNPs must be prepared to lead the process of selection and implementation of information technology products by being versed in the activities of each system's life cycle. They must understand the current evaluative literature on informatics implementation and outcomes. They must also know how to use informatics tools to manage and analyze the data for knowledge discovery (Jenkins, Wilson, & Ozbolt, 2007).

Several studies acknowledged the barriers to implementation of information technology in health-care practices, but they also found that the benefits can far outweigh the difficulties. Hillestad et al. (2005) found that national implementation of EHRs could save the health-care system more than $81 billion annually by improving health-care efficiency and safety. These authors posited that with the added implementation of health information technology to improve disease prevention and to manage chronic diseases, the savings could be much greater than $150 billion annually.

Miller et al. (2005) found that the initial costs of implementing an EHR in a private practice would be about $44,000, with an additional $9000 needed annually to maintain and update the system. These authors also estimated that the savings attributable to the implementation of this type of system could be recouped entirely by the practice within 3 years and that such a system would increase profit thereafter. This study reviewed 14 physician offices and found that the financial benefits averaged $33,000 per physician per year. These savings came from two main sources: increased coding levels that led to improved billing and greater efficiency from a decrease in personnel costs. All practices reported some savings, ranging from $1000 to $42,500 per physician (or nurse practitioner) per year.

The Agency for Healthcare Research and Quality (2010) reviewed studies on the effect of health-care technology use in practice. The findings of this review showed that once providers become well versed in technology use, there are improvements in provider performance when clinical information management decision support tools are used. CDS systems form a significant part of the field of clinical knowledge management technologies through their capacity to support the clinical process and use knowledge to create diagnoses and recommend treatments and other interventions. CDS systems are typically designed to integrate medical knowledge, patient data, and an inference engine to generate case-specific advice.

The researchers found that the EHR was able to make data easily accessible so that information could be used to empower providers in their work. An example is a system that provides an overview of laboratory reports for a patient over the last 5 years that would allow the provider to determine how function has changed during that time. Informatics could also point out the changes that were the most dramatic and that might be indications of impending health problems. Another example is a computer that flagged items that should be addressed at the patient visit, such as smoking cessation, weight loss, immunizations, and other prevention issues. These would be individualized based on the patient history. The conclusion the Agency for Healthcare Research and Quality drew from its review of research was that health information technology was worth the "trouble" to implement; it has the ability to transform the delivery of health care, making it safer, more effective, and more efficient.

For nurses to use technology and informatics successfully and to help overcome the barriers to implementing technology, nurses must be educated and feel at home with this type of technology. The Technology Informatics Guiding Education Reform (TIGER) Initiative was initiated to move nursing education forward in the area of technology (TIGER, 2010). The TIGER Initiative is focused on using informatics tools, principles, theories, and practices to enable nurses to make health care safer, more effective, efficient, patient-centered, timely, and equitable. This goal can be achieved only if such technologies are integrated transparently into nursing practice and education. The TIGER Initiative has created nine collaborative teams to work on improving the understanding and use of technology and informatics in nursing education and practice: (1) standards and interoperability, (2) national health information and technology agenda,

(3) informatics competencies, (4) education and faculty development, (5) staff development, (6) usability and clinical application design, (7) virtual demonstration center, (8) leadership development, and (9) consumer empowerment and personal health records. The TIGER Initiative has identified strategies to increase nursing knowledge in the area of informatics and information technology and to help combat the barriers to technology implementation. Box 7-4 presents these strategies.

Box 7-4

TIGER Strategies for Transforming Nursing Education

- Expand collaborations by maximizing the Alliance for Nursing informatics and entering into national and international efforts as key partners. (This strategy would bring nurses to the table where discussions of information management are held and allow nursing knowledge and values to be included in planning and implementing information technology systems.)
- Interweave enabling technologies transparently into nursing practice and education, making information technology the stethoscope for the 21st century. (This strategy calls for information systems and technology to be a routine and fully integrated aspect of all levels of nursing education so that nursing students become comfortable and skilled in the use of these technologies in the same way as using a stethoscope.)
- Bring evidence-based knowledge to the practice setting, taking translation research from bench to bed and then into the home.
- Bridge the gap between practice and education, establishing new models for collaboration between academic and practice settings. (This strategy calls for new ways of educating advanced practice nurses whereby the clinical faculty and the lecture faculty both determine the competence and evaluate the performance of the student in the practice setting.)
- Transform standards for the use of enabling technologies, defining educational and licensure requirements for students, practitioners, and faculty. (This strategy would make informatics and information technology knowledge part of the tests for certification and licensure for all nurses.)
- Seek empowerment as knowledge broker and coach, using enabling technologies to support patients in self-directed management. (This strategy would use information technologies to provide patients with individualized health information so that they are aware of and can better manage their health-related issues—telemedicine is included in this area of information technology.)
- Reform the classroom to incorporate virtual continuous learning and clinical experiences for students, faculty, and practitioners. (This strategy would encourage the use of simulation technologies to provide experiences for students and determine their competence in a given situation.)

Source: TIGER Initiative. (2010). Technology Information Guiding Educational Reform. Retrieved from http://www.tigersummit.com/

Advancing Your Knowledge

S.M. has received her DNP and works as an advanced practice nurse. She works in a large multidisciplinary practice with more than 50,000 patients. There are 12 physicians of different specialties, 6 nurse practitioners, 1 social worker, 2 physical therapists, 1 acupuncturist, 5 medical assistants, 5 billing and insurance staff members, and 8 front-office staff members. At a monthly staff meeting of providers, questions about the institution of an EHR are discussed. Many of the providers are skeptical about the benefits of EHR and are very concerned about the costs involved in the purchase and implementation of such a system. The group asks for a volunteer to develop a presentation for the next meeting on the benefits and cost of such a system and what financial assistance the practice could get from stimulus monies. They are also interested in finding out how the work flow in the office might change based on the use of an EHR. Based on the knowledge that S.M. has about informatics, she volunteers to put together a short presentation for the next meeting.

1. What are the pros and cons of implementing an EHR for this group?
2. What are the important issues regarding choosing and implementing a system for this type of practice?
3. What changes in work flow might be needed for the implementation of an EHR system?
4. How would a system improve patient care, communication, and collaboration among providers and use of evidence-based practice?
5. How might an EHR system assist the practice with billing and reaping the rewards of pay for performance incentives?
6. What would your overall recommendation be?

Adopting Technology in Advanced Nursing Practice

Some of the difficulties expressed by advanced practice nurses in adopting technology include feeling incompetent in the area of information technology, lack of support to develop knowledge in this area, and the perception that information technology will not improve the advanced practice nurse's ability to do a good job (Gaumer et al., 2007). Certain types of technology have been shown to be important for advanced practice nurses. Blackberries and other smart phones offer nurses a way to access information in real time; these devices can provide knowledge and improved evidence-based decision making for nurse practitioners. These devices are used by many health-care providers and have been shown to improve patient outcomes and provide alerts and warnings in the areas of pharmaceuticals and medical devices (Rothchild, Fang, Liu, Litvak, Yoon, & Bates, 2006). In practices where EHR computerized charting is used, each provider may have a handheld computer or a computer on wheels to complete EHRs in the room. Robots are being developed that can deliver charts, medications, and x-rays and complete other tasks that save nurses time to allow for better patient-focused care.

Phases of Technology Adoption

Even though research has shown the increased time savings and the improvements in patient safety and efficiency of electronic information and documentation, there is often a lag between availability of technology and its widespread use. *Diffusion-innovation theory* (Rogers, 2003) is one framework that describes the lag time between technology development and its widespread use. This theory has five phases: (1) knowledge phase, (2) persuasion phase, (3) decision phase, (4) implementation phase, and (5) confirmation phase.

The *knowledge phase* is where an individual is first exposed to the innovation. Understanding and information about the innovation must still be acquired before the decision to adopt. During the *persuasion phase,* the individual seeks to learn more details about the innovation, including barriers to use, cost, and benefits of using the innovation. The *decision phase* is when an individual decides whether the benefits outweigh the barriers and decides to adopt or reject the innovation. Rogers stated that because individuals make decisions in different ways, the decision stage is difficult to predict. The *implementation phase* is when an individual starts to use the innovation and evaluates the usefulness of the innovation. During this period, the individual may require more information about the use of the innovation. In the *confirmation phase,* the individual decides whether to continue using the innovation and may begin to move toward using the innovation to its fullest potential.

To describe the people involved in the process of innovation acceptance, Rogers (2003) presented five adopter categories, as follows:

1. Risk-taking innovators are the first to adopt an innovation; usually these people are younger and have the closest contact with scientific sources or are acquainted with other innovators who have had success in adopting new innovations.
2. Early adopters are second in line to adopt new innovations and are usually opinion leaders.
3. The early majority represents a group who over time adopt innovations; they are not as eager as the innovators or early adopters to adopt new innovations.
4. The late majority represents the average members of society who have a high degree of skepticism about new innovations and often wait until others have adopted an innovation and been successful.
5. Laggards have an aversion to change and focus on traditions rather than innovation.

Acceptance of technology in nursing care is a process that must be thoroughly understood and then integrated into general practice.

Technology in Nursing Care: Classifications and Telehealth

Technologic innovations and the use of information technology have created new skills for nurses and enlarged the scope of nursing practice (Sandelowski, 2000). The past 50 years have seen the transition from the industrial age to the information age. In the past 25 years, changes in regulatory agency requirements, legal issues, and guidelines that create standards of care have been instrumental in increasing and changing the responsibility of nurses (Meiner, 1999, p. 17). Two of the major changes include learning documentation systems and using telehealth. Nursing itself has been experimenting with various documentation systems, including streamlining documentation systems, bedside charting, multidisciplinary charting, and using critical pathways and computerized documentation (Monsen, Fitzsimmons, Lescenski, Lytton, Schwichtenberg, & Martin, 2006). The challenge of charting is painting an accurate and complete picture of the care provided to patients while passing onto other providers the patient's story. Various formats for capturing and storing this information are in use, including focus charting, charting by exception, problem-implementation-evaluation, subjective-objective-assessment-plan, problem-oriented medical record, outcome-based charting, and others (Meiner, 1999).

Classification of Nursing Language and Taxonomy

To simplify and improve charting, nursing began developing a standardized taxonomy of nursing diagnoses in the 1970s through the North American Nursing Diagnosis Association (NANDA). In the 1990s, NANDA developed further standardized taxonomies, known as *Nursing Intervention Classifications* and *Nursing Outcome Classifications*. Even though standardizations exist, not all health-care organizations participate in using standardized documentation. The reason these classifications are not used in all settings may be lack of education regarding their value. Until a standardized classification system can be developed that is consistently used by providers of nursing care, informatics will be unable to capture the importance and usefulness of nursing interventions in populations across the United States.

The U.S. government supports and funds SNOMED CT (International Health Terminology Standards Development Organisation, 2004), as mentioned earlier in the chapter. SNOMED CT will include the following:

1. More than 1000 nursing intervention concepts modeled from the Georgetown Home Health Care Classification, the Omaha System, and the Nursing Interventions Classification.
2. Intervention concepts from the Perioperative Nursing Data Set.

3. Nursing diagnosis and problem concepts from NANDA, the Perioperative Nursing Data Set, the Georgetown Home Health Care Classification, and the Omaha System.

Despite numerous attempts, no single taxonomy that describes all of nursing practice in all settings is available (Averil, Zielstorff, Delaney, Carty, & Ferrell, 1998). The goal of all electronic documentation should be to represent nursing practice in all settings, not merely classification of the practice. The SNOWMED CT system is closest to meeting this goal, but nursing interventions differ across settings and across populations. At the present time, the SNOWMED CT system does not include many nursing interventions that are commonly used and that affect the outcomes of patient care; this is especially true in advanced practice nursing where nursing and medical care comingle in one practice.

At the present time, advanced practice nurses use medical charting and nomenclature to document, evaluate, and create plans of care for patients. Nurse practitioners use *Current Procedural Terminology* (CPT) codes and International Classification of Diseases, 9th Revision, Clinical Modification (ICD-9) codes to bill for services and create a diagnostic history. However, new codes should be developed to track and document the efforts and benefits of nurse practitioner care involving counseling, education, and discussion of a problem with the patient. As the focus of health care shifts to health promotion and disease prevention, it will be necessary to expand classifications to include effective therapies for changing health behaviors.

Privacy as an Issue in Health-Care Information and Technology

The Health Insurance Portability and Accountability Act of 1996 (HIPAA) is the first major federal policy to address privacy of health information. HIPAA covers what is termed *protected health information,* whether in paper, verbal, or electronic sources. There are 18 identified elements considered to be protected health information: (a) name; (b) date of birth (except year); (c) addresses other than state (street, city, county, and zip code); (d) telephone or fax numbers; (e) e-mail addresses; (f) medical record numbers; (g) Social Security number; (h) health plan beneficiary; (i) account numbers; (j) certificate or license numbers; (k) vehicle identification numbers; (l) vehicle serial numbers; (m) worldwide Web Uniform Resource Locators (URLs); (n) Internet Protocol (IP) addresses; (o) biometric identifiers (fingerprints and voice prints); (p) full face photographs; (q) device identifiers; and (r) any other unique identifying numbers, characteristics, or codes. Under HIPAA, the use of any one, or combination, of the patient data from any of these 18 elements in any format is protected from disclosure to anyone other than the appropriate health-care provider under HIPAA (Swinderman, 2003).

The rapid advance of technology over the past decade has threatened the essential security of personal information and is a barrier to the implementation and use of EHRs. The right to individual privacy is a social norm that has been a cornerstone of the American life. Computer technology has challenged that right. Social Web sites such as Facebook have challenged the American idea of privacy, and online purchasing has created a valuable vault of purchase records, purchase habits, and personal financial information on the Web.

Although advances in technology promote and improve the current state of health care by improving quality and efficiency and by providing more personalized service, there are concerns for privacy and the security of data stored on the Web. Not only are individuals concerned because their medical information is placed in permanent storage in a computer, but also they are concerned because information can easily be transferred to other persons and institutions. Many individuals are reluctant to share personal and medical information with employers and even insurance companies, but these entities can obtain information from computer databases that are outside of individual control. Individuals do not want information about their personal lives sold to advertisers, drug companies, or other groups. Policies such as those accompanying HIPAA regarding health-care information rights, security, and the maintenance of privacy for personal information are essential.

Although HIPAA laws protect written and verbal communications, there is an increased need for privacy protection of computer data because the data are stored and can be accessed through computers rather than in hard copy form. In 2008, the U.S. Department of Health and Human Services proposed specific regulations to protect privacy and create a framework for security within EHRs. Although these regulations are broad, they are meant to serve as a guide for patients, providers, and insurers as to the safety and security of personal health information. Table 7-4 presents the principles outlined in this document.

Although these principles are very general in nature, they are meant to protect Americans from the indiscriminate use of their private medical information and provide them with an avenue for redress if these principles are violated. Implications for DNPs in the area of computer security and individual privacy rights include maintaining adequate computer security for patient data, allowing patients access to their medical records, and obtaining permission to use any patient information from EHRs.

Conclusion

Information technology is a fast-growing and important component of health care today. Administrators and advanced practice nurses are challenged to become leaders in the acceptance and use of information technology and in the creation and implementation of computer systems. Such systems provide information for patient care, disease management, billing, and population-based care. The advanced practice nurse educated at the DNP level is charged with

Table 7-4

Nationwide Privacy and Security Framework for Electronic Exchange of Individual Identifiable Health Information

1. Individuals should be provided with a simple and timely means to access and obtain their individually identifiable health information in a readable form and format. Individuals should be able to obtain this information easily, consistent with security needs for authentication of the individual, and such information should be provided promptly so as to be useful for managing their health.
2. Individuals should be provided with a timely means to dispute the accuracy or integrity of their individually identifiable health information and to have erroneous information corrected or to have a dispute documented if their requests are denied.
3. There should be openness and transparency about policies, procedures, and technologies that directly affect individuals or their individually identifiable health information.
4. Individuals should be provided a reasonable opportunity and capability to make informed decisions about the collection, use, and disclosure of their individually identifiable health information.
5. Individually identifiable health information should be collected, used, or disclosed only to the extent necessary to accomplish a specified purpose and never to discriminate inappropriately. Establishing appropriate limits on the type and amount of information collected, used, or disclosed increases privacy protections and is essential to building trust in electronic exchange of individually identifiable health information because it minimizes potential misuse and abuse.
6. Persons and entities should take reasonable steps to ensure that individually identifiable health information is complete, accurate, and up-to-date to the extent necessary for the person's or entity's intended purposes and has not been altered or destroyed in an unauthorized manner.
7. Individually identifiable health information should be protected with reasonable administrative, technical, and physical safeguards to ensure its confidentiality, integrity, and availability and to prevent unauthorized or inappropriate access, use, or disclosure.
8. These principles should be implemented and adherence to them assured through appropriate monitoring, and other means and methods should be in place to report and mitigate nonadherence and breaches. This includes monitoring for internal compliance including authentication and authorizations for access to or disclosure of individually identifiable health information; the ability to receive and act on complaints, including taking corrective measures; and the provision of reasonable mitigation measures, including notice to individuals of privacy violations or security breaches that pose substantial risk of harm to such individuals.

Source: U.S. Department of Health and Human Services. (2008). The nationwide privacy and security framework for electronic exchange of individual identifiable health information. Retrieved from http://healthit.hhs.gov/portal/server.pt/gateway/PTARGS_0_10731_848088_0_0_18/NationwidePS_Framework-5.pdf

becoming a leader in the area of informatics and developing the knowledge necessary to improve the use of this technology for improved patient care, management of patient populations, and patient safety.

Different types of information and technology used in advanced practice nursing include EHRs, robotics, and telehealth. Personal privacy issues are still a concern when medical records and patient information are documented and stored electronically. Sharing patient information and using patient information for population-based inquiry is important, but regulations require shielding the privacy of personal health information. Governmental agencies including the U.S. Department of Health and Human Services have developed guidelines for allowing individuals to access their medical records and maintain personal privacy within EHRs.

The DNP-prepared advanced practice nurse with increased knowledge can assume leadership positions in the use of information technology. No other group of health-care providers has as broad an understanding of the different aspects of health care from community practice to hospitals, to diagnosic centers, to treatment facilities and the coordination that is required to maintain patient safety and satisfaction with servcies.

References

Abraham, S. (2010). Technological trends in health care: Electronic health record. *Health Care Manager, 29*(4), 318–323.

Agency for Healthcare Research and Quality. (2002). Medical informatics for better and safer health care. Summary, *Research in Action*, Issue 6. AHRQ Publication Number 02-0031. Rockville , MD: Agency for Healthcare Research and Quality. Retrieved from http://www.ahrq.gov/data/informatics/informatria.htm

Agency for HealthCare Research and Quality (AHRQ). (2010). The impact of consumer health informatics applications. Retrieved from http://www.ahrq.gov/about/annualconf10/finkelstein_gibbons/Gibbons.HTM.

American Association of Colleges of Nursing. (2004). AACN position paper on the practice doctorate in nursing. Retrieved from http://www.aacn.nche.edu/DNP/pdf/DNP.pdf

American Hospital Association. (2009). Resources: Availability of Web sites for hospitals. Retrieved from http://www.aha.org/aha/resource-center/Statistics-and-Studies/index.html

American Nurses Association. (1994). *The scope of practice for nursing informatics.* Washington, DC: American Nurses Publishing, NP-90 7.5M 5/94.

American Nurses Association. (2008). *Nursing informatics: Scope and standards of nursing practice.* Silver Springs, MD: Nursebooks.org.

Averil, C. B., Zielstorff, R., Delaney, C., Carty, B., & Ferrell, M. J. (1998). Setting standards for nursing data sets in information systems. Nursing Information and Data Set Evaluation Center (NIDSEC). Retrieved from http://www.ncbi.nlm.nih.gov/pubmed/9929318

Ball, M. J., Hannah, K. J., & Douglas, J. V. (2000). Nursing and informatics. In M. J. Ball, K. J. Hannah, S. K. Newbold, & J. V. Douglas (Eds.). *Nursing informatics: Where caring and technology meet* (3rd ed.). New York, NY: Springer.

Curran, C. R. & Abbot P. (2003). Informatics competencies for nurse practitioners. *AACN Clinical Issues, 14*(3), 320–330.

de Veer, J. E., & Francke, A. L. (2009). Attitudes of nursing staff towards electronic patient records: A questionnaire survey. *International Journal of International Nursing Studies, 47*(7), 846–854.

Ekeland, A., Bowes, A., & Flottorp, S. (2010). Effectivenss of telemedicine: A systemic review of reviews. *International Journal of Medical Informatics, 79*(11), 736–771.

Elford, R. (1998). Telemedicine activities at Memorial University of Newfoundland: A historical review, 1975–1997. *Telemedicine Journal, 4*(3), 207–227. Retrieved from http://www.liebertonline.com/doi/abs/10.1089/tmj.1.1998.4.207

Francis, P. (2006). Medical robotics and the impact on perioperative nursing practice. *Urological Nursing, 26*(2), 109–111.

Freeman, L. (2010). The digital office: Choosing and using integrated electronic medical records, billing and managmement systems. *Medical News*. Retrieved from http://www.birminghammedicalnews.com/news.php?viewStory=998

Gaumer, G., Koeniger-Donohue, R., Friel, C., & Sudbay, M. (2007). Use of information technology by advanced practice nurses. *Computers, Informatics, Nursing, 25*(6), 344–352.

Hatch, O. (2010). It is time to address the costs of defensive medicine: Comment on physicians views on defensive medicine: A national survey. *Archives of Internal Medicine, 170*(12), 1083–1084.

Health Level Seven International. (2004). About HL7. Retrieved from http://www.hl7.org/about/

Healthcare IT News. (2010). VA launches fourth data exchange pilot with NHIN. Retrieved from http://www.healthcareitnews.com/news/va-launches-fourth-data-exchange-pilot-nhin

Hillestad, R., Bigelow, J., Bower, A., Girosi, F., Meili, R., Scoville, R., & Taylor, R. (2005). Can electronic medical records systems transform healthcare? Potential health benefits, savings, and costs. *Health Affiliations, 24*(5), 1124–1126.

Hunter, K. M. (2001). Nursing informatics theory. In V. K. Saba & K. A. McCormick (Eds.), *Essentials of computers for nurses* (3rd ed., pp. 179–190). New York, NY: McGraw-Hill.

Institute of Medicine. (2001). Crossing the quality chasm: A new healthcare system for the 21st century. Retrieved from http://www.iom.edu/~/media/Files/Report%20Files/2001/Crossing-the-Quality-Chasm/Quality%20Chasm%202001%20%20report%20brief.pdf.

International Health Terminology Standards Development Organisation. (2004). Retrieved from http://www.snomed.org/

Jenkins, M., Wilson, M., & Ozbolt, J. (2007). Informatics in the doctor of nursing practice curriculum. *AMIA Symposium Proceeding Archives,* 364–368.

Jordan, T. J. (2002). *Understanding medical information: A user's guide to informatics and decision making*. New York, NY: McGraw-Hill.

Laramee, A., Bosek, M., Kasprisin, C., & Powers-Phaneuf, T. (2010). Learning from within to ensure a successful implementation of an electronic health record. *Computers, Informatics, Nursing, 29*(8) 478–479.

Meiner, S. E. (1999). Current approaches in charting. In S. E. Meiner (Ed.), *Nursing documentation: Legal focus across practice settings* (pp. 15–27) Thousand Oaks, CA: Sage Publications.

Miller, R. H., & Sim, I. (2004). Physicians' use of electronic medical records: Barriers and solutions. *Health Affairs, 23*(2), 116–126.

Miller, R., West, C., & Brown, T. (2005). The value of electronic medical records in solo or small group practices. *Health Affairs, 24*(5), 1127–1137.

Miller, R.H., & Sim, I. (2004). *Physicians' use of electronic medical records: Barriers and solutions, Health Affairs, 23*(2), 116–126.

Monsen, K. A., Fitzsimmons, L. L., Lescenski, B. A., Lytton, A. B., Schwichtenberg, L. D., & Martin, K. S. (2006). A public health nursing informatics data and practice quality project. *Computers, Informatics Nursing, 24*(3), 152–158.

Patel, V., & Currie, L. (2005). Clinical cognition and biomedical informatics: Issues of patient safety. *International Journal of Medical Informatics, 74,* 869–885.

Patel, V. L., Kushniruk, A. W., Yang, S., & Yale, J. (2000). Impact of a computer-based patient record system on data collection, knowledge organization, and reasoning. *Journal of the American Medical Informatics Association, 7*(6), 569–585.

Rogers, E. M. (2003). *Diffusion of Innovations.* (5th ed.). New York, NY: Free Press.

Rohan Academic Computing. (2010). Glossary of academic information technology terms. Retrieved from http://www-rohan.sdsu.edu/glossary.shtml

Rothschild, J. M., Fang, E., Liu, V., Litvak, I., Yoon, C., & Bates, D. (2006). Use and perceived benefits of handheld computer-based clinical references. *Journal of the American Medical Informatics Association, 1,* 619–626.

Saba, V. K. (2001a). Historical perspectives of nursing and the computer. In V. K. Saba & K. A. McCormick (Eds.), *Essentials of computers for nurses: Informatics for the new millennium* (3rd ed., pp. 9–45). New York, NY: McGraw-Hill.

Saba, V. K. (2001b). Nursing informatics: Yesterday, today and tomorrow. International Council of Nurses. *International Nursing Review, 48,* 177–187.

Sandelowski, M. (2000). *Devices and desires: Gender, technology and American nursing.* Chapel Hill, NC: The University of North Carolina Press.

Shortliffe, E. H. (2006). *Biomedical informatics: Computer applications in health care and biomedicine.* New York, NY: Springer Publications.

Sim, I., Gorman, P., Greenes, R. A., Haynes, R. B., Kaplan, B., Lehman, H., & Tang, P. C. (2001). Clinical decision support systems for the practice of evidence-based medicine. *Journal of the American Medical Informatics Association, 8*(6), 527–534.

Staggers, N., Thompson, C. B., & Snyder-Halpern, R. (2001). History and trends in clinical information systems in the United States. *Journal of Nursing Scholarship, 33*(1), 75–81.

Swinderman, T. D. (2003). The Health Insurance Portability and Accountability Act of 1996 (HIPAA). *FAU Research and Graduate Studies News, 2*(9), 4.

Thede, L. Q. (2003). *Informatics and nursing: Opportunities and challenges* (2nd ed.). Philadelphia, PA: Lippincott Williams & Wilkins.

TIGER Initiative. (2010). Technology Information Guiding Educational Reform. Retrieved from http://www.tigersummit.com/.

U.S. Census Bureau. (2010). Computer Use in Households in the United States. Available at http://www.census.gov/prod/2001pubs/p23-207.pdf. First accessed on February 12, 2010.

U.S. Department of Health and Human Services. (2008). The nationwide privacy and security framework for electronic exchange of individual identifiable health information. Retrieved from http://healthit.hhs.gov/portal/server.pt/gateway/PTARGS_0_10731_848088_0_0_18/NationwidePS_Framework-5.pdf

CHAPTER 8

INTERPROFESSIONAL COLLABORATION AND COMMUNICATION

Objectives:

By the end of the chapter, students should be able to:

1. Discuss the need and ways to increase teamwork and collaboration among health professionals in the complex health-care system by
   - b. Analyzing how interdisciplinary teams work
   - c. Discussing methods for monitoring team performance, and
   - d. Exploring barriers and challenges to team development and teamwork.
2. Discuss ways to design team structures and leadership roles.
3. Support the need for care coordination and patient-centered, culturally competent interdisciplinary health care.
4. Discuss the development of the medical home concept versus primary health care as examples of interdisciplinary teamwork.
5. Illustrate methods and key components of positive communication, and understand the need for positive communication among health-care professionals.
6. Discuss peer review for the advanced practice nurse as a component of interdisciplinary work.
7. Illustrate and describe the role of the advanced practice nurse as team leader in interdisciplinary team situations and as a doctor of nursing practice (DNP) in consultation.

To facilitate a changing and developing health-care system, the United States requires coordinated and comprehensive health care replete with patient-centered, multidisciplinary services. To institute such a system, there is a need for interdisciplinary teamwork and positive communication between and within teams. Effective teamwork requires not only leadership but also collaboration and positive styles of communication to provide a framework for the advancement of patient care. Nurses who have achieved a doctor of nursing practice (DNP) degree can provide the leadership, can support others in the leadership required for team development, and can bring a depth of clinical knowledge and person-centered values to the collaboration.

The American Association of Colleges of Nursing (AACN) essentials for DNP education address the need for communication and collaboration among professions. The AACN document states that the DNP program should prepare graduates to do the following (AACN, 2006, pp. 14–15):

- Employ effective communication and collaborative skills in the development and implementation of practice models, peer review, practice guidelines, health policy, standards of care, and other scholarly products.
- Lead interprofessional teams in the analysis of complex practice and organizational issues.
- Employ consultative and leadership skills with intraprofessional and interprofessional teams to create change in health care and the complex health-care delivery system.

To implement a team approach to health care, institutions should partner with other health-care providers, social welfare agencies, and communities to increase professional support for patients, families, and communities. Cross-setting work will become more essential as the pay-for-performance goal of the Centers for Medicare and Medicaid Services (CMS) is realized across all care settings. For example, when a patient is discharged from a hospital, more at-home follow-up will be necessary to meet the CMS goal of reducing readmissions within 30 days of discharge. An increase in home-care services provided to patients would be cost-effective and would increase care coordination between settings. Also, evidence suggests that teamwork, with contributions of multiple sources, skills, and knowledge, can reduce morbidity and mortality rates (Erickson, Ditomassi, & Jones, 2008).

This chapter presents information regarding interprofessional teamwork, effective strategies for communication and collaboration, and ideas to move toward more patient-centered and population-based care through collaboration with other professionals. Teamwork and collaboration with other health-care professionals is an especially important topic for DNP students and graduates. The DNP-prepared advanced practice nurse must coordinate the care provided by the many different professionals who play a role in the health and well-being of patients. To achieve an adequate level of care coordination, collaborative practice, teamwork, and positive communication are essential.

Teamwork and Collaboration Among Health Professionals

The Institute of Medicine (IOM) at the National Institutes of Health was created by the National Academy of Science to serve as an advisor to the United States in areas of health and wellness and health-care policy. The IOM publication entitled *To Err Is Human: Building a Safer Health System* noted that the systemic failures in the health-care system are due largely to the deficiencies in team performance (Kohn, Corrigan, & Donaldson, 2000). Other health-care quality groups have said that health care is or at least should be a "team sport" (Clancy, 2005). Inclusive membership of health-care professionals, a common team goal, and adequate nonaggressive leadership are driving forces in teamwork. Researchers found many positive outcomes from the use of interdisciplinary teams, including lower patient mortality, fewer and shorter hospitalizations, reduced drug prescriptions, improved patient satisfaction, improved morale, and improved functional status in elderly patients (Solheim, McElmurry, & Kim, 2007). In the medical office setting, teamwork was shown to enhance compliance, reduce the number of missed appointments, and improve physician expertise (Baker & Heitkemper, 2005). Teamwork was also shown to improve the delivery of comprehensive and continuous care to underserved populations. The IOM mandated the use of fully collaborative teams of health-care professionals to provide safe, timely, effective, efficient, equitable, and patient-centered care (AACN, 2004; IOM, 2003).

People interact with the health-care system at many levels and across a continuum of care, including primary care, specialty care, emergent care, hospital care, long-term care, outpatient care, pharmaceutical care, and therapeutic care including physical and occupational therapy. In each of these settings, patients are cared for by multiple professionals who have knowledge and skill in a specialized area. Each of the individual portions of a patient's plan of care provides its own interventions and resolution, and the health-care system in its current state lacks coordination of care across the multiple levels of the health-care continuum (Peikes, Chen, Schore, & Brown, 2009). A team approach allows groups of health-care professionals to enhance health promotion, public health, interdisciplinary research, community-based participatory research, and many other health-related activities.

Health-care professionals have been slow to work on collaboration and teamwork in providing health care. Many health-care professionals seem to think that preserving their own unique specialty area will enable them to continue to command the respect and reimbursement that they now receive. With an aging population and expanded health insurance coverage, however, most health-care professionals recognize that the increase in demand for care will exceed their capabilities. It is estimated that there could be a deficit of up to 200,000 physicians over the next 15 years (Cohen, 2010). With a likely deficit, it is important to learn how to use most efficiently the health-care practitioners that we do have.

Interprofessional health-care teamwork can facilitate more effective and efficient care because patients benefit from interaction with health-care professionals that boast different types of expertise. Efficiency can be achieved through removing duplication in assessment and evaluation, creating a positive dialogue regarding possible diagnoses and coordinating the testing process to establish and treat the problem in a coordinated fashion. In the current health-care system, if the primary care provider orders a test to determine the cause of a physical complaint and determines that the patient requires examination by a specialist, the specialist often repeats the test regardless of the findings from the original test. Test results are not always shared between health-care providers, which makes duplication necessary, decreases efficiency within the system, and adds cost to the diagnostic process. Teamwork can provide the coordination that prevents patient needs from being overlooked or shortchanged. Practitioners who participate in a team approach demonstrate higher levels of professional growth and job satisfaction than members of practices in which one group makes most health-care and practice decisions (Newhouse, 2008).

Team Structures

The structure of health-care teams is usually fluid, and membership often depends on the people involved in patient care, care planning, and decision making. As the situation changes for any patient or group of patients, team membership may change. If a team is formed to reduce childhood obesity, teachers, nutritionists, nurses, and others may be members of the team; if the team assesses a lack of adequate areas for after-school exercise, the team may invite city leaders and planners to become members of the group. The success of team efforts is based on the ability of the team to anticipate the needs of the individuals the team is attempting to assist; the ability of the team to adjust to changing objectives, actions, and environments; and the ability of the team to reach common goals. General attributes of successful teams include good leadership, mutual support among team members, adaptability of the team as a whole and of individual members, shared organization and outcome models, and effective communication.

Leadership Roles

Team leadership may also be fluid as the goals and objectives of the team change. Leaders must be active members of any team. The definition of *team leadership* includes the ability to direct and coordinate activities of team members, assess team performance, assign tasks, motivate team members, and create a positive team atmosphere (Association for Healthcare Research and Quality, 2010). Some of the main roles of the team leader are to foster communication between members, create an atmosphere in which all members feel they have a role in decision making, and ensure that ideas and team decisions are communicated to all members. Team leaders are also responsible for coordinating the efforts of the team and reducing duplication of team members. Team leaders must be able to do the following (Baker, Gustafson, Beaubien, Salas, & Barach, 2003):

- Facilitate team problem solving
- Develop performance expectations and acceptable interaction patterns
- Synchronize and combine work of individual team members
- Clarify team member roles
- Engage in preparatory meetings and feedback sessions with the team
- Evaluate team performance

Leadership is discussed in more detail later in this chapter.

Methods for Monitoring Team Performance and Outcomes

Finding or creating a method to measure team performance is a first step in understanding the elements of successful teamwork (Murray & Enarson, 2007). A richer understanding of team dynamics and effectiveness can benefit patient safety by assisting in team training and development and can boost individual and team competencies in nontechnical aspects of care, such as prioritization, leadership, and decision making. Team competencies that can be measured include the following:

- *Communication:* The quality and exchange of information
- *Coordination:* The management and timing of activities
- *Cooperation:* The assistance and support of others
- *Leadership:* The provision of directions and assertiveness behind decisions
- *Monitoring:* The awareness of ongoing processes and team observation

Ultimately, measuring team performance is the responsibility of the team leader and the organization within which the team functions. Setting team goals and determining whether goals were met is a joint effort between all team members and should be an ongoing team function. Measurement of team performance can be completed by developing team goals and determining when and if these goals are achieved. Measurable goals may look like the following: By the end of the second month, a team created to develop and provide services to older adults will have (1) a brochure of offered services in the community, (2) developed a mailing list of older adults who might benefit from services, (3) met at least once with town council members to discuss possible meeting times and spaces for the older adult group, and (4) a meeting with the subcommittee for program development to discuss programs that might benefit older adults in the community.

Barriers to Teamwork

Kim, Barnato, Angus, Fleisher, and Kahn (2010) surveyed 112 hospitals and reviewed 324 patient records and, after adjusting for hospital characteristics, discovered that the lowest mortality rates among patients in the intensive care unit (ICU) were found in hospitals where multidisciplinary rounds were made on patients daily. Nevertheless, Jansen (2008) speculated that the health-care system in its present form is incapable of true teamwork. In a review of the literature regarding teamwork in health care, this author found that as long as the physician is in control of patient treatment from the standpoint of authority and financial compensation, compartmentalization and fragmentation within patient care will continue to be the norm. Jansen found that although policy makers espouse teamwork as beneficial to patients and cost, they have not examined the current state of teamwork, and they have not developed methodologies to instill the need for teamwork in health-care providers or institutions. Historically, the compartmentalization of health services caused fragmented care, prioritization of provider needs over needs of the patient, and poor communication between providers and patients. Many professional organizations outside of nursing still impede the development of a team approach to patient care by promoting professional protectionism and attempting to monopolize reimbursement (Jansen, 2008).

There are many major barriers to developing a team approach in health care, including professional protectionism, differences in values between professions, blurred role boundaries, and professional rivalry. As health-care reform evolves, these barriers create a level of mistrust in advancing the ideas of teamwork in health care. Once teams have formed, there are still boundaries standing in the way of their success.

Professional Protectionism and Rivalry

Many professional organizations seem to dismiss the need for a team approach to health care, with each organization holding onto the authority it possesses and being unwilling to share authority or individual practices. The members of the organizations fear loss of professional identity. Professional cultures have evolved through historic factors, social class, gender, and financial issues and have created values, attitudes, and behaviors that are not conducive to collaboration. The education of each group of health-care professionals usually occurs in isolation from the others and instills the values, attitudes, and behaviors of the profession rather than fostering interprofessional understanding. Increasing specialization has immersed each group further in the knowledge and culture of its own profession. These professional cultures contribute to the challenges of effective interprofessional teamwork (Hall, 2005).

Blurred boundaries occur between physicians and advanced practice nurses when both have prescriptive authority and the authority to assess, diagnose, and treat patients. Rivalry has developed between these two groups, and the American Medical Association (AMA) created documents to regulate advanced nursing practice even though nursing is a distinct profession with its own regulatory bodies. The AMA questioned the ability of nurse practitioners to care adequately for patients and improve patient safety. The AMA passed a resolution stating that only medical doctors and osteopaths may be called *doctor* and that only these two groups can call parts of the education process a *residency* (AMA, 2008). In response, the American Nurses Association (ANA) stated that the term *doctor* is in common use for individuals who have achieved the highest level of education in a field (ANA, 2008). The ANA (2008) also stated that the term *resident* or *residency* is used for many different types of students who are increasing their knowledge through a concentrated study in one place and that physicians have a medical residency and DNP students have an advanced practice nursing residency.

Differences in Professional Values

Another restraint to teamwork is the difference in value systems between professions. Medicine has a set of values that are based on science and technology, whereas the values of nursing are more whole person–centered and come from both science and social science. When working together, physicians and nurses often do not see the patient and treatment through the same lens and define success or failure in patients differently. Hall et al. (2009) identified that although expert nurses understand patient knowledge and beliefs, they experience difficulty with the cultures of other professionals.

Compartmentalized professional education may contribute to these differences; recommendations have been made to encourage interdisciplinary education that includes learning on collaboration; team decision making; and an appreciation of values, roles, and competencies of other professions (D'Amour & Oandasan, 2004). Barriers and challenges to effective teamwork remain, and efforts to overcome barriers provide a challenge to advanced practice nurses in their attempts to address the complex needs of patients and families.

Once teams are in place, there are other barriers to their effective use. One such barrier is lack of accountability and role confusion. Lack of accountability can cause team members to be unable to determine their role within the team framework and be unsure of how and when to act. Lack of commitment or lack of education about the team environment likewise can derail the ability of professionals to act as a team, as can lack of trust. The willingness and motivation to work with someone or a group collaboratively do not exist in the absence of trust and respect. Actively striving to collaborate with many different types of health-care providers is essential to success in the present health-care system. DNP-prepared nurses, with their knowledge of leadership and communications skills, can advocate for teams and provide the necessary leadership and encouragement for teams to improve patient care.

Critical Thinking Questions

1. What are the traditional barriers to collaboration between health-care professionals, such as physicians, nurses, pharmacists, and social workers?
2. When should the notion of collaboration between health-care professions begin? How could this happen?
3. How could interprofessional collaboration be accomplished when the financial aspects of care are still linked to the physician?
4. How can collaboration be monitored within health care to determine whether improvements in collaboration and care coordination have been made?
5. If you were setting up a comprehensive health-care practice, how would you establish a collaborative model for the workers in the practice? How would you monitor this model's success?

Designing Teams and Team Leaders

Before turning our focus on designing an effective team, it is important first to discuss collaboration between health-care professionals as a foundational concept of effective teamwork.

Collaboration Between Health-Care Professionals

Collaboration has been defined as the process of joint decision making among independent parties, involving joint ownership of decisions and collective responsibility for outcomes (Boyle & Kochinda, 2004). The collaborative process involves a synthesis of different perspectives to understand complex problems. A collaborative outcome is the development of integrative solutions that go beyond an individual vision to a productive resolution that could not be accomplished by any single person or organization. Collaboration includes supporting sustained teamwork by creating a culture that values personal integrity, giving power and respect to each person's voice, integrating individual differences, resolving competing interests, and safeguarding the essential contribution each must make to achieve optimal outcomes.

To provide the most effective patient care possible, nurses must collaborate with other health-care professionals, including physicians (Boyle & Kochinda, 2004). Collaboration is a core value of nursing professionalism that must be taught and realized (Apker, Propp, Ford, & Hofmeister, 2006).

Advancing Your Knowledge

A multidisciplinary team practice, which includes a hospitalist, advanced practice nurses, nurses, physical therapists, social workers, and pharmacists, cares for 38,000 patients. The practice has set high standards for collaboration and teamwork, uses positive communication skills to establish patient safety and efficient care, and has a peer review system in which it evaluates and attempts to improve the care provided. The practice has benchmarked for patient outcomes, compliance, cost, and efficiency against other practices of similar size that do not use the team approach. At least 1 day a month is spent in meetings and peer review for each professional on the team; the practice has superior patient outcomes, has increased the revenue coming into the practice, has improved patient compliance with treatment plans, and has demonstrated high levels of patient satisfaction with services provided.

1. It takes time and increased costs to develop and implement this type of team practice. Is it worth it? Why?
2. What other services might this multidisciplinary team consider adding to "grow" the practice further?
3. How would you set up a team practice in which health promotion and disease prevention would be the emphasis?

Collaboration requires mutual respect, competence, and caring among collaborators. Collaborative practice between all health-care professionals and workers creates a positive work environment, decreases costs, improves job satisfaction among nurses, and improves patient care (Schmalenberg, Kramer, King, Krugman, Lund, Poduska, & Rapp, 2005). It also decreases patient morbidity and mortality (Aiken, Clark, Sloane, Sochalski, & Seiber, 2002; Dietrich, Kornet, Lawson, Major, May, Rich & Reily-Wasserman et al., 2010). Studies revealed that nurses who work in environments that foster collaboration among health professionals experience improved job satisfaction, which improves recruitment and retention rates compared with noncollaborative environments (Aiken, Sloane, Lake, Sochalski, & Weber, 1999; Nelson, King, & Brodine, 2008). Evidence showed that interprofessional collaboration between physicians, medical residents, and nurses is important to ensure quality clinical outcomes (Hojat, Nasca, Cohen, Fields, Rattner, & Griffiths, 2001; Sterchi, 2007; Thomson, 2008).

The ANA and the IOM both supported shared decision making and collaboration among professionals (ANA, 2005; IOM, 2004). The ANA proposed positive collaboration as a means of improving nurses' job satisfaction and autonomy. The IOM (2004) recommended that organizations adopt a structure that supports collaboration by encouraging interdisciplinary patient care rounds and providing ongoing education in the collaborative process and training for all staff.

In a pivotal study, Baggs, Schmitt, Mushlin, Mitchell, Eldredge, Oakes, and Hutson (1999) determined the effect of collaborative practice on outcomes of patients in the ICU. These researchers identified a perfect rank order correlation between organization collaboration on the unit and patient outcomes: Higher levels of collaboration between the health-care team created better patient outcomes. In another study in two hospitals, Hanson, Bull, and Gross (1998) found that when discharge planning and education were undertaken by a collaborative group that included social workers, physicians, and nurses, levels of patient satisfaction and success in follow-up care increased. This study also found that nursing satisfaction increased when nurses were able to provide adequate discharge education and planning for patients. In the area of discharge planning, collaboration may become even more important as pay-for-performance measures penalize hospitals when patients return for treatment within 30 days of discharge.

Bryan-Brown and Dracup (2002) posited that collaborative practice between different health-care professionals could meet the need for expanding health-care needs. These authors emphasized, however, that collaboration must be substantive and meaningful. The fundamental nature of collaboration is working together on a task. The aim of collaboration is to combine the skills and knowledge of more than one person to improve the outcome of a specific venture more than if the individuals were working on their own. In other words, the whole becomes greater than the sum of its parts.

Thompson (2008) studied the attitudes of nurses and physicians regarding collaboration on a medical surgical hospital unit. Using the Jefferson Scale of Attitudes toward physician-nurse collaboration (Hojat, Nasca, Cohen, Fields, Rattner, & Griffiths, 2001), this researcher found that nurses had a more positive attitude toward collaboration than physicians. Findings from this study showed that there were no significant differences in either nurse or physician attitudes according to gender. Hojat et al. (2001) compared U.S., Israeli, Italian, and Mexican nurse and physician responses related to questions regarding attitudes of nurse-physician collaboration. Findings revealed that, overall, nurses desired collaborative nurse-physician relationships more than physicians, regardless of cultural background and independent of gender and age. These researchers concluded that there is a great deal of role ambiguity between nurses and physicians in complementary practice environments and that this ambiguity makes collaboration more difficult.

Collaboration requires active participation at all health-care team levels to solve problems. From the nursing or medical assistant to the physician or advanced practice nurse, all team members must actively collaborate to improve health-care outcomes. If a patient tells the medical assistant that he is not taking his medication because it makes him nauseous, but he does not tell his health-care provider, collaboration between the medical assistant and the health-care provider could help the patient make needed changes in medications to improve health.

Cohn (2003) provided the following checklist of behaviors that are important for true collaboration to occur:

- Actively listen and participate
- Openly exchange ideas and viewpoints
- Build on one another's ideas
- Refrain from personal criticism
- Remain focused on the tasks for which one is responsible
- Monitor team progress at regular intervals
- Share responsibility for deadlines and ownership of results
- Develop win-win solutions
- Respect members' confidentiality

To be effective in collaboration, building trust and shared meanings is essential. Developing true partnerships takes time and patience to rise above simple information exchange toward true collaboration with shared ideas and creative solutions. As DNP-prepared advanced practice nurses continue to learn and grow as collaborators, their role as collaborators will identify them as essential to the health and well-being of their patients. Continuing to push for collaboration, even in the face of obstacles, is worthwhile. As trust in the expertise of others and willingness to understand different perspectives grow, collaboration will be easier to achieve. There is no one profession that has all of the answers, and there is no one group that even understands all of the questions that require answers. Therein lies the strength of collaboration.

Team Building

There are methods for developing collaboration that have proven successful (Dietrich et al., 2010). Team building is an important first step to establishing a collaborative environment among health-care workers. Mann (2008) proposed a five-step process to create effective teams. These steps are focused on building teams that achieve results. To produce results, strong interteam relationships must be developed and sustained. Step 1 is to measure the current effectiveness of the team in place; this serves as a benchmark to measure the team's increasing effectiveness. Measuring current effectiveness can be accomplished through individual team member interviews, asking team members to rate on a scale of 1 to 10 how effective the team is currently, or use of a valid and reliable assessment tool.

Step 2 is to create an idea of what a successful team would look like. The team should brainstorm to envision the most successful, productive, and cohesive team possible by discussing the following:

- The team's values, priorities, and desired results and the organization's values, priorities, and desired results for this team
- Each member's own values, priorities, and desired results for this team
- Productivity goals
- Productivity factors—factors that support the team in achieving results, accomplishing tasks, and staying on course to reach goals and objectives; these include strengths such as accountability, decision making, and goal setting
- Positivity factors—factors that focus on the interrelationships between team members and the spirit or tone of the team as a system; these include strengths such as trust, respect, clear communication, handling conflict, and camaraderie

Step 3 is to communicate effectively. Everyone hears information differently. To be effective, it is important to ensure that information and discussions are understood by everyone on the team in the same way; the best way to accomplish this is to have team members discuss what was said and determine if mutual understanding has been achieved.

Step 4 is to develop a plan to turn the team vision into reality; this requires goal setting by team members. Goals must be specific, measurable, attainable, realistic, and time oriented or have a deadline. Each member of the team must be aware of his or her responsibilities in meeting the goals set.

Step 5 in creating a well-functioning team is to encourage team support. Whether you are the team leader or simply a member of the team, being a cheerleader and supporter of team goals helps the team come together and be effective in its efforts.

Using the common goal of positive patient outcomes as a starting point to enhance unity among collaborators, an initial matter in team development is to agree on a definition of patient well-being (Calendrillo, 2009). Although this definition may originally differ among health-care providers and even among patients and families, the team members must establish common ground to move forward in a collaborative way. In any definition of well-being, the patient's wishes and desires should rest at the core of the discussion. One way to come to a common definition of patient well-being is through respectful negotiation. To neutralize the levels of power and authority in a group discussion, dropping titles and using names is useful. Calendrillo (2009) stated that nurses should not strive for dominance in collaboration but should derive strength in discussion from innovations and integrity. Advanced practice nurses have substantial power and influence in patient care settings because of their knowledge. Understanding the power they possess by virtue of this knowledge can create the freedom to become meaningful contributors in collaborative situations. Even with power, it is important to work within the hierarchical structure of institutions and health-care settings. It is best to use the chain of command set up to make ideas known. Nevertheless, when mutual goals and respect exist in a team, issues of hierarchy become secondary to innovation and sharing knowledge.

Conflict in a collaborative setting is unavoidable. Conflict can be a positive aspect of collaboration and can enable the group to make better overall decisions. Managing conflict is one of the cornerstones of collaborative practice. One of the best ways to manage conflict is to allow all ideas to be expressed and discussed openly and then to allow for compromise among members of the group. This takes active and strong leadership and a willingness among group members to be accepting of the ideas and values of others.

Negativity and negative behaviors can adversely affect collaboration. When in collaboration with other health-care providers, developing the ability to understand the perspective of others is crucial (McNamara, Lepage, & Boileau, 2011). Seeking to understand before attempting to be understood enhances team leadership skills and collaborative abilities.

Advancing Your Knowledge

When a group of advanced practice nurses initially attempts to collaborate with several physician specialists to develop a multidisciplinary practice, they are rebuffed and told that they do not have the knowledge or expertise to participate in a collaborative practice with physicians. To attempt to establish some collaboration with these physicians, the nurse practitioners asked the physicians if they could bring lunch to their offices and discuss how they could more effectively refer patients when necessary. During this lunch, the nurses not only used assertive skills to let the physicians know their level of knowledge and their use of evidence-based practice but also presented ways that collaboration could benefit the physicians financially. They presented their perspective of the other benefits of collaboration and acknowledged the physicians' perspectives in working with advanced practice nurses. Several days after the lunch, the nurse practitioners received a call from the office of three of the specialists who wanted to reconsider the collaboration agreement proposed by the nurses. The advanced practice nurses told the physicians that they would be delighted to discuss options for collaboration further.

1. Which aspects in this scenario do you think enhanced the physicians' willingness to work collaboratively with the advanced practice nurses?

2. What are the next steps that should be taken by the nurse practitioners?
3. How would collaboration benefit both groups? How would the advanced practice nurses remain autonomous in this collaboration?
4. What conflicts do you foresee as time goes on? How should they be handled?

Example of Effective Team Building Using TeamSTEPPS

To support attempts to develop and implement an interdisciplinary team approach to health care, Clancy and Tornberg (2009) created an educational program called the *STEPPS (Strategies and Tools to Enhance Performance and Patient Safety) program*. This program is available to the public through the Association for Healthcare Research and Quality (AHRQ) Publications Clearinghouse. The purpose of this program is to improve patient safety, create an evidence-based team approach to patient care, and improve communication and teamwork skills among health professionals. The program is a joint effort between AHRQ and the U.S. Department of Defense.

The TeamSTEPPS program has four core areas, as follows (Clancy & Tornberg, 2009):

- *Team leadership* requires an ability to direct and coordinate activities of team members, assess team performance, assign tasks, develop team knowledge and skills, motivate team members, plan and organize, and establish a positive team atmosphere.
- *Situation monitoring* is the capacity to develop common understandings of the team environment and apply appropriate strategies to monitor teammate performance accurately.
- *Mutual support* is the ability to anticipate other team members' needs and to shift workload among members to achieve balance.
- *Communication* is the ability to provide efficient exchange of information and consultation with other team members, including the patient.

There are also three phases to the TeamSTEPPS system. Phase 1 is to assess the readiness of the organization to undertake a team approach and the need for changes in the system to accommodate this new model. Phase 2 is planning and education of team members regarding the use of the TeamSTEPPS approach. This step also includes implementation of the team approach to health-care provision within the institution. Phase 3 is to sustain and spread the improvements in teamwork performance, clinical processes, and outcomes that result from implementing the TeamSTEPPS approach.

Using the TeamSTEPPS program has created higher quality and safer patient care through the establishment of effective teams that strive to achieve the best clinical outcomes. Improvements gained through the use of TeamSTEPPS include optimizing the use of information, people, and resources. The educational portion of the TeamSTEPPS system creates team awareness through clarification of team roles and responsibilities, reduces conflict through information sharing, and attempts to eliminate barriers to quality and safety.

Communication in TeamSTEPPS

There has been much discussion about communication in the "high-tech" and fast-paced acute care setting to reduce medical errors and improve patient safety. Communication is discussed in greater detail later on. AHRQ has developed tools in the TeamSTEPPS model to improve communications and ensure patient safety. These tools are aimed at increasing mutual trust between professionals and providing a team orientation to care. AHRQ has defined safe and effective communication as the process by which information is clearly and accurately exchanged between team members.

Communication in the TeamSTEPPS model begins with understanding your role in communicating patient information. Communications that advocate for the patient should be firm and respectful but should clearly state the concern, offer a solution to resolve the concern, and obtain agreement. Suppose a patient is being discharged home; the nurse leader does not think the patient has adequate support at home, and the physician does not order home health services. The nurse leader should make a statement such as, "Mrs. Smith is getting ready to be discharged, but I am concerned that she will not be able to care for herself adequately at home. She is unable to drive and get her medications and other essentials, and she has trouble remembering how to take her medications. I would like you to order home health services for Mrs. Smith to assist her in either getting needed help at home or getting placed in an assisted living facility where she can get the help she needs. Can I write an order for home health?"

If the physician ignores the initial request, the nursing leader should voice the concern at least two more times to be sure it has been heard and understood. Each time, the nurse should ask the physician to acknowledge that he or she has heard what has been said. If the outcome is still unacceptable, a stronger course of action should be taken, such as notifying individuals in the chain of command. Interprofessional relationships may be strained when actions are taken to ensure that patients receive what they need; however, patient safety is the number one priority of all health-care providers and must take precedence. Interprofessional relationships are not friendships but rather relationships that create optimal environments to provide excellent patient care. The nurse may go back to the physician after the fact and explain why she felt so strongly about the issue that she took up the chain of command.

The acronym *CUS* is used in this approach as a method for positive communication. *C* stands for "I am *c*oncerned," *U* stands for "I am *u*ncomfortable," and *S* stands for "This is a *s*afety issue." In the above-described scenario, the nurse might say, "I am concerned because Mrs. Smith is leaving today, and she does not have sufficient help at home. I am uncomfortable with letting her go home with no home health to evaluate her home situation and her ability to

Box 8-1

SBAR

SBAR is a process that fosters communication and ensures that necessary and vital information is communicated properly (Pope, Rodzen, & Spross, 2008). SBAR was developed by Kaiser Permanente of Colorado and has been increasingly adopted by hospitals throughout the United States. SBAR is used to report to a health-care provider a situation that requires immediate action; to define the elements of a handoff of a patient from one caregiver to another, such as during transfers from one unit to another or during shift report; and in quality improvement reports. SBAR stands for: *S*ituation, *B*ackground, *A*ssessment, and *R*ecommendation.

- *Situation:* This is Sally Smith, the nurse practitioner with Family Practice Associates, and I have called to let you know that Mrs. Jones has fallen at home and has been admitted to the hospital with a fractured femur.
- *Background:* Mrs. Jones is an 83-year-old woman who has Alzheimer's dementia, coronary artery disease, and angina and who lives with her son and his wife. She fell yesterday and was on the bathroom floor for several hours before her daughter-in-law arrived home from work. Her vital signs are stable, and she is comfortable now in the hospital. The family would like her to be seen by an orthopedic surgeon to determine what is best for her.
- *Assessment:* I believe that because of Mrs. Jones' age, cognitive status, and comorbid conditions that she is not a candidate for surgery but perhaps is a candidate for a procedure to immobilize the hip for comfort.
- *Recommendation:* I would like to put Mrs. Jones in traction and give her appropriate pain medications to reduce her discomfort. When she is stable, I would like to have a meeting with you, Mrs. Jones, and her family to discuss the surgical options and develop a plan that is the best and safest for her.

Advancing Your Knowledge *Continued from page 349*

D.I. calls the emergency response team, and the team calls Mr. Thomas' physician. The office says he is with a patient and will call back. After 15 minutes, when there is no call from the physician, the nurse calls again and states, "We are concerned. Mr. Thomas has become very unstable, and we think he should be transferred to ICU for further observation and care. This is a safety issue and I need to hear from the physician immediately." The office person tells the physician, and he comes to the phone immediately and provides appropriate orders for Mr. Thomas' transfer and care. Mr. Thomas is diagnosed with an extension of the myocardial infarction from 3 days ago. The physician has asked to be called that evening with an update of Mr. Thomas' condition. D.I. calls and uses SBAR to tell the physician that Mr. Thomas' situation is stable and tells the physician what the most recent vital signs were. D.I. tells the physician that Mr. Thomas is currently receiving a nitroglycerin drip and oxygen and is

care for herself after she leaves the hospital. This is a safety issue b
is not able to get her medications and seems confused about how t
medications."

Communication to Ensure Safe Patient Handoffs in TeamSTEPPS

When the responsibility for patient care is shifted from one team member to another, a handoff occurs, such as during change of shift, when transferring to a new physician or physician group, or when the patient is transferred to a new level of care within the facility or to a different facility. Box 8-1 presents an alternative to the TeamSTEPPS system, called *SBAR* (Situation, Background, Assessment, Recommendation). In the TeamSTEPPS system, the acronym *I PASS the BATON* is used when the nurse transfers the care of the patient to another nurse or health-care provider. This acronym could be used when the advanced practice nurse shifts responsibility of patient care to a specialist or other health-care provider, such as a physical therapist:

I	Introduction	Introduce yourself and your role/job (include the patient).
P	Patient	Name, identifiers, age, sex, location.
A	Assessment	Present chief complaint, vital signs, symptoms, and diagnosis.
S	Situation	Current status/circumstances including code status, level of uncertainty, recent changes, and response to treatment.
THE		
B	Background	Comorbidities, previous episodes, current medications, and family history.
A	Actions	What actions were taken or are required? Provide brief rationale.
T	Timing	Level of urgency and explicit timing and prioritization of actions.
O	Ownership	Who is responsible (person/team), including patient/family.
N	Next	What will happen next? Anticipated changes? What is the plan? Are there contingency plans?

More information about TeamSTEPPS is provided at the AHRQ website (http://www.ahrq.gov/qual/teamstepps).

Advancing Your Knowledge

D.I. is a nurse who is caring for Mr. Thomas. Mr. Thomas has been in the hospital for 3 days following a myocardial infarction. On the morning of the fourth day, Mr. Thomas begins to experience chest pain and his blood pressure decreases. He is diaphoretic and states that he has some nausea and feels like he has to throw up. His EKG shows some T wave elevation in the anterior leads.

Continued on page 350

resting comfortably; D.I. assesses that the patient should continue to be monitored but that for the moment he is stable. D.I. suggests that some medication for anxiety for Mr. Thomas would help him sleep and have a good night. Both the physician and D.I. are pleased that Mr. Thomas is stable, and the physician tells D.I. he will call Mr. Thomas' wife and tell her that he is stable.

1. Were the communication tools used in this scenario appropriate?
2. How did they help to protect Mr. Thomas?
3. How did they provide a method for interdisciplinary communication that was satisfying to both the physician and the nurse?

Team Leadership

Team leadership is a challenging responsibility, especially when the team has members from different professional disciplines who may have differing objectives for the care they provide. In some situations, the leadership role is fluid and can shift from one team member to another; this is especially the case when the team is more informal, and team members represent different health-care professionals. When the team comprises nurse practitioners, physicians, pharmacists, and a physical therapist, each individual could be the leader at a given time when his or her expertise in caring for the patient is required. The challenge in this type of team is for members to assert their leadership at appropriate times and to listen and be guided by members with the knowledge required to improve patient outcomes at other times.

De Pree (1989) stated that true leadership is a matter of character. Leadership is an art rather than a set of techniques (Anderson, Manno, O'Connor, & Gallagher, 2010). Managing health-care teams requires effective communication and collaboration skills. Another essential skill required of an effective team leader is the ability to encourage a positive attitude in each team member. Ensuring that people know what their role is within the team structure and providing clear guidelines so that everyone has the same goals and objectives for team success help with team member self-esteem. Additional attributes of successful team leaders include enthusiasm for the team goals and missions and confidence in the team and the care it provides. Good leaders in multidisciplinary teams provide necessary resources for team success and training to help each member reach his or her fullest potential. Listening to each member of the team with full attention allows members to know that their input is appreciated and that they are considered to be important members of the team. Providing feedback is another job for the team leader. Praise for a job well done and discussion when things could be better are both essential to team spirit and meeting team objectives and goals. A more complex role of the team leader is guiding the analysis of complex practice and organizational issues within the team organization and work. Important qualities and responsibilities of a team leader are listed in Table 8-1. Chapter 5 provides a complete discussion of leadership for the DNP-prepared advanced practice nurse.

Table 8-1

Qualities and Responsibilities of a Team Leader

1. Good communication skills
2. Ability to inspire trust
3. Make decisions with the input of others
4. Act consistently
5. Provide team members with the information they need to be successful
6. Create SMART (specific, measurable, achievable, realistic, timed) goals
7. Ability to keep the team focused
8. Ability to listen to feedback and ask questions
9. Show loyalty to team members
10. Ability to create an atmosphere of growth
11. Have vision
12. Provide support, praise, and recognition; reward team success
13. Ability to criticize constructively and address problems
14. Display tolerance and flexibility
15. Exhibit a willingness to change
16. Treat all team members with respect
17. Be accessible and available
18. Have a sense of humor
19. Create motivation for all team members

Advancing Your Knowledge

You are asked to form a team within a large office practice setting to improve working conditions within the office and improve the flow of patient care. You choose two medical assistants, one front desk person, the office manager, and yourself to be on the team. You are the team leader.

1. What would be the priorities at the first team meeting?
2. How would the team meet the goals of improving working conditions and the flow of patients?
3. How would existing problems be identified?
4. What team leader qualities would be important in this situation? How would you infuse your leadership with these qualities?

Advancing Your Knowledge

M.T. is an advanced practice nurse in a small practice in a suburban area. She works with one physician. Many patients in this practice are older adults with typical chronic conditions. M.T. has worked hard to develop an interdisciplinary team to assist these older adults with their health and treatment plans. This formal team consists of home health nurses, a pharmacist, a physical therapist, and the nurse practitioner. The team members work together to ensure these older adults are safe and understand their medications. When an older patient has a new diagnosis of a chronic disease or when a chronic disease escalates to a higher level, M.T. activates the team by ordering a home health evaluation and notifying the pharmacists of new medications. The home health nurse evaluates the patient's ability to conform to the medication or treatment regimen and his or her understanding of when to call the nurse practitioner. The pharmacists make a quick call to the patient several days after the change in medication dosage or addition of new medication to ask how things are going and to determine whether the medication is being taken correctly. M.T., the home health nurse, and the pharmacist have a conference call on Friday mornings to discuss all the patients they jointly treated that week. When needed, the physical therapist also gets involved and is consulted on the Friday telephone calls.

These team interactions take less than 20 minutes per week per patient. M.T. keeps a log of these interactions and phone conversations and estimates that this teamwork has prevented many hospitalizations and has even reduced mortality among these older adults. For example, one patient who was receiving warfarin (Coumadin) had her international normalized ratio checked by a cardiology office. She was called the next day and told to take "5 of Coumadin" daily. Because this was a new onset of atrial fibrillation for this patient, the pharmacist called to ensure the patient knew how to take the medication. The orders from the physician were to take 5 mg of Coumadin daily. The patient stated to the pharmacist that the physician wanted her to take 5 tablets of Coumadin a day. The pharmacist was able to explain that this was not correct and that she was to take one 5-mg tablet a day. The pharmacist notified M.T. of the confusion, and M.T. called the next day to ensure the patient understood how to take her medication. This action averted what could have been a disaster for the patient.

1. How can teams such as this one be formed in other practice areas?
2. What are the overall benefits of the team approach to care?
3. The professionals in this situation are not being paid for their time interacting with the patients as a team. What other ways are they benefiting? How can practices benefit from these types of team associations?

Primary Health Care

Primary health care (PHC) is care that encompasses the physical, psychosocial, environmental, and spiritual aspects of health. PHC is a concept that was first described in 1978 by the World Health Organization (WHO) in a document entitled the Declaration of Alma Ata (1978). The Alma Ata was ratified by 134 countries around the world. This document described PHC as the best framework for health systems in both highly developed and less developed countries. The definition of PHC differs from primary care because it includes social issues and is meant to create the capacity to meet all of the health-care needs of patients, families, and communities in one place. Traditional primary care organizational health-care delivery has many gaps that reduce the efficacy and efficiency of care for patients. The primary care model continues to divide the provider from the front office staff, creating a lack of communication, collaboration, and coordination of care. The fee-for-service structure within the current system also offers incentives for providers to increase the number of billable services rather than increase the quality of care rendered.

The focus of traditional primary care is on the individual, whereas the focus of PHC is on both the individual and the community. Primary care is a component of PHC, but PHC is broader in scope. PHC involves engaging the community in dialogue concerning the health-care needs specific to that group (Solheim, McElmurry, & Kim, 2007). The framers of the Alma Ata believed that active community participation in health matters increases knowledge, promoting health and reducing the burden of disease. For example, health-care providers should know that children living in a certain area of a community have a higher-than-average level of upper respiratory infections, which could come from environmental issues such as industrial smoke or waste. This knowledge can promote action by the health-care provider in alerting community leaders to this problem and, it is hoped, leading to a change in environmental regulations and healthier children.

To create PHC skills, teamwork, collaboration, and communication are required. The Alma Ata document stated, "Primary health care relies … on health workers, including physicians, nurses, midwives, auxiliaries and community workers as well as social workers to work as a health care team and to respond to the expressed health needs of the community" (Declaration of Alma Ata, Article VII, Number 7 (1978). Within the concept of PHC, the team takes an interdisciplinary approach that emphasizes increased interdependence, jointly defined goals, and patient-focused plans of care. The WHO predicted that this broad-based type of inclusive interdisciplinary teamwork would promote success in providing personal and community-based health care. The key concepts included in PHC as defined by the WHO are listed in Box 8-2.

In one study, a PHC setting was developed at Midwestern University (Solheim, McElmurry, & Kim, 2007). The team used in this PHC setting included physicians, nurses, advanced practice nurses, community members, social workers, pharmacists, psychologists, nutritionists, and physical therapists. Nursing faculty members who provided care at the clinic were surveyed to determine their satisfaction with this model and where they thought that the model had the highest impact on the health and well-being of patients and the community. The survey was administered to 94 nurses and had a response rate of 26%. The study found that the problems that benefited most from an interdisciplinary team approach included nutrition and obesity, diabetes, hypertension, heart disease, women's health issues, dental health, depression, and sexually transmitted infections. The study revealed that PHC contributed positively in the areas of medication management, screening, preventive care, and referral

Box 8-2

Key Concepts Within Primary Health Care

- Essential health care based on practical, scientifically sound, and socially acceptable methods and technology, made universally accessible and through communities' full participation and at a cost that the community and country can afford to maintain at every stage of individuals' development in the spirit of self-reliance and self-determination
- An integral part both of the U.S. health system and of the overall social and economic development of the country
- The first level of contact of individuals, the family, and community with the health system bringing health care as close as possible to where people live and work
- Focus on prevention of disease and health promotion
- Multidisciplinary approach integrating social and economic development with health programs

Source: McElmurry, R., & Keeney, T. (2006). Setting a foundation: underlying values and structures of health promotion in primary health care settings. *Primary Health Care Research, 7* 172–182.

services. The main motivations for the nurses in this study to become involved in PHC were professional values; an ability to address health disparities, access, and injustice; and the efficacy of the PHC model. In this study, the participants found that the most effective work was centered around health promotion and disease prevention, rather than highly technical illness management.

Barriers to the Development of Primary Health Care

In the U.S. health-care system, barriers exist to the development of true PHC. These barriers include the following:

- *Inadequate and cumbersome financial coverage for health care:* Specialist care receives a higher level of reimbursement than PHC, where tests and diagnosis are the only reimbursable actions, and other aspects of care such as education, counseling, and an assessment of factors that could contribute to health problems (and health promotion and disease prevention) are not reimbursable actions (Pho, 2010).
- *Physician training:* Medical schools are very slow to embrace the need to prepare primary care physicians to provide true PHC with all its components (Glied, Prabhu, & Edelman, 2009).
- *Inadequate understanding of PHC:* Americans are slow to move toward behavior change as a method of health promotion. Many people still want a "pill" to "fix" them and are unwilling to become active partners in their own health (Gillam, 2008).
- *Lack of political support:* There is little political support for improving access to PHC (Gillam, 2008).

Care Coordination

An important function of PHC is care coordination. Care coordination helps to ensure that a patient's needs and preferences for care are understood and that those needs and preferences are shared between providers, patients, and families as a patient moves from one health-care setting to another (Bodenheimer, 2008).

The following are important outcomes of patient-centered primary care coordination:

- Improved quality and timeliness of care
- Patient and family involvement in health-care decision making
- Increased peer support and information sharing within the provider community
- Improved health outcomes
- Reduced health-care costs

Care among many different providers must be well coordinated to avoid waste; overuse, underuse, or misuse of prescribed medications; and conflicting plans of care. Care coordination is an approach in which all of a patient's needs are coordinated with the assistance of a primary point of contact. The point-of-contact person provides information to other health-care providers, the patient, and the patient's caregivers. The primary point-of-contact person works with the patient to ensure that the patient gets the most appropriate treatment, while ensuring that health care is not accidentally duplicated. This process appears to save money on health-care costs and improves the quality of care and patient satisfaction (McAllister, Presler, & Cooley, 2007). Table 8-2 presents the objectives of care coordination.

The Commonwealth Fund (2009) found that one-third of Americans had experienced health-care and medical errors as a result of lack of care coordination. Without the ability to support care coordination, barriers to positive patient outcomes continue to exist. One example concerns older adults and polypharmacy. When older adults are prescribed medications from different health-care providers and no one coordinates the use of these medications, drug interactions or drug reactions can occur. Care coordination requires adequate personnel and time and is often limited in primary care by lack of necessary

Table 8-2

Objectives of Care Coordination

- Ensure a locus of ongoing, proactive, planned care activities
- Build and use effective communication strategies among family, the medical home, schools, specialists, and community professionals and community connections
- Help improve, measure, monitor, and sustain quality outcomes (clinical, functional, satisfaction, and cost)

Source: McAllister, J., Presler, E., & Cooley, W. C. (2007). Medical home practice based care coordination. Retrieved from http://www.medicalhomeimprovement.org/pdf/MHPracticeBasedCC-Workbook_7-16-07.pdf

resources. Some states have begun to reimburse physicians, nurse practitioners, and physician assistants for care coordination activities (Commonwealth Fund, 2009).

Medical Home

The concept of the medical home, an example of PHC, was created by the American Academy of Family Physicians (2007) and other physician groups and is focused on providing comprehensive primary care and care coordination. In this new model, the medical office is transformed into the central point where health care is organized and coordinated based on patient needs and priorities. The home boasts modern conveniences, such as e-mail communication and same-day appointments; quality ratings and pricing information; and secure online tools to help consumers manage their health information, review the latest medical findings, and make informed decisions. Consumers receive reminders about necessary appointments and screenings and other support to help them and their families manage chronic conditions such as diabetes or heart disease. The health-care provider helps each person to obtain the services of medical specialists and other health-care providers, such as nutritionists and physical trainers. The consumer decides who is on his or her team, and the health-care provider ensures they are working together to meet all of the patient's needs in an integrated, "whole person" fashion (Backer, 2007). The medical home is an optimal setting for family-centered care coordination (Weissman & Fratantoni, 2010). Box 8-3 presents the objectives of a patient-centered medical home.

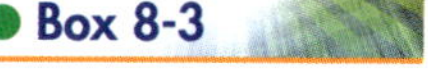

Objectives of Patient-Centered Medical Homes

- *Ongoing care:* A sustained patient/clinician partnership is established, and care is provided in the context of family and community. The practice is able to address most personal health care needs.
- *Comprehensive:* The practice care team takes responsibility for all care needed by the patient across the patient's life span.
- *Interdisciplinary team approach:* Communication and collaboration occur across disciplines for the benefit of the patient. Referrals are made when needed care falls outside the scope of the provider.
- *Coordinated:* Care is integrated and coordinated across the health-care system to include referrals to specialists, therapists, hospitalization, home health care, and long-term care as determined by the patient's needs.
- *Enhanced access:* Systems are employed to ensure that patients can be seen in a timely manner, including same-day appointments, expanded hours, and a wider array of communication options.

Continued on page 358

Box 8-3

Objectives of Patient-Centered Medical Homes *Continued from page 357*

- *Quality and safety:* The care team uses evidence-based clinical decision making. There is active participation in continuous quality improvement. Issues of quality and safety are addressed by multiple mechanisms, including electronic health records and an ongoing quality improvement program.
- *Added value:* Provider reimbursement reflects the added value provided to patients within a practice that incorporates all the criteria of coordinated primary care.

Source: Garnica, M. (2009). Coordinated primary care: Medical home model. *Clinical Scholars Review, 2*(2), 60–65.

The concept of the medical home is one way in which the United States is beginning to develop a PHC model for individuals and communities. The American Academy of Pediatrics (AAP) introduced the medical home concept in 1967 as a central location for archiving a child's medical record. In its 2002 policy statement, the AAP expanded the medical home concept to include the following operational characteristics: accessible, continuous, comprehensive, family-centered, coordinated, compassionate, and culturally effective care. The American Academy of Family Physicians and the American College of Physicians subsequently developed their own models for improving patient care, called the *medical home* (American Academy of Family Physicians, 2007) or *advanced medical home* (American College of Physicians, 2006). The Medicare Improvement and Extension Act of 2006 funded pilot medical home demonstration projects.

These organizations define patient-centered medical homes as health-care settings that facilitate partnerships between individual patients, their personal physicians, and, when appropriate, the patient's family. The model facilitates care through registries, information technology, health information exchange, and other means to ensure that patients get the indicated care when and where they need and want it, in a culturally and linguistically appropriate manner.

Although many states are establishing pilot medical homes, there are gaps between the model proposed by the American Academy of Family Physicians and other physicians groups and the concept of the PHC created by the WHO. The two most glaring differences are that the medical home is physician-dominated, whereas the PHC is a collaborative team approach to health, and the fact that the medical home is still focused exclusively on the individual rather than on the individual and the community.

At the present time, most state pilot medical home project legislation and Medicare legislation provide only for physicians to be patient care providers in medical homes. Many advanced practice nursing groups, including the American Association of Nurse Practitioners and the National Organization of Nurse Practitioner Faculty, assert that as chronic disease and health-care costs escalate, nurse practitioners are in a pivotal position to participate in the Medicare medical home demonstration projects. In 2009, the American College of Physicians and the National Committee on Quality Assurance endorsed the inclusion of a nurse practitioner–led medical home within the Medicare demonstration project (National Committee on Quality Assurance, 2010).

Other tasks for the medical home include reducing health-care costs; providing timely, efficient, and equitable care across a continuum of patient types and settings; and improving patient safety within the health-care system. All of these objectives are incorporated in advanced practice and DNP educational programs, making the DNP a logical professional to organize and manage medical homes.

One of the most challenging issues in primary care is the amount of nonreimbursable time that a primary care provider and staff must spend on patient education, assistance with reimbursement issues, and other care coordination issues. In one medical home demonstration project aimed at Medicaid patients, health-care providers were paid an additional amount per patient per month to provide care coordination. The outcome of this project revealed a cost savings for Medicaid of between $66 million and $220 million compared with traditional Medicaid fee-for-service costs (Abrams, 2008).

Hasmiller and Span (2010) speculated that because of the shortage of primary care physicians and the poor communication between physicians and patients—studies showed that one-third of patients leave the physician's office not understanding their disease or the treatment instructions—nurse practitioners should be included in the organization and management of medical homes in the United States. Advanced practice nurses are essential not only because of physician shortages but also because their experience dovetails with the daily work of medical homes—person-centered and family-centered care and care coordination.

The idea of a medical home that provides PHC would entail redesigning health care using an interdisciplinary approach to meet the needs of communities and individuals. As chronic conditions, health promotion, and disease prevention become the main emphasis of health, and increased health literacy and patient involvement in self-management become essential, the advanced practice nurse with skills in patient-centered care is well placed to be an effective coordinator of Medicare medical home demonstration projects. DNPs have added knowledge and abilities in the areas of communication, collaboration, leadership, health-care finance, and policy that propel them to leadership positions in medical home management and primary health care.

Advancing Your Knowledge

T.M. is a DNP-prepared nurse practitioner who has opened a medical home for young adults with mental disabilities, such as Asperger's disorder, autism, depression, and Down syndrome. Many practices care for children with these

Continued on page 360

Advancing Your Knowledge *Continued from page 359*

problems, but there are few practices for young adults. Although these young adults still need parental involvement, many of them face typical young adult health and social issues, such as nutrition, sexual health, stress, and support for health promotion activities. To meet the needs of these young adults, T.M. includes psychologists, social workers and community members who assist with housing and applying for financial assistance, and a women's health nurse practitioner to help female patients who are sexually active. The medical home has 1500 patients from one town. Classes are held at the medical home on safe sexual practices, nutrition, applying for and interviewing for a job, living independently, and dental health. Both parents and young adult children are welcome to attend these classes. The social worker helps patients to live independently if they are able, to manage finances, and to obtain financial assistance for health insurance and other needs. One of the community members assists these young adults to find living quarters away from home, ensures they are safe, and helps them learn to live independently and pay their bills. All of the professionals at the medical home keep abreast of legislation for young adults with disabilities and advocate for their clients at the local, state, and federal levels. The medical home works closely with the families of these young adults to support independence while keeping the patients safe.

1. What other services could the medical home provide for these patients and their families?
2. Why is the DNP the "right" professional to manage and lead in the medical home and PHC movements?
3. How can PHC create opportunities for health promotion and disease prevention and create a situation where the community comes together to meet the health needs for all members?

Communication

The bedrock of effective patient care is clear and appropriate communication. Likewise, the bedrock of collaboration is communication (Arford, 2005). Despite communication between professionals being one of the most important aspects of patient care, clear and meaningful communication between health-care professionals remains problematic (Manojlovich & Antonakos, 2008). Communication plays a primary role in establishing a trusting relationship with patients, working with other professionals to establish safe and effective care strategies, enabling patients to become self-reliant, and creating understanding with families regarding patient health and well-being.

Better communication between health professionals has been proven to result in better conflict resolution (Dixson, Larison, & Zabari, 2006). These researchers showed that unambiguous and respectful communication between health-care professionals increased nursing job satisfaction, increased physician satisfaction, reduced length of stay for patients, and improved patient satisfaction with the hospital stay. The same study and a similar one completed in 2008 revealed that more effective communication continued to improve job satisfaction among nursing staff members, yielded improvements in patient outcomes, and resulted in fewer medical errors (Dixson, Larison, & Zabari, 2006; Manojlovich & Antonakos, 2008).

The designation of Magnet Hospitals by the American Nurses Credentialing Center means that the health-care institution so designated has provided an atmosphere of nursing excellence (American Nurses Credentialing Center, 2006). Magnet Hospitals have better patient safety and outcomes records than other hospitals. Positive and open communication is such an important part of health care that it is one of the attributes of Magnet Hospitals (American Nurses Credentialing Center, 2006).

Effective communication is the cornerstone of interdisciplinary collaboration. It is especially crucial where two different professions with different values, such as medicine and nursing, are working together to care for patients. Kennedy, Ferri, and Sofer (2004) studied the effect of participation in an educational program on leadership skills, teamwork, and collaborative communication. The educational program was provided over an 8-month period and included 23 hours of meetings and educational dialogue. The post–educational session evaluations showed that all participants communicated better and reported increased satisfaction with their communication and leadership skills. Nurses were queried again 6 months after the educational session, and it was found that staff nurses perceived better collaboration and problem solving on the units and reported a decrease in personal stress. When provided with the appropriate tools and education, nurses are able to communicate effectively with physicians and are able to have a collaborative role in patient care.

Researchers found that little attention is given to professional communication skills in nursing and medical education programs or during physicians' residency years (Thomson, 2008). In several other studies, nurses cited goals worksheets and patient conferences as effective ways to communicate patient care issues, whereas physicians preferred abbreviated discussions pertaining to medical issues as effective communication (Baggs, et al., 1999; Gionta, Harlow, Litman, & Leeman, 2005). Manojlovich and Antonakos (2008) also found that nurses and physicians differ in their ideas about what constitutes effective communication. In this study, 462 nurses and 78 physicians were surveyed and asked to describe openness, understanding, and accuracy as components of effective communication. Physicians described the need to spend little time on communication; the abilities of the nurse to anticipate the physician's needs and take orders correctly were important to them. Physicians did not identify information obtained from nurses as particularly useful or important and often described it as bothersome. Findings from this study highlight the need to identify effective communication techniques as perceived by each health-care profession.

Components of Positive Communication

Components of positive, productive communication include the following (Arford, 2005):

- *Trust:* Individuals with whom you communicate must trust that their communication will be kept confidential if they ask it to be, trust that they will be heard with an unbiased ear, and that the listener will be honest and fair in his or her response.
- *Common understanding of the responsibilities and accountabilities of each party in the communication:* This aspect of communication requires that all persons in the communication are aware of the responsibilities and accountabilities of all others in the group and that ideas and thoughts presented are regarded with respect to individual responsibilities and accountabilities.
- *Listening:* It is crucial to be authentically present and listen to each communicator with an open mind and an attempt to understand what he or she is saying and why he or she is saying it.
- *Ability to compromise:* This means giving in to some ideas that are different from your own to achieve consensus among the group and a greater probability that the end product will be accepted by all.
- *Common goal for the communication:* There should be no "hidden agenda," and the goal of the communication experience should be the same for all participants.

Skilled communication focuses on critical communication proficiencies, including self-awareness, inquiry and dialogue, conflict management, negotiation, advocacy, and listening. Before effective communication can occur, it is important to understand the basic components of communication.

McKay, Davis, and Fanning (1995) outlined four essential components of good communication among health-care professionals: collaboration, credibility, compassion, and coordination. The first is to adopt a framework of collaboration as the underlying goal of communication. *Collaboration* is evident when the advanced practice nurse solicits information; organizes what is to be said; and provides information to other team members in an organized fashion, engaging in dialogue to identify solutions and participate in decision making.

The second component of positive communication is credibility. *Credibility* can be established by avoiding jargon and vague terminology and entering into a conversation with all the facts at hand. Credibility is established when communication to team members is adjusted to meet the level of understanding and needs of each based on role, personality, and context. One way to prepare for credible communication with other health-care professionals is by using the SBAR tool that was mentioned earlier. Originating from the nuclear submarine service, *SBAR* is defined as follows (Hamilton, Gemeinhardt, Mancuso, Sahlin & Lea (2006):

S—Situation: What is happening at the present time?
B—Background: What are the circumstances leading up to this situation?

A—Assessment: What do I think the problem is?
R—Recommendation: What should we do to correct the problem?

SBAR creates a credible mental model for effective information transfer by providing a standardized structure for concise, factual communications among clinicians.

The third component of communication is compassion. *Compassion* is used not only to care for patients and families but also for team members. Compassion mandates that the nurse communicate in ways that advocate for the patient and team members. The advanced practice nurse demonstrates compassion when he or she displays caring and consideration for all team members and shows respect and affiliation both verbally and nonverbally. Covey (1989) in his book, *The Seven Habits of Highly Effective People,* said that to be effective you must listen and strive to understand before you speak and try to be understood. The Greek philosopher Epictetus said, "God gave man two ears but only one mouth that he might hear twice as much as he speaks." Compassion begins with effective listening skills.

There are four different types of listening: active listening, as in a discussion; listening with empathy, when someone else just needs your time and patience; listening with awareness to learn new information; and listening with openness when someone provides ideas for changes or improvements. Tips for promoting effective listening include the following:

- Listen with an open mind and an open heart.
- Be authentically present with the person you are listening to; avoid the temptation to begin formulating a reply while the other is speaking.
- Do not interrupt the person while speaking, and do not try to fill the silence; allow the speaker to think about what he or she wants to say.
- Understand the context from which the person is speaking. Is the speaker asking for advice, just venting, or trying to sort things out by speaking to you? Ask questions to clarify what is being said.

The final communication component is coordination. Using *coordination,* the person speaking organizes what is going to happen while encouraging team members and valuing their input. Coordination means ensuring everyone is aware of and agreeable to their assignments as members of the team. Coordination occurs when the advanced practice nurse mentors others and encourages input from team members. Techniques to infuse your communication with the four essential components of good communication are listed in Table 8-3.

Nonverbal Communication

Nonverbal communication is an important aspect of the overall communication experience. There are times when verbal communication is secondary to nonverbal communication, and without a clear understanding of nonverbal communication, the exchange is unsuccessful. Each party is left with differing ideas of what was said and of the meaning of the conversation.

Table 8-3

Techniques for Positive Communication

Collaboration
Actively listen to team members' ideas by summarizing what was heard and seeking clarification when needed.
Offer ideas and opinions using professional advanced nursing practice rationale.
Ask open-ended questions where appropriate, and follow up with probing questions for more information.
Present information to team members in a concise and organized manner.
Credibility
Speak in a clear and confident tone of voice.
Use specific and accurate language when conveying information.
State respect for others' viewpoints, but address points of disagreement directly.
Show calm and detached manner in conflict situations—focus on objective data rather than personal feelings.
Compassion
Use facial expressions and body language that invite others to communicate, such as facing others, smiling, nodding head, open stance.
Use touch when appropriate to provide reassurance, esteem, and belonging.
Express respect and appreciation for the contributions to patient care made by other team members.
Respond with positive feedback and support when others share feelings and uncertainties.
Speak up for team members when they are intimidated by others.
Coordination
Clearly delegate tasks to subordinates and provide clarification regarding expectations.
Offer guidance to team members when needed or solicited.
Ask team members for their input and positively reinforce their information sharing.
Serve as liaison between team members who have limited contact with one another.

Source: Apker, J., Propp, K., Ford, W. Z., & Hofmeister, N. (2006). Collaboration, credibility, compassion and coordination: Professional nurse communication skills sets in health care team interactions. *Journal of Professional Nursing, 22*(3), 180–189.

Body Language

Body language is an important aspect of nonverbal communication. When the person speaking is in a relaxed stance and has a calm demeanor, his or her message is interpreted quite differently then when the speaker is sitting on the edge of the chair, wringing his or her hands. When you are in a relaxed position when speaking to patients, they perceive that you are interested in what they have to say and are not thinking of other things.

Eye Contact

Eye contact can be crucial in communication efforts. In some cultures, it is improper to make eye contact with someone who is of a different gender or in a higher professional position. Eye contact signals that the speaker is engaged and that the listener is listening. Eye contact can build rapport and shows respect for the speaker and the listener. Eye contact can be taken as a sign of respect for the other person engaged in the communication experience.

Personal Space

Personal space is the invisible zone of physical space that provides psychological comfort when we interact with others. This buffer zone creates a bubble of personal safety even with individuals who are our friends. When people "invade" your personal space, it creates an uncomfortable feeling that can hinder communication. Personal space needs vary depending on whom we are talking to and the situation that we are in. If you are attentive to nonverbal communication issues, you will know when you are invading someone's personal space. When someone invades your personal space and does not seem to realize he or she doing so, it is possible to decrease your own discomfort by moving or sitting down in a space that cannot be physically invaded.

Posture, Pitch, Rate of Speech

A person's posture or stance communicates a rich variety of messages. Certain postures convey a negative attitude. Folded arms or crossed legs usually send the message that the listener is defensive or not interested in what is happening. This posture often indicates withdrawal from the entire situation and an unwillingness to embrace any new idea. If the speaker droops while standing or keeps the head bent downward or looks at the floor, he or she is more likely to be ignored or not taken seriously. It is best to stand up straight and face the person you are communicating with to demonstrate confidence and surety.

The pitch of the voice also communicates meaning. The rate at which the person is speaking (e.g., rapid, slow), the intensity of the voice (e.g., loud, soft), and the tone of voice (e.g., whining, growling) all have connotation in communication and meaning. Speaking rapidly can indicate nervousness or anxiety. People who speak very softly may be shy or lack self-confidence. Whining or growling may be evidence of fear or anger.

Facial Expressions and Gestures

The human face is able to express countless emotions without the person saying a word. In contrast to some forms of nonverbal communication, facial expressions can be universal. The facial expressions for happiness, sadness, anger, surprise, fear, and disgust are the same across cultures. Facial expressions can reveal feelings and emotions that may not even be intended during communicational exchanges. Expressions that are sad, anxious, confused, startled, warning, or barely tolerant all give meaning to (or can change the meaning of) the words spoken.

Gestures are woven into the fabric of our daily lives. We wave, point, beckon, and use our hands when we are arguing or speaking animatedly. Expressing ourselves with gestures is a natural way to communicate, often without thinking. Shaking a finger, folded arms, looking away, raising eyebrows, or clenching hands all add meaning to a conversation. However, the meaning of gestures can be very different across cultures and regions; it is important to be aware of personal gesturing and attempt to understand the gestures of others on the team.

Gender and Communication

Gender differences play a role in communication. Effective communication between men and women requires understanding the perspective and the role of gender. Although the ways in which men and women communicate overlap, there are distinct differences. Men tend to want a more factual and problem-solving approach to communication, whereas women often want to discuss and investigate options in communication. Christen, Alder, and Bitzer (2008) listed the differences in communication styles between men and women:

Men	Women
Live in a world of status	Live in a world of connection
Conversations are negotiations for power	Conversations are negotiations for closeness
Want to preserve independence	Want to preserve intimacy
Seek to win, avoid failure	Seek closeness, avoid isolation
Avoid taking orders (because that means low status and loss of independence)	Okay with taking orders (if it is perceived as forming a connection)
Seek control	Seek understanding
Prefer inequality and asymmetry	Prefer equality and symmetry
Are adversarial (with conflicting goals)	Are synergistic (with common goals)
Value differences	Value similarities
Goal of conversation: Transmit information	Goal of conversation: Maintain interaction
Offer advice	Seek connection and understanding

Nursing has been a primarily female profession and historically comes from a feminine perspective. Medicine has been historically a male-dominated profession and comes from the masculine perspective of communication. Collaboration and conflict resolution between these groups can be difficult, even from a gender perspective. Realizing the differences in communication styles that exist and creating methods to bridge the gap can stimulate better communication techniques and better understanding between these groups. For example, understanding the male need to win and the female need to seek closeness, a communicator could praise ideas provided and gently work toward a compromise where everyone wins and no one feels as though they have not been heard. When men seek to give advice and women seek understanding, the team involved could allow the men to provide their advice and the women to delve further into the ideas provided in that advice to seek understanding and resolution to problems. Often, when it is evident that gender differences in communication are creating tension or miscommunication, simply stopping the discussion and reiterating the end goal of the communication may resolve many differences.

Advancing Your Knowledge

A DNP-prepared advanced practice nurse is communicating with a gastroenterologist regarding a patient she is referring. The advanced practice nurse wants to share information about the patient, who is 70 years old and is scheduled to undergo a colonoscopy. The DNP wants to share that the patient lives alone and has no caregivers in the area. She is concerned that the patient will have difficulty with the preparation required for the procedure. She also wants to share with the gastroenterologist that this patient has mild cognitive impairment and often is frightened in new situations. The gastroenterologist simply wants to schedule the patient for the procedure. He says, "I am a medical man, and that is information for a social worker."

1. How can the advanced practice nurse make these important facts known to the gastroenterologist?
2. How does the information that the DNP wants to pass on affect the outcomes of this patient's care?
3. How can the separation between scientific knowledge and social information be mitigated so that patients are viewed as whole and unique?
4. Are gender differences in communication insurmountable?

Cultural and Language Differences in Communication

There are also cultural differences in communication techniques and styles. Culture infuses everything people do, including how they communicate. For communication to be effective, all of the parties involved must understand its contents and intent. When patients and providers speak different languages, there are two factors that can deter good communication and a complete understanding on both sides. The first is the language difference itself, and the second is the cultural differences associated with language. The understanding of a word or phrase might be different in different languages. Some cultural groups find it inappropriate for women to speak with an assertive tone, even in a professional context. Communication among team members from different cultures is affected by many dimensions, including the following:

- *Directness:* Making a point or getting a point across. *Example:* In some cultural groups, directness is thought to be rude; a roundabout discussion of issues leading to making a point is a better method of communication.
- *Hierarchy:* Following orders versus engaging in debate. *Example:* In some cultures, it is disrespectful to question someone of higher authority in any way. In others, respectful questioning is seen as being interested or being a critical thinker.
- *Consensus:* Accepting dissent. *Example:* In some cultures, expressing dissent is seen as inappropriate, whereas in others it is seen as being interested in the task at hand.

- *Individuality:* Individual winners versus team effectiveness. *Example:* In some cultures, team membership is valued above individuality; in others, the opposite is true.

Advancing Your Knowledge

An Islamic family, new to the United States from Oman, visits a primary care provider. The family members speak some English and bring an uncle who is fluent in English as an interpreter. The wife is dressed with a scarf covering her head and part of her face. She tells the male physician that she has pain but will not tell him or the uncle the location of the pain. The physician becomes frustrated and walks out of the room. Hearing the discussion, the female nurse practitioner walks by and asks if she can help. The wife says that she will speak to a woman about her problem. The nurse practitioner and physician work together and find out that the woman has breast pain and a lump in her right breast.

1. How can the nurse practitioner work effectively with this woman to help her get the diagnostic tests and the care she needs?
2. Why is adequate communication essential in this situation? How will counseling be affected by the cultural aspects of communication?

Advancing Your Knowledge

M.T. is an advanced practice nurse who has an independent practice of about 5000 patients. One of her patients with a diagnosis of hypertension comes to her and says that she cannot afford the medication that was prescribed by her cardiologist for her high blood pressure. This medication costs $150 a month and she cannot afford that and her other medications. M.T. would like to put the patient on a less expensive medication that is similar in classification and action as the one used by the cardiologist. She calls the cardiologist and tells him that the patient cannot afford the medication he prescribed and that rather than have her take no medication for her hypertension, M.T. would like to have her take this less expensive, similar medication. The cardiologist gets angry, says that he is not worried about the patient's financial issues, that he is a physician and not a social worker, and that if the patient does not follow his orders she can just go somewhere else.

1. What are the issues in communication here?
2. How can M.T. handle this situation so that the patient can continue to go to this cardiologist she has been seeing for some time?
3. How could communication be fixed to meet the needs of patients?

Advancing Your Knowledge

S.T. is an advanced practice nurse with many years of experience in primary care. She is sending a patient to see a cardiologist, but S.T. wants to speak with the cardiologist before he sees the patient. She wants to explain some of the patient's history and important health information that she wants the cardiologist to know. The cardiologist is an older physician who does not like speaking to anyone but other physicians. He is often less than collegial when called by an advanced practice nurse, but he is the only cardiologist who will accept the patient's insurance. As S.T. prepares to call this physician, she creates an SBAR for the conversation. She begins with the fact that the patient is a 62-year-old woman who has been a patient in her practice for only 3 months. The patient experiences episodes of near syncope and tachycardia (most likely premature atrial contractions). She has had these symptoms for at least 1 year and has tried beta blockers and other medications without success. These intermittent episodes often correspond to increased levels of stress in the patient's life. She has never had a syncopal episode. Her blood pressure has been normal on each of her four visits to the office with the last blood pressure measurement 128/72 mm Hg. Her laboratory work is all within normal limits, and her cholesterol levels from 1 week ago are total cholesterol 204, HDL 42, LDL 145, and triglycerides 148. The patient is taking rosuvastatin (Crestor) 10 mg for hyperlipidemia, which she has taken for 5 years; 81 mg of aspirin daily; and acetaminophen with diphenhydramine (Tylenol PM) for occasional insomnia. Once when she was out of town, the patient experienced an episode of paroxysmal atrial tachycardia that would not resolve, and she had to be given medication to convert her to sinus rhythm. She is being sent to the cardiologist for a thorough work-up to determine the cause of this problem and treat it. Because stress appears to be a significant trigger for the problem, the nurse practitioner has also sent the patient for stress reduction classes and counseling. S.T. tells the cardiologist she would like the patient to have a stress test, an echocardiogram, and a thorough examination to rule out any cardiovascular issues other than the paroxysmal atrial tachycardia.

1. What other information would be useful for S.T. to share with this physician?
2. How can she overcome any remarks made by the physician that are not collegial in nature?
3. How can S.T. work with this physician and get the best care for the patient?
4. How should S.T. end this conversation?

Advancing Your Knowledge

Mrs. Sikes is a 54-year-old female patient in a primary care office. She comes in for her annual physical examination. She is handed a clipboard with forms for her to update. She is placed in an examination room, and the health-care provider comes in. The provider sits with his back to the patient and asks questions. As she answers the questions, the provider is typing into the computer. One of the most important reasons for this visit today is that Mrs. Sikes has

Continued on page 370

Advancing Your Knowledge *Continued from page 369*

recently been laid off from her job. She cries a lot and feels very depressed and hopeless. She is also worried about so many things all the time. She wants to discuss this with her provider, but the short-answer questions being asked and the fact that the provider does not face her prevents her from talking about these things. The provider leaves the room telling her to undress and put on the provided gown. When the provider returns, Mrs. Sikes begins to speak and the provider asks her to be quiet so he can hear her heart and other "important" things. At the end of the visit, the provider quickly tells Mrs. Sikes that she is fine and to come back in 1 year or sooner if needed. He quickly leaves the room. Mrs. Sikes tries to speak again as the physician is leaving, but before she can the door is closed. She leaves the office confused and upset that she was unable to talk about her feelings. Being "dismissed" by her health-care provider increases her feelings of helplessness and hopelessness.

1. How could the outcome of this office visit have been different?
2. Why are some health-care providers poor or unwilling listeners?
3. What skills does this particular provider need to learn?

Peer Review

Peer review is an important aspect of advanced practice because it helps to demonstrate professionalism and clinical competency. Peer review addresses the competency of advanced practice nurses through methods such as mandatory continuing education, national nursing or specialty certification, practice requirements, and independent record review. The ANA (1988) defined peer review as "an organized effort whereby practicing professionals review the quality and appropriateness of services ordered or performed by their professional peers." To institute and use a peer review system appropriately to improve care, nurses must use effective communication skills, team-building skills, and collaboration techniques. Peer review is not meant as a punitive exercise but rather to strengthen practice and improve patient care through the use of communication and collaboration. One goal of peer review is self-regulation. Through peer review, the performance of advanced practice nurses is measured against standards of care, as codified by national guidelines and local benchmarks. Briggs, Heath, and Kelley (2005) stated that the most important aspect of peer review is to improve care through individual professional growth or by improving systems and quality.

For advanced practice nurses who work in health-care settings, peer review can be approached as part of quality review and improvement. Health-care settings should institute formal peer review mechanisms whereby advanced practice nurses may review charts and patient outcome measures for each other. The process must be seen as one that fosters growth rather than one that is punitive.

For advanced practice nurses in smaller practices or for nurses who work as the only advanced practice nurse in a practice setting, peer review can be more difficult. Physicians may perform chart review for the advanced practice nurse in small practices, especially where the physician is the owner of the practice. When a physician performs the chart review, however, it is not considered peer review because physicians and advanced practice nurses have different professional standards and ideas of positive patient outcomes. One method to provide for peer review may be to work within local nurse practitioner councils or groups to develop peer review strategies for smaller practices. This type of activity not only strengthens the professional status of advanced practice nurses but also creates a stronger bond between advanced practice nurses within a community.

Review should include substantive outcomes and should include aggregate data as well as chart reviews to measure items such as patient satisfaction, ease of obtaining appointments, and willingness to provide appropriate referrals to specialists. Before implementing a peer review process, advanced nursing groups must address issues such as patient confidentiality, practice confidentiality, and adequate education for persons who participate in peer review processes.

DNP-prepared advanced practice nurses should be well equipped based on their knowledge of evidence-based practice, leadership, collaboration, and communication skills to design and implement peer review systems within health-care organizations or individual practices. As health-care reform and other new initiatives progress toward using a multidisciplinary approach to providing increased access to health care for more Americans, the advanced practice nurse must meet all levels of professional responsibility. As advanced practice nurses assume increasing authority and accountability, peer review will help to highlight the benefits these nurses provide to the health-care system.

The DNP and Teamwork, Collaboration, and Communication

DNP-educated members of teams have advanced preparation in the interprofessional dimension of health care, such as communication, collaboration, and team building, which enables them to facilitate collaborative team functioning and overcome impediments to interprofessional practice. Because effective interprofessional teams function in a highly collaborative fashion and are fluid depending on the patients' needs, the leadership of high-performance teams can change. The DNP graduate has preparation in methods of effective team membership and is prepared to play a central role in establishing interprofessional teams, participating in the work of the team, and assuming leadership of the team when appropriate.

Nursing leaders are well placed to foster this collaborative approach to health care based on their holistic view of health and their ability to communicate effectively with people at different levels of the health-care continuum. Nurses are more likely to accept and use the input from multiple health-care providers, the patient, and family members to develop the plan of care (Powell & Hohenhaus, 2006). This type of collaboration provides acceptable, efficient, and effective care strategies at the lowest possible cost (Baker & Heitkemper (2005).

Examples in the literature demonstrate the role of advanced practice nurses in effective teams that improve patient care. In a study on the use of interprofessional teams to combat elder mistreatment, Baker and Heitkemper (2005) found that nursing professionals played key roles in a multidisciplinary team that included social workers, law enforcement personnel, and medical professionals charged with identifying abuse victims and providing services to stop the abuse and care for the older adults. Horan and Timmins (2009) found that advanced practice nurses played a key role in a community-based multidisciplinary team for osteoporosis treatment and prevention. Felber, Madigan, and Narasavage (2003) determined that patients with chronic obstructive pulmonary disease who were treated in a multidisciplinary fashion, including home visits by an advanced practice nurse team member, had fewer rehospitalizations, fewer depressive symptoms, and increased functional ability compared with patients treated in the usual care model.

Team Leadership and Participation for DNP-Prepared Nurses

Advanced practice nurses will be called on to participate in many different types of interdisciplinary teams and to take a leadership position within health-care teams. Advanced practice nurses have great team leadership potential because nursing has a long history of working with different disciplines to meet the needs of patients, families, and communities effectively.

Leading teams of professionals who have traditionally worked autonomously is challenging and requires a person who (1) has the ability to allow each professional to be valuable to the team and (2) can inspire professionals to work together in a coordinated and efficient fashion toward better patient care. An essential aspect of team leadership is respecting each individual on the team and valuing his or her patient care knowledge and efforts. Likewise, the ability to create efficient work flow, negotiate and resolve differences of opinion, and keep the patient as the focus of teamwork are tasks for interdisciplinary health-care team leaders. These skills, along with expert health-care knowledge and skills, have been engrained in DNP-prepared advanced practice nurses by DNP educators.

Differences in goals and objectives for patient care arise among health-care professionals because of the differences in professional focus. Physicians concentrate treatments toward a cure or at least the best physical status possible for a patient. However, a patient and family may be unwilling to comply with the rigors of a care plan to achieve these goals. The nurse practitioner team leader may be able to intervene and facilitate dialogue between the family members, patient, and physician to set jointly approved goals that meet the needs of all persons involved. This is a very different idea for many physicians, who have been taught that they know what is best for the patient and that their role is to provide this information and facilitate orders to see that the patient complies. Nurses have long identified themselves as patient advocates, and true advocacy involves leading negotiation with other health-care professionals, patients, and family members to keep care patient-centered and create meaningful change in patient safety and care.

Consultative Skills

Nurses who are educated in clinical practice at the doctoral level will be in demand as consultants for health-care institutions and for community and outpatient care settings. These nurses may consult on the design for practice development, creation of practice protocols, and methods to meet the needs of regulatory bodies.

Health-care consultants are used to design and implement new product lines, new strategies, or new practices in a health-care setting. Consultants work with practices to develop and implement electronic medical records, open a new practice, and develop plans for a community health-care center. The DNP-prepared advanced practice nurse with experience and knowledge in informatics, leadership, communication, team building, collaboration, and translating knowledge into practice is well positioned to be a leader in this area.

Conclusion

As the health-care system becomes more complex and the focus of care shifts to health promotion and disease prevention, the DNP will play a pivotal role. Creating interdisciplinary teams of professionals is challenging because of the tradition within each health-care profession to be educated and work separately without understanding the goals and objectives of the other professions. Nonetheless, creating these teams is necessary to reduce medical errors, improve health-care quality, decrease costs, and enhance the safety of health-care practice. Nurses have the broadest understanding of the health professions because of their view of the patient as whole and complete. They work with medicine, physical therapy, pharmacy, social work, and other disciplines to provide a complete care plan for patients. Advanced practice nurses will be called on to be leaders in the creation and running of interdisciplinary teams.

Collaboration and communication are two of the bedrocks of effective interdisciplinary teams of professionals. The need to be open to collaboration and willingness to learn skills to foster collaboration are part of DNP education. Positive communication is the most important aspect of effective collaboration. Communication skills must be learned and used even in the face of challenges from team members who do not use positive communication styles. The advanced practice nurse, educated in positive communication skills, must set the example of how to communicate effectively within a team.

References

Abrams, M. K. (2008). *Achieving person-centered primary care: The patient-centered medical home*. New York, NY: The Commonwealth Fund.

Aiken, L., Sloane, D., Lake, E., Sochalski, J., & Weber, A. (1999). Organization and outcomes of inpatients with aids. *Medical Care 37*(8). 760-772.

Aiken, L., Clarke, S., Sloane, D., Sochalski, J., & Siber, J., (2002) Hospital nurse staffing and patient mortality, nurse burnout, and job dissatisfaction. *Journal of the American Medical Association, 306*(20), 2187–2283.

American Academy of Family Physicians. (2007). Joint principles of the patient centered medical home. Retrieved from http://www.medicalhomeinfo.org/downloads/pdfs/jointstatement.pdf

American Association of Colleges of Nursing. (2004). Position statement on the practice doctorate in nursing. Retrieved from www.aacn.nche.edu/DNP/DNPPositionStatement.htm

American Association of Colleges of Nursing. (2006). The essentials of doctoral education for advanced nursing practice. Retrieved from http://www.aacn.nche.edu/dnp/pdf/essentials.pdf

American College of Physicians. (2006). Patient centered medical home. Retrieved from http://www.acponline.org/advocacy/where_we_stand/medical_home/

American Medical Association. (2008). Title protection resolution 303(A-08). Retrieved from http://forums.studentdoctor.net/showthread.php?t=531549

American Nurses Association. (1988). Peer review guidelines. *Journal of Advanced Nursing*, (NP-13), i–iv, 1–14.

American Nurses Assocation. (2005). Partnerships and collaboration: What skills are needed. *Online Journals of Issues in Nursing.* Retrieved from http://www.nursingworld.org/MainMenuCategories/ANAMarketplace/ANAPeriodicals/OJIN/TableofContents/Volume102005/No1Jan05/tpc26lnx16004.html

American Nurses Association. (2008). Response to American Medical Association House of Delegates Resolution 303(A-08) Protection of Titles Doctor, Resident and Residency. Retrieved from http://www.njsna.org/displaycommon.cfm?an=1&subarticlenbr=414

American Nurses Credentialing Center. (2006). Forces of magnetism. Retrieved from http://nursecredentialing.org/Magnet/ProgramOverview/HistoryoftheMagnetProgram/ForcesofMagnetism.aspx

Anderson, B., Manno, M., O'Connor, P., & Gallagher, E. (2010). Listening to nursing leaders: Using national database of nursing quality indicators data to study excellence in nursing leadership. *Journal of Nursing Administration, 40*(4), 182–187.

Apker, J., Propp, K., Ford, W. Z., & Hofmeister, N. (2006). Collaboration, credibility, compassion and coordination: Professional nurse communication skills sets in health care team interactions. *Journal of Professional Nursing, 22*(3), 180–189.

Arford, P. (2005). Nurse physician communication: An organizational accountability. *Nursing Economics, 23*(2), 72–77.

Association for Healthcare Research and Quality. (2010). Team STEPPES national implementation. Retrieved from http://teamstepps.ahrq.gov/

Backer, L. A. (2007). The medical home: An idea whose time has come … again. *AAFP Journal, 14*(8), 38–41.

Baggs, J., Schmitt, M., Mushlin, A., Mitchell, P., Eldredge, D., Oakes, D., & Hutson, A. (1999). Association between nurse-physician collaboration and patient outcomes in three intensive care units. *Critical Care Medicine, 27*(9), 1991–1998.

Baker, D., Gustafson, J., Beaubien, J., Salas, E., & Barach, P. (2003). Medical teamwork and patient safety: The evidence-based relation. American Institutes for Research. Retrieved from http://www.air.org/

Baker, M., & Heitkemper, M. (2005). The roles of nurses on interprofessional teams to combat elder abuse. *Nursing Outlook, 53,* 253–259.

Bodenheimer, T. (2008). Coordinating care: A perilous journey through the health care system. *New England Journal of Medicine, 358,* 1064–1071.

Boyle, D. K., & Kochinda, C. (2004). Enhancing collaborative communication of nurse and physician leadership in two intensive care units. *Journal of Nursing Administration, 34,* 60–70.

Briggs, L. A., Heath, J., & Kelley, J. (2005). Peer review for advanced practice nurses: What does it really mean. *AACN Clinical Issues, 16*(10), 3–15.

Bryan-Brown, C., & Dracup, K. (2002). Keeping the turf (wars) trimmed. *American Journal of Critical Care, 11,* 408–411.

Calendrillo, T. (2009). Team building for a healthy work environment. *Nursing Management, 40*(2), 9–12.

Christen, R. N., Alder, J., & Bitzer, J. (2008). Gender differences in communication skills. *Social Science and Medicine, 66*(7), 1474–1483.

Clancy, C. M. (2005). Quality is the goal for patient safety and health IT. Presented at the Annual Patient Safety and Health IT Conference, Washington, DC. Retrieved from http://news.yale.edu/

Clancy, M., & Tornberg, T. (2009). Team STEEPS: Assuring optimal teamwork in clinical settings. *American Journal of Medical Quality, 22*(3), 209–218.

Cohen, R. (2010). Health insurance coverage: Early release of estimates from the National Interview survey. Retrieved from http://www.cdc.gov/nchs/data/nhis/earlyrelease/insur201109.pdf

Cohn, K. (2003). Surgeon frustration: Contemporary problems, practice solutions. *Contemporary Surgery, 59*(2), 76–85.

Commonwealth Fund. (2009). Health care coordination: A cost saving and quality initiative. Retrieved from http://www.commonwealthfund.org/

Covey, S. (1989). *The seven habits of highly effective people.* New York, NY: Free Press.

D'Amour, D., & Oandasan, I. (2004). Interprofessionality as the field of interprofessional practice and interprofessional education: An emerging concept. *Journal of Interprofessional Care, 1,* 8–20.

DePree, M. (1989). *Leadership is an art.* New York, NY: Dell Publications.

Dixon, J., Larison, K., & Zabari, M., (2006). Skilled communication: Making it real. *Advances in Critical Care, 17*(4), 376–382.

Dietrich, S., Kornet, T., Lawon, D., Major, K., May, L., Rich, V., & Reily-Wasserman, E. (2010). Collaboration to partnership. *Nursing Administration Quarterly, 34*(1), 49–55.

Erickson, J., Ditomassi, M., & Jones, D. (2008). Interdisciplinary institute for patient care: Advancing clinical excellence. *Journal of Nursing Administration, 38*(6), 308–314.

Felber, D., Madigan, E., & Narasavage, G. (2003). APN-directed transitional home care model: Achieving positive outcomes for patients with COPD. *Home Healthcare Nurse, 21*(8), 543–550.

Garnica, M. (2009). Coordinated primary care: Medical home model. *Clinical Scholars Review, 2*(2), 60–65.

Gillam, S. (2008). Is the declaration of alma ata still relevant to primary health care? *British Medical Journal, 336*(7543), 536–538.

Gionta, D., Harlow, L., Loitman, J., & Leeman, J. (2005). Testing a mediational model of communication among medical staff and families of cancer patients. *Medical Care, 12,* 454–470.

Glied, S., Prabhu, A., & Edelman, N. (2009). The cost of primary care doctors. Retrieved from http://www.bepress.com/fhep/12/1/4/

Hall, L., Headrick, L., Cox, K., Deane, K., Gay, J., & Brandt, J. (2009). Linking health professional learners and health care workers on action-based improvement teams. *Quality Management in Health Care, 18*(3), 194–201.

Hall, P. (2005). Interprofessional teamwork: Professional cultures as barriers. *Journal of Interprofessional Care, 19*(S1), 188–195.

Hamilton, P., Gemeinhardt, G., Mancuso, P., Sahlin, C., & Lea, I. (2006). SBAR and nurse-physician communication: Pilot testing an educational intervention. *Nursing Administration 30*(30), 295–299.

Hansen, H., Bull, M., & Gross, C. (1998). Interdisciplinary collaboration and discharge planning communication for elders. *Journal of Nursing Administration, 29,* 37–46.

Hasmiller, S., & Span, T. (2010). Physician communication and patient satisfaction. Robert Wood Johnson Blog Retrieved from http://rwjfblogs.typepad.com/healthreform/2009/04/index.html

Hojat, M., Nasca, T., Cohen, M., Fields, S., Rattner, S., & Griffiths, M. (2001). Attitudes toward physician-nurse collaboration: A cross-cultural study of male and female physicians and nurses in the United States and Mexico. *Nursing Research, 50*(2), 123–128.

Horan, A., & Timmins, F. (2009). The role of community multidisciplinary teams in osteoporosis treatment and prevention. *Journal of Orthopaedic Nursing, 13,* 85–96.

Institute of Medicine. (2003). *Patient safety: Achieving a new standard of care.* Washington, DC: National Academy Press.

Institute of Medicine. (2004). *Keeping patients safe: Transforming the work environment of nurses.* Washington, DC: National Academy Press.

Jansen, L. (2008). Collaborative and interdisciplinary healthcare teams: Ready or not? *Journal of Professional Nursing, 24,* 218–227.

Kennedy, S., Ferri, R., & Sofer, D. (2004). Collaboration between ICU nurses and physicians: An educational program can improve the work environment. *American Journal of Nursing, 104*(6), 18.

Kim, M., Barnato, A., Angus, D., Fleisher, L., & Kahn, J. (2010). The effect of multidisciplinary care teams on intensive care unit mortality. *Archives of Internal Medicine, 170*(4), 369–376.

Kohn, L. T., Corrigan, J. M., & Donaldson, M. S. (Eds.). (2000). *To err is human: Building a safer health system.* Washington, DC: National Academy Press.

Mann, C. (2008). Five steps to effective team building. Retrieved from http://ezinearticles.com/?5-Steps-to-Building-a-Successful-Team&id=509105

Manojlovich, M., & Antonakos, C. (2008). Satisfaction of intensive care unit nurses with nurse-physician communication. *Journal of Nursing Administration, 38*(5), 237–243.

McAllister, J., Presler, E., & Cooley, W. C. (2007). Medical home practice based care coordination. Retrieved from http://www.medicalhomeimprovement.org/pdf/MHPracticeBasedCC-Workbook_7-16-07.pdf

McElmurry, R., & Kenney, T. (2006). Setting a foundation: underlying values and structures of health promotion in primary health care settings. *Primary Health Care Research, 7* 172–182.

McKay, M., Davis, M. & Fanning, P. (1995). *Messages: The communication skills book.* (2nd ed.). Oakland, CA: New Harbinger Pub. Inc.

McNamara, S., Lepage, K., & Boileau, J. (2011). Bridging the gap: Interprofessional collaboration. *Clinical Nurse Specialist, 25*(1), 33–40.

Murray, D., & Enarson, C. (2007). Communication and teamwork: Essential to learn but difficult to measure. *Anesthesiology, 106,* 895–896.

National Committee on Quality Assurance. (2010). Medical homes: Promoting quality and cost effective care. Retrieved from http://www.ncqa.org/tabid/1300/Default.aspx

Nelson, G. A., King, M., & Brodine, S. (2008). Nurse-physician collaboration on medical/surgical units. *Journal of Medical Surgical Nursing,* October 2008.

Newhouse, R. (2008). Evidence-based behavioral practice: An advancing your knowledge of interprofessional collaboration. *Journal of the Organization of Nurse Executives, 38*(10), 414–416.

Peikes, D., Chen, A., Schore, J., & Brown, R. (2009). Effects of care coordination on hospitalization, quality of care, and health care expenditures among Medicare beneficiaries. *Journal of the American Medical Association, 301*(6), 603–618.

Pho, K. (2010). Specialists and primary care pay per hour. Retrieved from http://www.kevinmd.com/blog/2010/10/specialist-primary-care-pay-hour.html

Pope, B., Rodzen, L., & Spross, G. (2008). Raising the SBAR: How better communication improves outcomes. *Nursing, 38*(3), 41–43.

Powell, S., & Hohenhaus, M. A. (2006). Multidisciplinary team training and the art of communication. *Clinical Pediatric Emergency Medicine, 7,* 238–240.

Schmalenberg, C., Kramer, M., King, C., Krugman, M., Lund, C., Poduska, D., & Rapp, D. (2005). Excellence through evidence: Securing collegial/collaborative nurse-physician relationships. *Journal of Nursing Administration, 35*(10), 450–458.

Solheim, K., McElmurry, B., & Kim, M. J. (2007). Multidisciplinary teamwork in US primary health care. *Social Science and Medicine, 65,* 622–634.

Sterchi, L. S. (2007). Perceptions that affect physician-nurse collaboration in the perioperative setting. *AORN, 86*(1), 45–57.

Thomson, S. (2008). Nurse-physician collaboration: A comparison of the attitudes of nurses and physicians in the medical surgical patient care setting. *MEDSURG Nursing, 16*(2), 87–91.

Weissman, M., & Fratantoni, K. (2010). Care coordination in the medical home: Better care for better pay. Retrieved from http://www.childrensnational.org/files/PDF/ForDoctors/cnhn/care-coordination-in-the-medical-home.pdf

World Health Organization. (1978). Declaration of Alma Alta. Retrieved from http://www.who.int/hpr/NPH/docs/declaration_almaata.pdf

CHAPTER

9

Kelly J. McCaffrey, PhD, and
Jamie M. Elfrank, MA candidate, Publishing

PROFESSIONAL WRITING AND PUBLISHING

Objectives:

By the end of the chapter, students should be able to:

1. Realize the importance of writing and publishing for nurses with doctor of nursing practice (DNP) degrees.
2. Describe the writing process and understand the differences between, and how to organize, informative and persuasive papers.
3. Discuss the use of writing as a critical thinking tool.
4. Identify the differences in publications and be able to evaluate a journal or publishing house for submission.
5. Recognize the different editorial roles.
6. Compare different writing styles and mechanics for writing textbooks, journals, query letters, and book proposals.

This chapter focuses on the importance of communication through writing for professionals in the nursing discipline. Writing skills are critical for nurses, especially nurses with advanced degrees. Writing not only helps to highlight the importance of advanced practice nurses in the health-care community but also is the best means to disseminate information gathered from research and practice. As advanced practice nurses with a doctor of nursing practice (DNP) degree become more autonomous within the health-care system, they will take on the responsibility to educate health-care consumers and other health-care providers. Practice-based ideas, population-based health-care needs, and outcomes from patient care translational research projects must be communicated in writing for them to have a lasting effect. As DNP-prepared advanced practice nurses seek out entrepreneurial opportunities, they need to have the ability to craft well-written business plans to persuade investors and to develop collaborative agreements with other providers. Under all circumstances, good writing skills not only get the word out more effectively, but they also engender confidence in the writer. Individuals who write well gain respect in almost every aspect of their professional lives. The following topics related to the importance of writing are examined more closely in this chapter:

- Purpose of writing
- Writing process
- Why good writing skills are essential to professionals
- Goals of clear and correct writing, including informative writing, persuasive writing, and writing for a specific audience
- Writing as a method of the critical thinking process
- Organizing writing and creating a logical flow of ideas in writing
- Correcting common writing errors
- Submitting manuscripts for publication
- What to expect from a publisher
- Web sites with information about good writing skills and publication

To achieve clarity and efficiency in writing, the following are necessary (Abdullah, 2009):

- *Clear objectives:* The purpose of your document is clear.
- *Adequate and effective organization:* Paragraphs are in a logical sequence. There is a transition between paragraphs to allow the reader to flow from one idea to another without confusion.
- *Clear, brief, and concise writing:* There is appropriate sentence development and the use of understandable language that is not burdened with extraneous adjectives and adverbs.
- *Appropriate language:* The complexity of language used and choice of words is appropriate for the audience you are attempting to reach.
- *Correct spelling and punctuation:* There are no spelling or punctuation errors to distract from your ideas.

Effective Writing Skills Are Essential

Effective writing skills are essential for many reasons, including the following (Marquette University, 2010):

- Writing is the primary basis on which your work and your intellect are judged in the workplace and in the community.
- Writing expresses who you are as a person.
- Writing is portable and permanent. It makes your thinking visible.
- Writing helps you move easily among facts, inferences, and opinions without getting confused—and without confusing your reader.
- Writing promotes your ability to pose worthwhile questions.
- Writing fosters your ability to explain a complex position to readers and to yourself.

- Writing helps others give you feedback.
- Writing helps you refine your ideas when you give others feedback.
- Writing requires that you anticipate your readers' needs. Your ability to do so demonstrates your intellectual flexibility and maturity.
- Writing ideas down preserves them so that you can reflect on them later. Writing out your ideas permits you to evaluate the adequacy of your argument.
- Writing stimulates you to extend a line of thought beyond your first impressions or gut responses.
- Writing helps you understand how truth is established in a given discipline.
- Writing is an essential job skill.

In all areas of practice, nurses are increasingly required to write clearly to convey ideas, thoughts, and the findings of evidence in the practice setting. Writing does not simply communicate ideas; it creates them. Good writing skills improve communication between nurses and between nurses and other health-care professionals. The ability to write clearly and organize thoughts and ideas into an appropriate written format advances nursing evidence, teaches others, and promotes critical thinking. Nurses must become and remain proficient with a variety of writing tasks, such as the following:

- Clinical writing, which includes charts, care plans, assessments, and clinical guidelines
- Academic writing, such as research projects and reports
- Professional writing, such as resumes, correspondence, and manuscripts for publication

The goals of clear and correct writing are as follows:

- Translate and materialize ideas and thoughts into accessible documents that are useful to others
- Report work performed in informative, concise, and professional formats
- Communicate via the written word accurately, not to be misunderstood, underestimated, or ignored

The Internet has changed professional communication. Put simply, because of Internet communication, we are relying far more on the written word. As a result, it has become more important than ever that we use language correctly and effectively. When relying on the written word alone, it is very easy to be misunderstood; it is important to be able to write succinctly and accurately what you mean and organize your writing in a way that effectively portrays your meaning to readers.

Writing Process

Writing is a process that requires you to make choices and consider alternatives. Because it is difficult to consider all the elements of writing all at once, experienced writers find it helpful to break the project up into separate stages.

Following these general steps in the writing process can assist you with almost any writing situation you may encounter. Although these steps may appear to be linear, experienced writers know that the writing process is recursive—meaning that the steps do not always proceed in an orderly fashion, one after the other. Often, you repeat certain steps in the writing process, doubling back before moving forward, then repeating some of the steps yet again. Several drafts are required to polish and perfect your writing, each draft filled with additions, deletions, and rearrangements.

Planning

Every writing situation is different, but every writing situation benefits from planning. As you approach a writing assignment, there are several factors to take into account. Identify your purpose and envision your audience to focus and shape your writing. Other elements of writing that you need to consider are your subject; the sources of information available to you; and special requirements, such as format, length, and deadlines.

Your subject, or topic, may be given to you, or you may be free to choose your own. If you can choose your own subject, select one you are curious to learn more about. Being interested in your topic makes the writing project more enjoyable. Also, be sure that you can tackle your subject in the amount of time and space that you have to complete the project. Depending on the number of pages you are limited to or when your deadlines are, you may have to revise your topic. These limitations may force you to narrow or broaden your topic appropriately.

Another step in the planning process is deciding where to procure your details, facts, and examples. The sources of information you use affect your topic and the entire writing project. Can you develop your subject using personal experience, or are you required to use information gathered from observation, interviews, or research? After you have determined what your sources of information might be, you need to determine whether these sources are readily available to you. Do you have time to conduct personal interviews or direct observations? Are there relevant subjects to interview or observe that are accessible to you? If you are doing secondary research, are the materials you need in your own library, or will you need to order them through interlibrary loan? Do you have time to order these materials, considering your deadline? All of these considerations also affect the selection and development of your topic.

Other important considerations include the length and format of your writing assignment. Is there a minimum or maximum number of pages required? Even if no strict length requirements are in place, you always want to be as concise as possible. More importantly, specific document designs will probably be required. For example, when writing for academic or professional purposes, nurses use American Psychological Association (APA) style. APA style regulates page format and documentation style. Elements such as headings, charts and graphs, lists, parenthetical citations, and the reference page all are standardized by APA.

Gathering Ideas

After your careful planning, do not jump into writing your first draft. You will benefit from exploring your subject in numerous different ways. If you are having difficulty getting started, these steps will guide you in developing your thoughts and ideas.

Talking and Listening

Often, when you are confronted with a challenge, conversing with someone helps to clarify your thoughts on the situation. The same is true of writing. When you are trying to come up with ideas to write about or trying to develop ideas you already have, talking and listening can be valuable tools. Before you ever write a word, conversation can focus and sharpen your thoughts. Talking and listening to others can also help you to discover what aspects of your topic others may find interesting or confusing. If you are writing a persuasive piece, talking and listening will allow you to explore a variety of different perspectives on the issue. Conversing with others also enhances the collaborative experience of the writing process. You might brainstorm aloud in a group of classmates, colleagues, or professors.

Annotating Texts and Taking Notes

Often when you write, it is in response to something you have read. One way of generating ideas to write about is to mark up the text you are reading. The notes you make when you read actively are a good source for new thoughts and ideas. Underline important concepts, mark questions you may have or contradictions you notice. After reading and annotating a piece of writing, you may notice patterns that lead to a topic.

Listing

Listing is the most recognizable of all the different forms of brainstorming. Listing is helpful in identifying what you know about a topic and what questions you may have. Write down ideas as they occur to you, and you can rearrange them into groups as patterns and themes emerge. After some thought, you can usually identify general categories, and after additional consideration, you may be able to add to, delete from, or rearrange your list into an outline.

Mapping

Also called *clustering,* mapping is a method of brainstorming that visually depicts the relationships between ideas. To map your ideas, place your topic in the center of your paper and put a circle around it. Draw lines to additional circles with ideas inside them as well. You can make your circles different sizes to represent bigger and smaller ideas, subdividing your topic and adding details. As more and more ideas occur to you, your map will expand. Figure 9-1 shows an example of mapping.

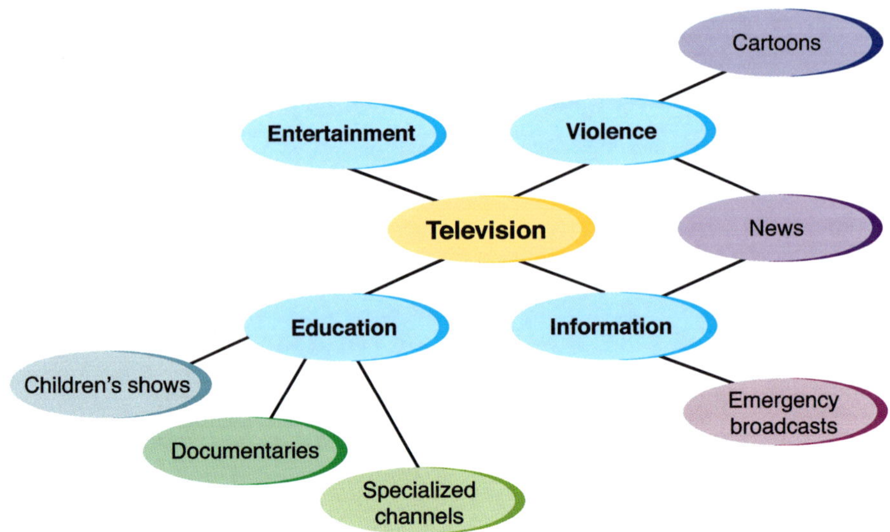

Figure 9-1 Mapping.

Freewriting

Freewriting is continuous, uninhibited writing. For a set amount of time, perhaps 5 or 10 minutes, write anything and everything that comes to mind, without worrying about word choice, grammar, or organization. Do not stop to rewrite, review, or delete anything; do not let anything interrupt the flow of your ideas. One suggestion when writing on a computer is to turn off the monitor and write. This allows you to concentrate solely on your ideas, without being distracted by the actual writing. Feel free to ask questions during your freewrite, without worrying about the answers. When you freewrite on a specific topic, the technique is often referred to as *focused freewriting*. The process is the same, but you are writing on a particular subject. With this type of freewriting, you should also try to observe emerging connections among your ideas.

Asking Questions

When journalists research a story, they generally ask a standard set of questions: *Who? What? When? Where? Why? How?* These same questions can help you form and refine ideas for writing. Often, the answers to these questions generate further questions that explore the topic more deeply. Often, academic writing is generated in response to a question. Posing a writing topic as a question helps keep you focused on trying to find the answer. The answer to your question may emerge as your thesis statement.

Journaling or Blogging

A journal is generally a place for private writing, but it can also provide an abundance of ideas to write about. Because a journal is private, you may feel free to explore and play around with different thoughts and language. A journal is an excellent place to record ideas and details because such ideas may disappear quickly if not written down. A journal is different from a diary in that a journal does not record your day-to-day activities. Instead, a journal contains responses to what you have read, observations you have made, questions you may have, and reflections on your own beliefs and opinions.

In a journal, you might use some of the brainstorming techniques already mentioned. You may make a list of questions that occurred to you during a lecture or a reading that you did. You might freewrite for one entry and then use mapping to connect various ideas in another entry. Keeping a journal allows you to explore issues and ideas in a variety of ways, without worrying about what other people think.

Writing daily in a journal also helps develop critical thinking and writing skills. Writing every day gets you in the habit of producing text. Words flow more easily and comfortably the more you write. Also, keeping a journal develops the skills of close observation and discovery, intellectual abilities that good writers possess.

Blogging is one type of journal, although it is public writing instead of private writing. A blog is a perfect place to post your opinions, summarize a reading selection or an event, record observations, and vent frustrations. Comments from readers may prompt new ideas and responses.

Developing a Thesis Statement

As you develop and gather your ideas about a topic, you must begin to consider ways of organizing your material. Try to identify a central idea or message; this is known as a *thesis statement*. A thesis statement announces the focus, or the essential idea, of your writing. It is an assertion of the point you want to make about your topic. It helps guide you as you write, and it communicates your central point to your readers.

Often, as your essay evolves, so will your thesis statement. Initial thesis statements are usually revised to reflect changes in the overall plan and main point of the essay, so do not feel tied to the first thesis statement you create.

Thesis statements are also usually one sentence—a succinct and focused announcement of the main point of your essay. Being able to summarize the central idea of your essay in one sentence demonstrates your critical thinking abilities. This one statement should shape and guide all of the other writing in your essay, report, or assignment.

Organizing an Outline

After you have developed ideas to write about, and after you have identified your main idea in an initial thesis statement, it is time to try to organize the material that you will use in support of your thesis statement. One way to do this is to create an outline. An outline displays the relationships among your ideas and provides a visual layout of your ideas. An outline can illustrate areas of your essay that are in need of further development and areas of your essay that might need to be edited or subdivided into smaller units.

There are many different types of outlines. The most basic is an *informal outline,* consisting of your thesis statement followed by a list of your major ideas. You do not need to write complete sentences within your outline; words or phrases may be enough. An outline written with just words and phrases is referred to as a *topic outline*. With an informal outline, you can organize your ideas, decide the order in which you will present each of your ideas, and add to or edit your ideas.

Another type of outline is a *formal outline*. This type of outline uses numbers and letters to represent the relationships among your ideas. Most formal outlines are written out in complete sentences, which makes drafting easier as a result. The APA style established an official system for the organization (hierarchy) of an outline, which is presented in Table 9-1.

There may be more than two subdivisions for each section. However, if you subdivide a section, there must be at least two entries: If there is an "A," there must be a "B." Likewise, if there is a "1," there must be a "2." Otherwise, there would be no need to subdivide. Another feature of a formal outline is parallelism. All the ideas within a specific section must be presented in the same grammatical form. Parallelism is discussed in more detail later.

Composing Paragraphs

After you have organized your material into an outline, you are ready to draft an initial version of your essay. Drafting means putting your ideas into sentences and putting sentences into paragraphs. Because you have planned and shaped your essay from the beginning, you already have an advantage when you begin to write or type.

Table 9-1

Formal Outline Format

I. Improving Diabetic Care
    A. Patient Access to Care
    B. Education
        1. Diet
        2. Medication
            a. Taking medication properly
            b. Side effects
II. Measuring Outcomes of Diabetic Care
    A. Compliance With Diabetic Diet and Medications
    B. Lab Values
        1. Hemoglobin A_{1C} levels
        2. Proteinuria
            a. Further lab testing ordered
            b. Referral to nephrology

The purpose of a first draft, or a rough draft, is to get your ideas out. During the drafting process, do not worry about grammar, punctuation, or spelling. You will address these issues at a later phase in the writing process. Part of the drafting process is simply to keep moving forward.

As you proceed and accumulate text, organize your sentences into manageable and logical units. A paragraph is a group of sentences that develops a single idea. This is a concept referred to as *unity*. The prefix *uni* means "one," which means there should be only one idea per paragraph. Unity strengthens the connection between the main idea of the paragraph and the supporting sentences that make up the body of the paragraph. Unity provides a single focus for you as you write and for readers as they read. Sentences that digress or distract from the single idea of the paragraph should be edited out. When you begin to address a new idea, start a new paragraph.

The first sentence of a paragraph, also known as the *topic sentence,* announces the main point of the paragraph. The topic sentence shapes and controls the content of the entire paragraph. All the sentences in that paragraph should support the main point. Likewise, all the topic sentences in an essay should support the thesis statement.

Another factor in effective paragraphs is the concept of *coherence*. Literally, the root of the word coherence means "to stick together." In a paragraph, coherence is achieved when all the sentences in the paragraph flow logically and smoothly from beginning to end. Without coherence, a paragraph is just a series of choppy sentences; coherence cements the structure of a paragraph.

One of the best techniques for improving the coherence of your paragraphs is to include transitions between sentences. Transitions are similar to road signs in that they guide your reader through the content of your paragraph, allowing the reader to follow along more easily. Another technique for improving the "tightness" of your paragraphs is to repeat a key word or phrase throughout. This deliberate repetition ties together the various sentences within your paragraph.

Just as a paragraph must be unified and coherent, so must your essay as a whole. In order for your whole essay to have unity, all the paragraphs must pertain to a single idea, known as the *thesis statement*. Just as your paragraphs must "stick together" from one sentence to the next, so too must your entire essay flow logically and smoothly from one paragraph to the next. Transitions between paragraphs help guide your reader through the entire essay.

Style and Tone

Style and tone are more difficult to define precisely because they do not follow a specific set of rules the way grammar does. Style and tone are more flexible and have more to do with the way you say something, rather than what you say. *Style* refers to the sentence structures you create, whereas *tone* refers to the mood or attitude of your writing demonstrated through word choice.

One way in which style and tone work together in your writing is in regulating the level of formality you express. Generally, there are three levels of formality: informal, semiformal, and formal. Informal writing is the type you might find in an e-mail to a friend; it is casual and conversational. Semiformal writing is the type most usually found in academic writing. Its style is clear and concise, and its tone is intelligent and fair. Formal writing is usually reserved for contracts and policy, where precision is a necessity.

Related to formality is the concept of personality in your writing. Sentence structure and word choice determine how much of yourself you reveal through your writing. There are three levels of familiarity that you might use to express yourself: subjective, familiar/polite, or objective. Subjective writing interjects the writer into the writing, using personal opinions and experiences. You would most likely use this type of writing to communicate with a close friend. A familiar/polite level of personality in your writing exemplifies a more professional relationship with your reader, one in which you reveal some personal thoughts but not so many as to interfere with the subject matter. An objective style leaves the writer out of the writing, focusing solely on the idea or topic being discussed. This type of writing is appropriate for scientific journals.

There are several ways to experiment with style. All of them require practice. Style does not usually emerge from a rough draft; rather, it comes from working and reworking a certain passage. For example, to keep your readers' attention, vary your sentence length. You might also try using different sentence types, which are discussed in the following section. Changing the pacing and rhythm of your sentences keeps your writing lively.

Tone is the mood that you express through your writing. For example, your writing might be serious, sarcastic, silly, or condescending. As with speaking, tone reflects the attitude of the speaker, but in writing, you cannot rely on volume or inflection. Tone is modulated through careful word choice. Using a thesaurus will allow you to experiment with different words, each having their own connotation. Connotation is a subtle yet powerful tool in writing, so it should be used with careful consideration. *Connotation* is the implied meaning of a word, the added meaning given to some words in particular. For example, consider the two words *house* and *home*. Both refer to a structure in which a family unit dwells, but *home* incorporates additional meaning, such as safety, comfort, and love.

When you use synonyms to affect the tone of your writing, be sure that the synonym has the correct connotation that you mean for it to have. Synonyms literally mean the same things, but some have additional meanings that can influence your reader. Words that are carefully and thoughtfully chosen can move your readers in various ways.

Sentence Variety

Using various sentence types can contribute to a more stylish way of writing. Experiment with the following four sentence types to create a more interesting and lively essay.

Simple Sentence

A simple sentence contains one subject and one verb (one independent clause): *I bought some bread.*

Simple sentences usually get a good deal of emphasis because there is not a lot of writing to interfere with the central message. A simple sentence is short and direct. However, do not use too many simple sentences. Otherwise, you will have lots of short, choppy sentences together.

Compound Sentence

A compound sentence contains two or more independent clauses: *I went to the store, and I bought some bread.*

A compound sentence combines two complete sentences. A compound sentence reflects the natural rhythm in which we think and speak. In that way, it is familiar and comfortable to us.

The two complete sentences can be combined in a number of ways. One way, as seen in the example, is with a comma and a coordinating conjunction. There are seven coordinating conjunctions in the English language: *and, but, or, nor, for, so, yet.* Each one of these conjunctions exemplifies a different relationship between the two sentences, so choose which conjunction you use carefully.

Another way to coordinate the two complete sentences is with a semicolon: *I went to the store; I bought some bread.*

A semicolon is correctly used to connect two complete sentences. A semicolon is usually used between two sentences that are short and are closely related in subject matter. To facilitate the transition between the two sentences, often a transition word is used in the second sentence: *I was late to the airport; however, I made my flight.*

Other transition words you may find useful are *moreover, nevertheless, furthermore,* and *thus.* There are many others you can find as well. A comma follows the transition word in the second sentence.

Complex Sentence

A complex sentence contains an independent clause and a dependent clause: *Because I was late to the airport, I almost missed my flight.*

A complex sentence contains a fragment attached to a complete sentence. If the fragment comes at the beginning of the sentence, it is set apart with a comma. If the fragment comes at the end of the sentence, it is not set apart by a comma: *I almost missed my flight because I was late to the airport.*

Dependent clauses (fragments) usually begin with a subordinating conjunction (e.g., *because, since, when, although*). Be thoughtful in choosing the subordinating conjunction you use because each demonstrates a different relationship between the dependent and the independent clause.

Compound-Complex Sentence

A compound-complex sentence combines a compound sentence with a complex sentence. Two or more independent clauses are combined with a dependent clause: *Because I was late to the airport, I almost missed my flight, and my luggage was lost.*

These sentences are longer and more complicated, so use them sparingly. However, they are effective in explaining concepts and should be used to increase sentence variety.

Parallelism

Parallelism refers to the consistency of grammatical form. Especially in lists and in outlines, all items should be the same part of speech. Look at the following sentence: *I like to sing, to dance, and teaching.*

This sentence is not parallel. How would you correct this sentence to make it parallel?

I like to sing, to dance, and to teach. In this example, all the items in the series are the same. They are all infinitives, or "to" verbs. The original sentence can also be corrected using all "-ing" words: *I like singing, dancing, and teaching.*

Both corrections are equally valid. When items in a list are parallel, each gets equal emphasis. When you create bulleted lists, parallelism is especially important. Each bullet must begin with the same part of speech:

- Imagine yourself on vacation.
- Plan activities you would enjoy.
- Avoid overexposure to the sun.
- Beware of pickpockets.
- Enjoy your trip.

All the items in the list begin with a present tense verb. You could rewrite this list using all "-ing" words:

- Imagining yourself on vacation
- Planning activities you would enjoy
- Avoiding overexposure to the sun
- Being aware of pickpockets
- Enjoying your trip

Either list is correct; consistency is key. Even when making slides for PowerPoint, remember to make bulleted lists parallel.

Writing is an essential skill for any professional, and the DNP student and graduate should strive to obtain the skills necessary to write clearly and concisely and to create informative and persuasive manuscripts for use in practice. Most universities have a writing center that can provide valuable assistance as you begin your professional writing and complete DNP assignments.

Critical Thinking Questions

One of the ways that the knowledge obtained from a DNP program can benefit the discipline of nursing is for DNP students to publish the findings from the capstone project or other projects undertaken while in school and after graduation. It is also important for DNPs to use their writing skills to remain active in legislation and health-care policy. DNP-prepared advanced practice nurses are qualified to create textbooks and other materials for new DNP students.

Advancing Your Knowledge

The community in which you practice has decided to fund a clinic for underinsured or uninsured persons to receive health care. The clinic will be funded partly by tax dollars, partly by hospitals that want to decrease the number of uninsured people who come to the emergency department for routine care, and partly by a private community-based funding organization. You believe that you are the right person to lead the effort to develop this health-care center and eventually run the center's day-to-day operations. You feel this way because of your leadership ability, your ability to understand culturally based person-centered care, and your understanding that the clinic could be staffed with advanced practice nurses and other types of providers to be cost-effective and provide patients with the care they require to stay healthy. The community has asked for a proposal from interested persons and a business plan for development and ongoing management of this center.

1. How will your writing skills influence your ability to be successful in developing your plan?
2. How would you develop clear objectives for this proposal? Why is clarity important?
3. The group has limited the length of the proposal to 5 pages; what are the challenges from this limitation? How will you meet those challenges?
4. As you create this business plan, how will your writing skills be influential in making the point that you are the best person for this project?

Purpose of Writing

Because writing is a lasting and concrete illustration of personal thoughts and ideas as well as a passing on of knowledge, it is vital to communicate clearly, concisely, and effectively when writing. The National Commission on Writing (2004) found that "individual opportunity for advancement in the United States depends critically on the ability to present one's thoughts coherently, cogently, and persuasively on paper."p 38. In the modern age of information overload, if written communication does not grab the attention of the reader and present information precisely and quickly, it could get lost or ignored. When sending a message to staff via e-mail, nursing managers who are able to provide important information in a few paragraphs rather than several pages get better attention from staff, and the information provided is read and retained longer (Ramirez, 2010).

Many professionals spend time and effort in writing and reading. Studies show that managers spend approximately 80% of their time communicating through the written word (Lehman & Defrene, 2008). Writing skills make an impression on the people around you, including your patients, your boss, and your colleagues. Writing skills correlate closely with success in the profession and the ability to be respected by peers and colleagues (Ramirez, 2010).

Effective writing conveys the intended message simply and immediately, meeting the main goal for effective communication, which is to send information to the reader. Readers should be able to comprehend the message within the first few sentences and should not have to probe or interpret what has been written to discover its meaning.

It is also helpful in drafting an effective message to keep the message limited in scope, covering just a few points in a single message. It is unwise to create a message that covers many different problems, conveys many different messages, or attempts to persuade the reader of many different ideas. If many different ideas must be conveyed, it might be best to send different distinct messages or create sections within the message so that the items do not run together.

Comprehension is fostered by carefully considering two central concepts in developing a message: purpose and audience. Generally, the purpose of writing is either to inform or to persuade. Think carefully about your intended objective writing. What do you want to occur when your reader is finished reading your writing? Do you simply want to disseminate information and have the reader understand something? Or is the goal to convince the reader to believe something or to take some course of action? Because writing takes time and effort, and because reading the intended message requires the reader's time and effort, writers must possess a clear, focused goal when planning to write.

Informative Writing

Informative writing, also known as *expository writing,* provides and explains information to readers. This type of writing sets forth detailed ideas, observations, facts, data, and statistics. Informative writing appears in textbooks, encyclopedias, reports, manuals, newspapers, and magazines. Its primary goal is to educate readers. To educate readers, the writing must be clear, accurate, and complete. Informative writing has the following characteristics:

- It has one subject, such as information about a new insulin protocol.
- It uses a specific type of language, such as terminology specific to the management of postoperative blood sugar.
- It contains new information, such as information regarding how to implement the new protocol and how to document the actions taken.
- It uses facts and data, such as providing the reason for instituting the new protocol and allowing the nurse to understand why tighter glucose control is important to postoperative patients.
- It teaches new information, such as the need for the new protocol and how to implement it in appropriate patients.

Critical Thinking Questions

Choose a topic that you feel is important for advanced practice nurses but about which they may not be as aware as they should be. Examples are barriers to independent practice, implementing guidelines, using evidence-based practice ideas, or collaborating with specialists. Or choose any other topic you think is important.

Using the bullet points that precede this box, create a 2- to 4-page document that could be used to educate advanced practice nurses on your topic.

Persuasive Writing

Persuasive writing, also known as *argumentative writing,* differs from informative writing in that it attempts to sway readers' opinions. It deals with debatable topics on which people may have differing views. A well-written persuasive piece is supported with a series of facts that help the author argue his or her point. Many authors also include counterpoint arguments in their pieces, which they can debunk, illustrating to readers that they have considered both sides of the argument at hand and have valid reasons to dismiss those on the other side. In addition to facts, authors may include anecdotes and hypothetical situations to build a stronger case.

Critical Thinking Questions

You are making an argument for allowing advanced practice nurses to direct medical homes throughout the United States.

1. What important facts would you include in this argument?
2. What counterpoint argument would you present, and how would you show the reader that this counterpoint argument against your ideas is not as important as the main argument for your ideas? (Read the original article by Backer [2007] on medical homes and primary care from the American Academy of Family Physicians at http://www.aafp.org/fpm/2007/0900/p38.html).
3. Develop a situation that could cement the value of your argument for allowing advanced practice nurses to become directors of medical homes.

Writing as a Reflection of Critical Thinking

Being educated means being able to communicate your ideas in written form. To translate ideas into writing, writers must possess intellectual skills of summary, analysis, inference, synthesis, and evaluation. Good writers understand the relationship between writing and learning, and they routinely use these skills involved with critical thinking to understand concepts at a deeper level and to improve their ability to communicate important ideas.

Critical reading often precedes critical writing. Many times you will be writing in response to something you have read or using what you have read as the basis for further ideas or as background for a presentation of project outcomes. The skills involved in critical thinking allow you to comprehend your reading more completely and communicate your responses more clearly.

Critical reading adds to your knowledge base, strengthens your intellectual abilities, and improves your communication skills. Critical reading means that the reader uses processes that result in enhanced clarity and comprehension of what they are reading. Processes that can enhance critical reading include reading with an open mind and reflecting on what is read, reading slowly and carefully so that the full meaning of the writing is absorbed, using a dictionary and other reference works to be able to understand what the writer means, making notes while reading, and keeping a journal of thoughts about what has been read (Cleveland Writing Center, 2011).

Critical writing requires the writer to examine ideas deeply and thoroughly, looking beneath the surface to the core and substance of an idea. It involves the careful analysis of a text, a presentation, or an image. It means identifying the strengths and weaknesses of an argument, assessing the quality of evidence, and considering implications. The steps in critical writing include the following:

- Gaining the main point of the document you want to write—determining the facts, claims, evidence, and arguments that will provide a clear and concise outline of your main point
- Critically piecing together knowledge and arguments that explain order and often provide predictive power for a position; critical thinking should result in writing that goes beyond stylistic appeal to convey a credible and significant message
- Comparing and contrasting your position with others on the same topic—list the facts that support or contradict your ideas
- Creating a final argument that supports the ideas you are attempting to assert
- Providing a final summary of your ideas

Steps in the Critical Writing Process

This section presents steps in the critical writing process: summary, analysis, inference, synthesis, and evaluation.

Creating a Summary

The first step in the critical writing process is creating a summary, being able to identify and restate the main idea and key points. In reading, this skill is essential to comprehension. In your course work as well as your professional work, you will often be asked to summarize a chapter or an entire book or a patient's case history. Your goal in summarizing is to articulate the main idea and key points; you should present them simply and briefly, without sacrificing accuracy. Summaries are usually short, so part of the intellectual task of summarizing is deciding what not to include. Understanding and identifying the most important features of the material demonstrate your higher-order thinking skills. In writing, being able to summarize is essential to your conclusion, your last chance to make an impression on your readers.

Analysis

The next step in the critical writing process is analysis. Analysis involves breaking the material into its component parts and understanding each part and how each contributes to the overall message. This skill is especially important in persuasive writing. To comprehend or construct an effective argument, you must be able to identify individual points and their overall effect. Similar to summary, analysis means selecting the most significant information; beyond summary, analysis inspects more closely the parts that make up the whole message.

Inference

The third step in the critical writing process is inference. Once you have identified the main idea and examined its individual parts, you should be able to infer what is suggested but not stated in the message. What are the implications of the passage? What does the author intend for you to comprehend without stating it explicitly? In critical reading and critical writing, you should be aware of tone and bias. These are clues to the writer's position, which affects the overall message.

Synthesis

Synthesis is the next step in the critical writing process. Synthesis means putting things together. Take the specific ideas you have analyzed and inferred, and connect them with knowledge you have gained from other readings, previous learning, or your own experiences. Critical thinking entails making connections beyond the reading itself. Synthesis works in writing as well. An effective piece of writing brings together different ideas and sources of information to further the knowledge in a field.

Evaluation

The last step in the critical writing process is evaluation. Evaluation involves making a judgment about the quality of the material and forming your own opinion about it. Evaluation requires an overall assessment of all of the aspects of the piece. Is the author reliable? Is the author's reasoning sound and fair? Is the evidence that is presented accurate and convincing? Does the author achieve his or her purpose? These are only a few of the questions you may ask. Just as you evaluate what you read, others will evaluate your writing, including your professors and your employer. Keeping evaluative questions in mind as you write results in a better final product.

Critical Thinking Questions

Read the following writing piece and answer the questions:

Yes, the DNP is the appropriate degree not only for nurses in advanced practice but also for clinical teaching positions at the basic and advanced practice levels,

Continued on page 396

Critical Thinking Questions *Continued on page 395*

clinical leadership positions such as nursing administration in health-care systems, and information technology management and nurse entrepreneurs. The academic preparation and skill sets included in DNP programs, delineated in the American Association of Colleges of Nursing (AACN) essentials document (AACN, 2006), provide core content necessary for the practice environment in which most nurse leaders work.

Although nursing needs clinical leaders prepared at the DNP level, this does not negate the need for some nurses to be prepared with research degrees (PhD or Doctor of Nursing Science). As an applied health discipline, nursing needs far fewer research prepared nurses and far more nurses prepared at the highest level of clinical practice and leadership: These nurses would receive the DNP. My own belief is that the balance in nursing should be similar to what is present in the medical discipline; only a small percentage of physicians are prepared at the MD/PhD level and therefore have a primary emphasis on basic research. All physicians, however, are prepared at the professional doctorate level, the MD. In nursing, we should also reserve the PhD in nursing as the preparation for basic science research.

There are other reasons why the DNP is the appropriate degree for clinical leadership in practice, education, and applied research. The current emphasis on master's level education for nurse leaders in clinical settings does not provide either the breadth or depth of knowledge and experiences in leadership, health systems design and evaluation, evidence-based practice, health policy, or applied research. DNP programs, on the other hand, are designed to broaden the knowledge base of the advanced practice clinician and provide the skills to participate as an equal member of the healthcare team. Some may argue that nurses are as well prepared as physicians and other healthcare professionals for healthcare team leadership, but these arguments fall short when educational preparation is compared. As leaders within the largest workforce in health care, nurses prepared at the DNP level will be in an ideal position to initiate efforts to improve the health of the nation at local clinical levels and within the health policy arenas. There has been support within the nursing leadership literature for the professional doctorate as entry level for practice for many years. The current movement for the DNP for advanced nursing avoids the entry-level debate, but some of the same arguments for parity with other healthcare professionals and better educational preparation for leadership and scholarship remain.

One of the most critical reasons for advancing the DNP degree in nursing is to provide nurse leaders with knowledge and skills to question current practices and change future practice. Questions related to Healthcare delivery and costs, clinical interventions for improved patient care, and more effective use of staff are ideal issues for inquiry of those prepared at the DNP level.

I have argued elsewhere that it is unethical for schools of nursing to prepare nurses at the PhD level when those nurses have no intent to focus their careers in research. The resources required to prepare PhD graduates are tremendous, and many graduates never pursue research beyond the dissertation. The DNP focus on applied research addresses the need within the discipline for integration of scholarship and practice and ultimately bridges the gap between academic and practice-based nursing.

—FITZPATRICK (2007).

1. Using critical writing skills, summarize the points that are made by the author in this piece.
2. Analyze what was said, and define the overall message that is presented.
3. What is inferred but not clearly stated within this message?
4. Connect the messages provided in this piece with what you know to be true and your ideas to support or refute the message presented.
5. Evaluate what the authors have stated and present your ideas of the truth of what has been said and your support or rebuttal of the ideas presented.

Creating Clear and Concise Policies and Documentation

Nursing policies and procedures are an integral part of nursing practice and are usually created by nursing leaders with the assistance of nurses at the bedside who actually perform the procedures and policies created. Each area of nursing may have guidelines that are unique to that area, but the entire group of policies and procedures is characterized by clarity, readability, and cohesive writing.

Nursing policies should be written with close attention to nursing values, the mission and vision of the organization, and the need for patient advocacy. Although the nursing leader may be the one writing the policy, input from people involved in the use of the policy helps to create a meaningful and appropriate version of the policy that is user-friendly and valid.

Creating Clear Documentation

Nursing professionals must document or write down (charting) findings from assessments, treatments, and procedures performed (including instructions given to the patient) and the reaction or outcomes of those procedures. Clear and careful use of words is an essential element of good documentation, and accurate written communication is vital to successful teamwork among professionals and positive patient outcomes (Quan, 2009). Other health-care providers must be able to read written documentation and understand exactly what was done and the outcomes of treatments. Many nurses regard documentation as a burden, but it is an essential element of patient care, and, similar to therapeutic interventions, documentation must be completed with skill. Nurses need to know how to write effectively.

Writing for a Specific Audience

Once the purpose for the writing has been identified, the writer must consider who will read what has been written. Identifying the audience also entails determining the best way to reach that audience. Tailoring the writing content and style to the intended audience increases the chances of achieving your purpose (i.e., to inform or persuade). Characteristics to consider when identifying your intended audience include age, gender, level of knowledge, professional position, and personal rapport. When addressing persons in positions of authority, the writing style may be more formal, clearly stating the purpose of your communication and providing necessary background information. When the audience contains colleagues or friends, less formal language may be used, and anecdotal evidence or stories may be the best way to make the point.

When writing to a predominantly male audience, short bursts of information such as bullet points may be the best way to get information across. Women are often more persuaded by stories and examples. When writing for an audience that is not composed entirely of medical people, such as when applying for institutional review board approval for a project, it is important to explain in "layman" terms what you are going to do and what you are trying to accomplish. Avoid using jargon or concepts that are not fully explained. Ultimately, your document should be as custom-tailored to the audience—in terms of language, complexity, style, substance, and writing vehicle—as possible. Put yourself in the reader's frame of mind to determine what his or her needs are and how best to meet them.

Collaborative Writing

Just as nursing is a team effort, writing is also enhanced when people work together. Collaboration encourages a more diverse spectrum of ideas. Collective intelligence is more likely to foster a greater number of new and different ideas than an individual working alone; this is especially true during the brainstorming phase of the writing process. In persuasive writing, different people can examine the different sides of a debatable topic.

Collaborative writing also distributes writing tasks among the group, allowing the workload to be shared. In addition, individual members of the group can work on specific areas according to their strengths. Writing with others also increases confidence when writers support one another.

One start toward collaborative writing could be to have someone else look over your writing after you have completed a draft. It often takes time for writers to become comfortable sharing their writing, but this is a vital step to improving your writing skills. A more direct form of collaborative writing entails two or more people completing a single writing project. Frequently, professional articles are co-authored or written by a number of people, which may increase the chances of being published.

Several qualities enhance the collaborative writing experience. First, careful planning is necessary to ensure smooth work flow. The group should agree on times and places to meet, due dates, software packages, and individual responsibilities. Everyone needs to commit to the plan. Second, the task should be divided equally among the members of the writing group. Fairness promotes efficiency and avoids ill will when everyone has an equal amount of work to complete. Finally, clear communication is essential to a productive work environment. Communication may take the form of regular updates on progress of group members, summaries of decisions made at meetings, or feedback on drafts. Group members must remember that open and honest communication is essential to all collaborative work, especially writing.

Publishing Your Work

Just as there are several reasons to hone your writing skills, there are several reasons to pursue publication. Personal and professional enrichment, sharing your research or expertise with the nursing community, and perfecting your practice are just a few reasons that nurses seek to publish their work. Navigating through the publishing process can be very intimidating. The next sections of this chapter take you through the publishing process and explain the different types of nursing publishers, how to choose the right publisher, how to navigate publisher guidelines, and how to create a proposal and query letter.

Many view the publishing process as a convoluted process, full of rejection and stress. One way to avoid this experience is to have an idea of how publishers work, what their objectives are, and the overall publishing process. The publishing process begins by contacting an editor. You will probably encounter several individuals with the word *editor* somewhere in their title. Table 9-2 outlines the different editorial roles a publishing house can have. Although each house and journal has its own defined roles, the roles typically fall into the categories delineated in Table 9-2.

Publishing in Nursing Journals

Perhaps you would like to write about a topic but are unsure if it is substantial enough to be a full textbook. Or perhaps you do not have the time to devote to writing a full-length book. One avenue you can explore is publishing your work in a nursing journal. There are two types of journals: peer-reviewed and non–peer-reviewed.

Peer-Reviewed Journals

Peer-reviewed journals publish high-quality academic works that go through a rigorous review process by other qualified professionals in the field. Some examples of peer-reviewed nursing journals are the *Journal of Nursing Education,* the *American Journal for Nursing Practitioners,* and the *Online Journal of Issues in*

Table 9-2

Editorial Roles

Role	Description
Acquisitions editor	Responsible for acquiring manuscript, negotiating author contracts, and overseeing the vision of the manuscript.
Project editor	Responsible for the schedule, ensuring all permissions have been obtained and preparing manuscript for production.
Developmental editor	Works hand in hand with the author to develop the manuscript from beginning to end (is *not* the same as a copy editor).
Managing editor	Oversees copy editing and ensures manuscript is properly prepared for production.
Assistant editor	Assists editors with various tasks (including sending manuscript out for review) and sometimes is primary contact for authors before their manuscript is accepted for publication.
Editor-in-chief	Oversees the entire editorial department; tasks can vary, such as deciding which articles will be published, determining which book projects to move forward, and developing a long-term plan for the journal or publishing house.

Nursing (OJIN). They are often supported by grants and have a high respectability in the academic community. The peer review process ensures that the material being published is of high academic standing. The downside of peer review is that the process is lengthy, so there is a risk of the material being dated by the time of publication. Authors also tend to have more responsibility in finalizing and editing the manuscript than in commercial or non–peer-reviewed journals.

Non–Peer-Reviewed Journals

Non–peer-reviewed journals are typically glossier and more visually appealing than peer-reviewed journals, targeting a mass consumer circle. Many are written in a less scholarly fashion, enabling the reader to read quickly and take away the main points without digging very deep. Peer-reviewed journals are supported by grants, whereas non–peer-reviewed journals are supported by advertising. The journals have a short-term plan (e.g., 6 months, 1 year) for their issues and use market research to determine issue themes and articles. The editorial staff members often write articles themselves and have greater input in the final copy than they would in a peer-review setting. Examples of non–peer-reviewed journals are *Nursing 2011* and *The American Nurse* (official journal of the American Nurses Association).

How to Evaluate a Journal for Article Fit

There are several questions an author should ask himself or herself when deciding where to send an article for publication. Table 9-3 presents a breakdown for how to evaluate a journal for the best fit. Before you submit to a journal, you should take time to read a few of its most recent issues. Choosing a journal should generally be one of the first decisions an author makes. Some authors

Table 9-3

Evaluating a Journal for Article Fit

Who is the audience of the journal?	Clinical practicing nurses, researchers, academics, clinical specialists, advanced practice registered nurses.
What is my message for this readership? Why would the journal audience read my article?	To update their knowledge; to learn about new research, guidelines, or algorithms; to read about a unique case study; to gain tips from an experienced nurse.
What do I have to contribute to this readership?	Are you a novice or an expert? Be realistic about your skills in communicating the message to the journal audience.
Would I be happy to be published in this journal?	Consider the following: • *Impact factor:* Are the authors and articles included in the journal highly quoted in other journals? • *Publishing schedule:* Monthly versus 2–6 issues a year. • *Indexing:* Is the journal indexed in the National Library of Medicine (PubMed)? • *Readership:* Is there a large readership? • *Additional outlets:* Is the journal online as well as in print media? • *Continuing education:* Does the journal have continuing education activities? • *Appearance:* Is the journal printed in black and white or color? Does it use graphics, illustrations, and photos? Does it have an attractive layout?
Have I examined the journal index? What impression do I have after closely examining several recent issues of the journal?	Has the journal published on my topic recently? Do they publish on related topics? Have any of my colleagues published in this journal? Would my article seem to "fit" here?

Source: From Edmunds, M. W. (2011). Publishing in nursing journals. In J. Stanley (Ed.), *Advanced practice nursing: Emphasizing common roles* (3rd ed., p. 281). Philadelphia, PA: F.A. Davis Company.

choose the journal before choosing the topic they are to write about it. By doing so, they tailor their article (as they are writing it) to the journal. One of the biggest challenges prospective authors face is determining and developing their manuscript to the audience the journal or publishing house is targeting.

Understanding Journal Guidelines

Each journal provides guidelines for the prospective author to follow. These guidelines include the page length, margins, if the journal is peer-reviewed and what standards the journal follows (e.g., the *American Journal of Nursing* follows the standards set by the International Committee of Medical Journal Editors, the World Association of Medical Editors, and the Committee on Publication Ethics [http://edmgr.ovid.com/ajn/accounts/ifauth.htm]), where to submit queries, if there should be a cover letter, and what should be included in the cover letter. It is very important to follow the guidelines outlined by the publication. Because many journals are flooded with submissions, a submission may not be considered at all if it does not meet the criteria, no matter how well the research is done (Table 9-4).

Evaluating Your Manuscript for Journal Publication

Many students (particularly DNP students) are encouraged to publish practice or clinical focused papers. There is a distinct difference, however, between an academic paper and a publishable paper. Although an academic paper may be very well written and researched, it may be rejected for publication because it was written from an academic perspective. It is very important to understand

Table 9-4

Summary of Major Problems That Discourage Editors From Accepting Articles

Problem	Comments and Examples
Missing the point	• Not understanding the audience of the journal, so article sent is inappropriate • Sending a student paper • Sending a whole thesis or dissertation • Abstract same as the first paragraph of the article
Not following guidelines	• Sending graphics in wrong format • Expect publisher to get permission to reprint illustrations, photos, or quotations • References in wrong format • Failure to keep paper to recommended length • Excessive number of references
Unethical behavior	• Having paper reviewed and revised and then withdrawing article and sending to another journal • Sending to several journals at the same time • Plagiarism, self-plagiarism • Failing to identify financial conflict of interest of author

"Little things"	• Not taking time to address editor personally with query letter telling editor:
	  • "You are a fool if you pass this up"
	  • "I got an A on this paper so I know you will want it"
	  • "I sent it to another journal but thought I'd give you first chance if you want it"
	  • "I worked really hard on this so I can't believe you rejected it"

Source: From: Edmunds, M. W. (2011). Publishing in nursing journals. In J. Stanley (Ed.), *Advanced practice nursing: Emphasizing common roles* (3rd ed., p. 283). Philadelphia, PA: F.A. Davis Company.

this distinction to develop your manuscript properly for submission. When writing an academic paper, the student is attempting to convey his or her understanding of a subject to faculty (i.e., a novice demonstrating a grasp of a concept to an expert); however, a published author is expected to be an expert already. Experience often is the best teacher for learning how to convert your student paper to publishable material. Editors generally do not have the time or the resources to give solid feedback regarding why your paper was rejected. One way to learn is to review the journal in detail, paying attention to the format, tone, style, and use of references.

Critical Thinking Questions

Compare a recent student paper with a published article (or chapter) on a similar topic. Create a list of ways that your paper illustrates a student mentality and ways the published manuscript illustrates an expert mentality. Do you think your paper is ready for publication in its current form? Why or why not? What would you change if you were going to send it out for publication?

Creating a Query Letter

Once you have your article idea and have determined the journal where you would like to attempt publication, you should compose a query letter to send to the editor of the journal. Query letters can be compared with a cover letter accompanying a resume and can be equally intimidating. Today, query letters and manuscript submissions occur online or through e-mail. For many publishers, it is the preferred method of submission.

The goal of a query letter is to grab the editor's attention and explain succinctly what your article is and why it is a fit for the journal. There are many articles online describing pitfalls unpublished authors often make when sending their work out to publishers. Following are some common mistakes:

- Sending your letter to the wrong editor. Always triple-check that the editor you are sending your letter to is the correct one. If you are unsure, call the publisher. You should be able to speak with an assistant who can confirm that the name and contact information you have is correct.
- Not explaining what the article is about clearly and concisely. This seems simple enough, but so many authors fail to execute this properly. Be sure to explain thoroughly what your article is about. Have colleagues, friends, or family read over your letter and ask them to repeat to you what your article is about. If they can't, go back and rework the letter.
- Forgetting the audience. Readers of your article need to be able to gain insight and information that can be applied to their work or life. Don't get so swept away by the research that you lose sight of how it can be applied.
- Not doing your homework. Many authors just send a query in without researching the publication first. As discussed earlier, this research is vitally

important. If you are familiar with the journal's audience, style, and content, this comes through in your query and catches notice.
- Not including a SASE (self-addressed stamped envelope). Nowadays, most queries and material are submitted online, but if you do decide to submit by post, be sure to include an SASE.

The key to a great query letter is to be precise, professional, and passionate. Be sure to show the editor you have something new to offer.

Advancing Your Knowledge

Examine the sample query letter found on davisplus.com. What mistakes do you see and what did the author do well? Attempt to write your own query letter. What journal would you submit it to? Which editor? Why?

Book Publishers

Writing a textbook is great way to gain recognition in your field. Often, faculty members commit to writing a textbook for their students because they believe the current books on the market do not do an adequate job. A nurse with a DNP degree may write a handbook for novice nurses to aid them in the transition from the classroom to a full-time clinical setting. There are key differences in writing a journal article versus writing a book manuscript (Table 9-5).

As you can see in Table 9-5, one of the main differences is the amount of time that must be committed to the project. Generally, once your contract is signed and your proposal (more about that in a moment) is accepted, your

Table 9-5

Writing a Journal Article Versus a Book Manuscript

Journal Article	Book Manuscript
Shorter time commitment (generally less than 1 year)	Can take a minimum of 1½–2 years to develop manuscript and another year for production; large books can take 5 years to develop.
Page length is shorter	Page length can range from 200–2000 pages depending on the project and topic.
Sole author of article	Depending on the project, may need to hire co-authors to contribute chapters; the main author would be required to manage and pay these co-authors.
Likely to be quickly outdated	Revisions allow a book to have sustainability, giving the author a chance to update the text with the latest research and findings; a well-received textbook can go through four or five editions.

manuscript will have at least 1 year to be developed. During this year, count on every spare moment you have being dedicated to writing the manuscript or communicating with the publisher. Although this commitment may seem daunting, many authors speak of how the research and writing helped them to be a better nurse or educator and fostered significant personal enrichment and reward.

Writing the Proposal

Every published book begins as a proposal (or idea) that is submitted to an acquisitions editor at a publishing house. Before you begin working on a proposal, you should review the proposal guidelines at the publishing house where you would like to submit your work. Major nursing publishers include (but are not limited to): F.A. Davis, Elsevier, Lippincott Williams & Wilkins, McGraw-Hill, and Springer Publishing Company. Each house has its own set of guidelines it would like prospective authors to use when submitting a proposal. F.A. Davis (which specializes in nursing education textbooks) encourages authors to start by considering three questions:

1. What are the needs of students and educators your book would be targeting?
2. What are competitors' strengths and weaknesses?
3. How can you create a better book than any of your competitors?

These questions are designed to get you thinking in terms of marketability and will help you convince the publisher or acquisitions editor to sign your book. Every publishing company has two goals: publish high-quality textbooks and sell those high-quality textbooks. Publishing is a business, and similar to any business, there is a bottom line. It is important to understand this when you begin creating your proposal. Authors also have a vested interest in the sales of the book because generally authors are paid by royalty checks (a percentage of every sale is given to the author in a lump sum twice a year).

A proposal generally consists of three parts: prospectus, table of contents, and sample material (or sample chapter). Not all publishers use these terms, and some may ask for more detail than others.

Prospectus

The prospectus is the description of the project. The amount of information required varies from publisher to publisher, but generally it should include subject matter, format, philosophy, tentative title, market, important features, and timetable. The prospectus is the author's chance to convince the publisher that the idea is worth publication.

- *Philosophy:* What is the philosophy or rationale the book would use? What is the purpose of the book? Explain your tentative title here and why you think it is appropriate.
- *Subject matter:* Will this be an educational book, a handbook, or reference book? What will you cover within the book? Generally, the more specific

you can be (e.g., pediatric acute care nursing), the better. Use this portion to begin brainstorming a table of contents.

- *Type of product:* What kind of product will you produce—a core textbook, a manual, electronic book, software, video? Describe the form the book will take and any additional components that would accompany it. For example, would there be online material (e.g., printable worksheets, PowerPoint, or instructional videos)? If your book will be used for educational purposes, what instructor and student ancillary material will you develop?
- *Market:* Who will read your book? Are there secondary markets? If you are writing a textbook, your market would be the faculty who are teaching the textbook as well as the students using it. Does your approach appeal to both equally? Is the reading level appropriate for the audience?
- *Important features:* What does your book feature that is unique? Be sure to describe which features you feel are most important and why you think this.
- *Mechanics:* How long will the book be? Give an estimated page number and what art and figures you will be including (art and figures are discussed later in the chapter). If this is a video product, how many discs will there be?
- *Timetable:* Estimate how long it will take you to complete. This will be a lengthy discussion between you and your publishers, but it is good to let them know up front what your tentative expectations are.

Table of Contents and Sample Material

Once you have outlined your idea, create a table of contents. How many chapters will it take for you to cover the material the way you envision? Outline each chapter as much as you can, and be as detailed as possible. A detailed table of contents allows the publisher to see how the prospectus will be translated into a manuscript.

After the table of contents is complete, begin working on a sample chapter. This sample will be used to judge your writing ability and determine if your tone and style match the market expectations.

After Your Proposal Is Accepted

After the publisher or acquisitions editor has decided to pursue your proposal, it will be sent out for review. The review process helps the publisher gauge how well received your book would be and if there is a need for it. Depending on what the reviewers say, the publisher may decide to move forward with presenting the proposal to the editorial board or publishing committee for approval, or the proposal may be returned to the author to add or delete material before presentation. During this time, the publisher discusses the contract terms. These terms include if the author will have a co-author, royalty payments, if there is an advance (payment in advance for the completion of the manuscript, which is deducted from the royalties) or grant (money allocated by the publisher for help with permissions or contributors, which is not taken from the royalties), timetable, page length, and other production details (e.g., if the book will be in color). Once the publisher receives approval from its in-house committee, the contract is sent to you for signature, and then the development work begins.

Critical Thinking Question

Think of an idea you would like to write about and create a sample prospectus and table of contents using the guidelines from a major publisher.

During the initial discussion, your editor will ask you whether you want to be the sole author or if you would like to work with a co-author (or several co-authors if your project is particularly ambitious). There are many points you should consider when deciding if you want to complete your project single-handedly or work as part of a team.

Sole Author

The benefit of being the only author of the manuscript is you receive full credit for the work and will not have to share royalties. You also will be able to make many key decisions with your publisher regarding formatting, deciding to cut a chapter, or adding new material. Still, you must also take on all the work yourself. Sole authors often reach out to individuals and ask them to contribute a chapter to the book. There is usually a fee involved, which is generally paid from the author's royalties. The author is responsible for communicating deadlines and ensuring the contributor stays on track and delivers the manuscript in a timely manner. After the manuscript is received, the author works with the contributor in making edits to finalize the chapter before sending it to the publisher.

Co-author

Many larger textbooks are written by multiple authors, allowing the work to be spread out evenly. If one author becomes overwhelmed by work or personal events, the co-authors can help pick up the slack to ensure the schedule is maintained. Royalties are typically split evenly; this is decided between parties before signing the contract. Co-authors also are useful if there are different specialties being covered in the book. For example, a book on maternity and pediatric nursing may have two authors—one who specializes in maternity and one who is a pediatric nurse. The downside to working with co-authors includes the possibility of a clash in personalities or vision for the book, managing busy schedules, and ensuring that each author fulfills his or her end of the bargain. Despite the downsides, co-authoring a book is a great way to have the opportunity to author a textbook and keep the time commitment manageable.

Ancillaries and Art

There are other requirements beside the manuscript that you must complete. One is developing an art program (art, photos, and figures to illustrate the text), securing permissions, and creating ancillary material for the text.

Art and Figures

Each book has an art program. The number of art pieces or figures is determined by the publisher. The author is always responsible for providing the materials to the publisher, regardless of whether or not the publisher is having the figures re-created. When your book is first signed, your publisher will review the art guidelines and what is required of you. It is very important to ask questions if anything is unclear to you. Ask for a sample art program so you can have an idea of what you should be submitting. Never save finding art or figures for the very end. This is one of the key components that can delay a book in meeting its schedule.

Permissions

When building their art program, many authors borrow art and figures from other references. It is generally the author's responsibility to secure permission from the source. Your publisher should guide you (typically there is a generic form they provide that you can fill in when submitting a request for reprint). Permissions are another huge hurdle when developing a manuscript and should never be put off until last. Authors are also responsible for paying the permission fee, although this is typically paid out of their royalties by the publisher. Most publishers encourage authors to adapt their material (either through redrawing or making significant changes) to avoid paying for permission. The material must look significantly different from the original—simply changing the title or the layout is not enough to be considered adapted. Some publishers require three different examples (called *scrap art*) to be provided for adapted material, which the art department uses to create a unique figure.

It is important to discuss with your publisher the permissions process and what permissions are required. In the past, print rights alone were acceptable but with the growing eBook market, most publishers require electronic rights as well. These are separate considerations, so you must be clear when requesting permission from the original source.

Ancillaries

As mentioned earlier, when writing an educational textbook, most publishers require you to outline the ancillary (additional) material that will accompany the text. Most instructors will not consider a book for adoption if it does not have instructor and student resources. These include (but are not limited to) PowerPoint slides, test banks, syllabus, case studies, interactive exercises, and suggestions for teaching the content. These materials should have just as much thought put into them as the manuscript. Because ancillary material takes less time to prepare and publish than the manuscript, it will have a different schedule. Discuss the ancillary schedule with your publisher at the same time you are discussing the manuscript schedule to avoid being blindsided when the manuscript is finalized and given to the publisher. It is easy to forget about the ancillaries when you are deep into development, but they are just as valuable as the core text. The last thing you want is to push hard through development and then realize the ancillaries are so far behind schedule they will not be available the day the book is published.

Conclusion

Writing and publishing your work is a great way to achieve personal and professional enrichment. As a DNP, it is likely that you will be required or encouraged to publish your work. Although this chapter gives you an outline of what the process is, there will still be curveballs thrown your way. The publishing industry is constantly growing and changing, which makes it very exciting and intimidating. Check out writing blogs and nursing blogs, and stay informed of the latest events and trends in the industry. You never know when a great idea will come to you. See Tables 9-6 for Web sites that offer tips for writing and publishing.

Table 9-6

Web Sites With Writing Tips

Web Site Name	URL
Purdue Online Writing Lab (OWL)	*http://owl.english.purdue.edu/*
Guide to Grammar and Writing	*http://grammar.ccc.commnet.edu/grammar/*
Essay Writing Help.com	*http://www.essaywritinghelp.com/*
Writing.com	*http://www.writing.com/page/writing_help/writing_help.html*

References

Abdullah, A. (2009). Scientific writing tips. *Sudanese Journal of Public Health, 4*(2), 308–315.

Backer, L, (2007). The medical home: An idea whose time has come,…again. *Family Practice Management 14*(8). 38-41. Retrived from http://www.aafp.org/fpm/2007/0900/p38.html

Cleveland Writing Center. (2011). Critical reading: What is it and why do I need it? Retrieved from http://www.csuohio.edu/academic/writingcenter/critread.html

Edmunds, M. W. (2011). Publishing in nursing journals. In J. Stanley (Ed.), *Advanced practice nursing: Emphasizing common roles* (3rd ed., pp. 279–291). Philadelphia, PA: F.A. Davis Company.

Fitzpatrick, J. (2007). Is the doctor of nursing practice (DNP) the appropriate doctoral degree for nurses? *American Journal of Maternal Child Nursing, 32*(3), 138.

Lehman, C., & Defrene, L. (2008). Business and profession communication. Madison, OH: South Western Cengage Learning.

Marquette University. (2010). What makes writing so important? Retrieved from http://www.marquette.edu/wac/WhatMakesWritingSoImportant.shtml

National Commission on Writing. (2004). Writing + modern technology = student success. Retrieved from http://www.nwp.org/cs/public/print/doc/about/press_releases.csp

Quan, R. (2009). What is a nurse. Retrieved from http://www.suite101.com/content/what-is-a-nurse--a7761

Ramirez, P. J. (2010). How to write great headlines that get people's attention and keep them reading. Retrieved from http://paulramirez.wordpress.com/2010/08/07/how-to-write-great-headlines-that-get-peoples-attention-and-keeps-them-reading/

CHAPTER 10

RESIDENCY AND FINAL PROJECT INFORMATION FOR THE DOCTOR OF NURSING PRACTICE STUDENT

Objectives:

By the end of the chapter, students should be able to:

1. Analyze methods for creating residency objectives.
2. Link residency objectives to the American Association of Colleges of Nursing essentials for doctor of nursing practice (DNP) education.
3. Develop outcome measures for the residency experience.
4. Describe the use of a portfolio in the DNP program both as a tool to determine readiness for DNP education and as a final project reflective of the elements within the DNP educational process.
5. Recognize the requirements for the capstone project.
6. Develop a capstone proposal.
7. Recognize the importance of protecting human subjects within a project.
8. Discuss the need for a theoretical framework for the capstone project.
9. Analyze methods of evaluation for the capstone project.
10. Discover what several DNP students and graduates discuss in exemplars of their work.
11. Examine roles for the DNP graduate in the future.

The doctor of nursing practice (DNP) degree was developed to prepare practice experts in the field of advanced practice nursing. Advanced practice may be in the area of nurse practitioner, midwife, nurse anesthetist, clinical nurse leader, or administrator. Based on the American Association of Colleges of Nursing (AACN) essentials, each student must complete 1000 clinical education hours at the graduate level to receive a DNP degree (AACN, 2006). These clinical hours are spent in hands-on practice where the student applies information obtained in the classroom or laboratory to the real-life practice setting. The curriculum of any DNP program is organized so that, on completion, the student is able to demonstrate attainment all of the competencies required in the DNP essentials.

Clinical hours for students enrolled in a post-master's DNP program are determined based on the clinical hours the student completed in the master's program. These hours are often divided between several clinical experiences that include the residency and capstone projects. In a BSN-to-DNP program, the 1000-hour requirement is divided into several clinical courses plus the residency and the capstone hours.

One of the components of the DNP educational program that allows the student to put into practice and document all of the competencies learned in classes is a final (capstone) project. In the capstone project, the student identifies a problem in the practice area, creates a program to solve the problem or improve care in the area identified, implements the program, and evaluates the success of the program in improving practice or patient outcomes.

The residency, portfolio, and final capstone project aspects of the DNP degree demonstrate the student's mastery of advanced practice nursing in the chosen specialty. The residency experience allows students to put into practice all aspects of what they have learned in the DNP program. The portfolio is a compilation of examples of student work and experience that demonstrates knowledge and proficiency in program objectives and the DNP essentials (AACN, 2006). The practice-based final project provides the DNP student with an experience of the scholarship of practice that will guide future scholarly endeavors. Each DNP program has different requirements for the residency and final capstone project, so it is important for students to investigate the requirements for each and plan ahead as they progress through the DNP program.

Residency

The overarching purpose of the DNP residency is to refine leadership skills, apply theoretical standards in nursing practice, create methods for using evidence-based findings to care for increasingly complex patients, improve skills in advanced nursing practice, and advocate for patients in the area of health-care policy and delivery. The term *residency* has been used in medical education programs to define the years of study after graduation from medical school that students complete in the practice setting under the supervision of an attending physician or specialist. These programs are designed to take the knowledge gained in medical school course work and prepare the graduate medical student in an area of practice. The medical residency programs in the United States are directed by the Accreditation Counsel for Graduate Medical Education (ACGME). The ACGME (2006) has identified six competencies for medical residents, as follows:

1. Medical knowledge
2. Patient care

3. Practice-based learning and improvement
4. Systems-based practice
5. Professionalism
6. Interprofessional communication and collaboration

Table 10-1 presents outcomes related to each of the residency objectives.

Table 10-1

Accreditation Counsel for Graduate Medical Education Medical Residency Objectives and Outcomes

Objective	Outcome Measures
Medical knowledge	**1.** Demonstrate an investigatory and analytical thinking approach to clinical situations. **2.** Know and apply the basic and clinically supportive sciences that are appropriate to their discipline.
Patient care	**1.** Communicate effectively and demonstrate caring and respectful behaviors when interacting with patients and their families. **2.** Gather essential and accurate information about their patients. **3.** Make informed decisions about diagnostic and therapeutic interventions based on patient information, preferences, up-to-date scientific evidence, and clinical judgment. **4.** Develop and carry out patient management plans. **5.** Counsel and educate patients and their families. **6.** Use information technology to support patient care decisions and patient education. **7.** Perform competently all medical and invasive procedures considered essential for the area of practice. **8.** Provide health-care services aimed at preventing health problems or maintaining health. **9.** Work with health-care professionals, including those from other disciplines, to provide patient-focused care.
Practice-based learning and improvement	**1.** Analyze practice experience and perform practice-based improvement activities using a systematic methodology. **2.** Obtain and use information about their own population of patients and the larger population from which their patients are drawn. **3.** Locate, appraise, and assimilate evidence from scientific studies related to their patients' health problems.

Continued on page 414

Continued from page 413 Table 10-1

Accreditation Counsel for Graduate Medical Education Medical Residency Objectives and Outcomes

Objective	Outcome Measures
	4. Apply knowledge of study designs and statistical methods to the appraisal of clinical studies and other information on diagnostic and therapeutic effectiveness. **5.** Use information technology to manage information, access online medical information, and support their own education. **6.** Facilitate the learning of students and other health-care professionals.
Systems-based practice	**1.** Know how types of medical practice and delivery systems differ from one another, including methods of controlling health-care costs and allocating resources. **2.** Practice cost-effective health care and resource allocation that do not compromise quality of care. **3.** Advocate for quality patient care and assist patients in dealing with system complexities. **4.** Partner with health-care managers and health-care providers to assess and coordinate.
Professionalism	**1.** Demonstrate respect, compassion, and integrity. **2.** Demonstrate a commitment to ethical principles. **3.** Demonstrate sensitivity and responsiveness to patients' culture, age, gender, and disabilities.
Interprofessional communication and collaboration	**1.** Create and sustain a therapeutic and ethically sound relationship with patients. **2.** Use effective listening skills and elicit and provide information using effective nonverbal, explanatory, questioning, and writing skills. **3.** Work effectively with others as a member or leader of a health-care team or other professional group.

Source: Accreditation Counsel for Graduate Medical Education (ACGME). (2006). Introduction to competency based residency education. Retrieved from http://www.acgme.org/acWebsite/home/home.asp

Many of the objectives and outcomes that are used for medical residents apply to the DNP residency and are similar to those listed in the DNP essentials (AACN, 2006). The DNP residency expands on these objectives to include nursing values such as holism, patient advocacy, provision or culturally competent care, and patient/family–centered ideas of care that allow for co-creation of ideas of health and well-being. Box 10-1 provides the objectives for the residency experience from the AACN.

One major difference between the DNP residency and the medical residency is that nurses in the DNP residency have wide-ranging experience as nurses in the BSN-to-DNP programs, and many have extensive experience in advanced

Box 10-1

American Association of Colleges of Nursing Description of Residency Objectives

DNP programs provide rich and varied opportunities for practice experiences aimed at helping graduates achieve the essential and specialty competencies on completion of the program. To achieve the DNP competencies, programs should provide a minimum of 1000 hours of practice post-baccalaureate as part of a supervised academic program. Practice experiences should be designed to help students achieve specific learning objectives related to the DNP essentials and specialty competencies. These experiences should be designed to provide systematic opportunities for feedback and reflection. Experiences include in-depth work with experts from nursing as well as other disciplines and provide opportunities for meaningful student engagement within practice environments. Given the intense practice focus of DNP programs, practice experiences are designed to help students build and assimilate knowledge for advanced specialty practice at a high level of complexity. End-of-program practice immersion experiences should be required to provide an opportunity for further synthesis and expansion of the learning developed to that point. These experiences also provide the context within which the final DNP product is completed. Practice immersion experiences afford the opportunity to integrate and synthesize the essentials and specialty requirements necessary to demonstrate competency in an area of specialized nursing practice. Proficiency may be acquired through a variety of methods, such as attaining case requirements, patient or practice contact hours, completing specified procedures, demonstrating experiential competencies, or a combination of these elements. Many specialty groups already extensively define various minimal experiences and requirements.

Source: American Association of Colleges of Nursing. (2006). The essentials of doctoral education for advanced nursing practice. Retrieved from http://www.aacn.nche.edu/dnp/pdf/essentials.pdf

practice as post-master's DNP students. Nurses in DNP programs approach residency with a firm knowledge base in the discipline and area of practice. Medical residencies focus on the medical diagnosis and treatment of individual patients and specialty training in an area of patient care, whereas the DNP residency provides experiences in broader areas of leadership, population-based care, advocacy, and health-care policy.

The DNP residency program comes at a time in the DNP program when the student has become comfortable with the basic tenets of practice, including assessment, diagnosis, treatment, and follow-up, and is ready to move toward higher-level practice. DNP students are ready to move beyond basic practice skills to integrate the nursing core values of dignity, integrity, autonomy, altruism, social justice, caring, and holism in the practice setting (Brown-Benedict, 2008). DNP students must practice being in the clinical setting in an advanced practice capacity as an autonomous health-care provider who advocates for patients and creates a person-centered approach to health care. DNP students must learn how to create patient-centered, holistic, evidence-based practice and how to guide individuals through the confusing maze of health-care choices. During the residency, DNP students should also experience ways to assist populations toward lifestyle changes and focus on removing the inequities in health-care delivery to people in the United States.

Aspects of the DNP Residency Program

The purpose of the DNP residency is to allow students to use and test new knowledge in the practice area. In many situations, the student, who is already an advanced practice nurse, can complete the residency hour requirement where he or she currently works as an advanced practice nurse. To meet the requirements, however, it is necessary to delineate residency hours as separate and distinct from regular work time and effort. One way to separate out residency hours from normal working hours is to create goals and objectives for the residency, list the steps and time required to meet these goals and objectives, and set aside the number of hours required. The goals and objectives should reflect the essentials for DNP education objectives from the AACN (2006).

The following are examples of experiences that may meet the objectives of the DNP residency.

- *Scientific underpinning of practice:* Linking theory, practice, and research; experiencing a new area of practice specialty
- *Systems leadership for quality improvement and systems thinking:* Instituting a quality improvement project in the clinical area, becoming a leader in quality improvement efforts that currently exist, creating a systems approach to patient care in the clinical setting
- *Clinical scholarship for evidence-based practice:* Using new knowledge to create clinical questions based on practice experience; exploring and analyzing evidence; testing the evidence in practice to support interventions and actions by the advanced practice nurse to improve patient outcomes
- *Information systems and technology to improve and transform health care:* Instituting the use of informatics and information technologies in the practice area; identifying systems and group uses for technology to increase care coordination, improve patient compliance with treatments, or identify populations with increased disease burdens and develop plans to work in a community to reduce this burden
- *Health-care policy for advocacy:* Becoming involved in the local, state, and national debate over health care; influencing health-care policy, speaking for underserved people, and advocating for better health care at a better cost
- *Interprofessional collaboration for improving patient and population outcomes:* Developing a collaborative interprofessional group to address health-care problems in a community; creating opportunities for all health-care professionals to work together to improve the health of a community, group, or individual

- *Clinical prevention and population health for improving health in the United States:* Developing a program to promote healthy behaviors and educate people in communities and individually regarding the dangers of unhealthy habits and behaviors, creating support programs for persons who are attempting to change health behaviors
- *Advanced practice nursing:* Working toward becoming an advanced practice nurse using evidence-based practice, listening and developing trusting relationships with patients or employees, experiencing different specialties within the advanced practice domain

For more detailed examples, see Box 10-2.

Box 10-2

Examples of Residency Objectives and Goals

Following are examples of objectives and goals that students could set for completion of residence hours:

1. Work with staff in a clinical setting to create a theoretical framework for their nursing practice; this could be done in a practice setting or at a hospital, developing a link between the theoretical framework chosen and practice. Choose methods to determine appropriate outcomes from this theoretically based practice, and measure whether these outcomes are truly the result of the theoretical framework for practice.
2. Assess a practice problem, such as patients not taking their medications as prescribed. Investigate the problem to determine the cause. Develop a plan to overcome the problem, and institute it in the practice setting—for instance, create a list of least expensive medications for general use in practice, create a list of drugs that can be taken only once or twice a day so the patient does not forget a dose, or call the patient at home after a new prescription has been issued to determine if the patient has obtained the prescription and has any problems with taking it as prescribed. Once the new practices have been instituted, follow up to determine if they have improved the problem.
3. Create guidelines for practice using evidence-based knowledge for common diseases seen in the practice setting, such as diabetes and hypertension. Create programs for health promotion in areas of obesity, smoking, or drug or alcohol abuse that are based on best practice evidence.
4. Work with office personnel, both providers and staff, to determine whether there is a need for increased information technology, how to use existing technology better, or how patients and the practice could benefit from the purchase and implementation of new technology such as Web pages and online educational information.
5. Become active in a local, state, or federal initiative to improve the health and well-being of citizens. Volunteer for local and state initiatives for health-care issues. Work on the campaign of a candidate who understands and values the nursing role in health care and who wants to work to improve the health of all people in the area.

Continued on page 418

Box 10-2

Examples of Residency Objectives and Goals *Continued from page 417*

6. Work collaboratively with other health-care providers including physicians, social workers, physical therapists, pharmacists, and others on a health-care issue such as care coordination, health-care transition from hospital to home or nursing facility, or health-care cost control for patients and families.
7. Work on developing programs that stress health promotion and disease prevention. Work with patients, families, and other health-care providers to identify interventions that can assist people to manage their own health and well-being.
8. Create new practice areas for advanced practice nurses, such as in the area of the medical home or developing a home visit practice.

Critical Thinking Questions

1. How would you plan a residency for yourself or another student?
2. What are the most important aspects of the residency experience for advanced practice nurses?
3. What nursing values and knowledge should be evident in a DNP residency?
4. How might these differ from the values and objectives of a medical residency?

Residency in BSN-to-DNP Programs

The AACN has set the transition date of 2015 for all advanced practice nurses to be educated at the doctoral level. An increasing number of students will obtain advanced practice education directly from the bachelor's degree to the DNP. One reason for the decision to require doctoral preparation for advanced practice nurses was to respond to an increasingly complex health-care system. As the health-care system becomes more complex, the advanced practice nurse will be required to have skills in many of the DNP essential areas, including information technology, health-care policy, population-based care, and evidence-based practice. Another reason for the transition of advanced practice nursing education to the DNP level is to create degree parity with other health-care professions, such as pharmacy, physical therapy, and psychology. A final reason for this transition is to assist graduates to assume leadership roles in clinical practice, clinical teaching, and policy development.

Students in the BSN-to-DNP programs will use the residency hours in a slightly different fashion because they have less previous hands-on experience in advanced practice nursing. It may take more time for these students to become comfortable with the basic responsibilities of advanced practice and to reach the higher-level competency goals of the DNP residency, such as patient advocacy and co-creating treatment plans with patients in the areas of health promotion, disease prevention, and disease management. Nevertheless, all of the essential competencies for the DNP should be integrated into the BSN-to-DNP residency experience.

Generally, BSN-to-DNP students will not be employed already in practices where they can complete their residency hours. Students should meet with the clinical preceptor in the practice to outline goals and objectives for the residency. Some of the residency hour time can be spent in routine patient care and treatment, especially if the student desires to gain experience in specialty areas of practice, such as cardiology, dermatology, or gastroenterology. Other hours should be spent in working on the DNP competencies as outlined in the AACN essentials document (AACN, 2006). To accomplish all of the goals and objectives for BSN-to-DNP residency, students may complete experiences at several different sites.

Advancing Your Knowledge

F.M. is an advanced practice nurse with a DNP degree. She has been a preceptor to a BSN-to-DNP student in her primary care practice over the course of the last year or so. The student asks F.M. if she can complete her residency hours in the practice.

1. What must F.M. know about the residency before she can say yes or no to the student?
2. If she agrees to work with the student, what is the first step in goal setting for the residency process?
3. What goals would be appropriate for a BSN-to-DNP student? Do these goals agree with the essentials for DNP education from the AACN?
4. How would F.M. and the student measure these goals?
5. How much independence could the student have in the practice?
6. How would F.M. and the student tie the goals of the residency to a possible final capstone project?

Measuring Outcomes of the Residency

One of the challenges for DNP educators and students will be to measure the outcomes of the residency program. In clinical residency programs for other healthcare professionals, each student has a clinical instructor on site. The situation would be similar for BSN-to-DNP students, but for some master's level DNP students, who are already experts in advanced practice, the instructor would not be present during all residency hours. Outcome goals should be mutually developed between the student and instructor and reviewed at regular intervals.

Advancing Your Knowledge

D.D. is a DNP student preparing for residency. D.D. has been an advanced practice nurse for 5 years and is attending a post-master's DNP program. The goals that D.D. has set for her residency experience are the following:

1. Identify a population of interest
2. Evaluate issues and needs within this population

Continued on page 420

Advancing Your Knowledge *Continued from page 419*

3. List methods for assisting this population in the area of identified needs via Web sites, information retrieval, education, policy advocacy, and development of evidence-based guidelines. D.D. will use 250 hours of her clinical time to accomplish these goals.

Choose a population that D.D. could work with.

1. What issues and needs might D.D. identify in this population?
2. How might the needs of this population be met through information technology, policy advocacy, or evidence-based guidelines?
3. Identify some methods that D.D. could use to accomplish her goals.
4. How could D.D. measure whether she reached her goals for the residency experience?

Portfolio

Some schools allow or require students to complete a professional portfolio. A portfolio is a collection of visual and written work that provides an opportunity for students to exhibit their work to support or provide evidence of meeting curriculum objectives. This portfolio may be in lieu of the final capstone project, may be required in addition to the final capstone project, or may be used to determine whether a student is ready for admittance to a DNP program in the first place. Portfolios may be used to determine the eligibility of students who wish to enter a DNP program but do not currently have certification in an area of advanced practice. This type of portfolio allows the student to present the experiences and knowledge he or she possesses that make the DNP an appropriate degree for the student. Portfolios used as a final product in DNP programs allow students to demonstrate the methods and accomplishment of the competencies developed by the National Organization of Nurse Practitioner Faculty, the American Organization of Nurse Executives, and the essentials from the AACN. The portfolio documents the formative (evaluating events as they happen) and summative (an overall evaluation of learning throughout the DNP program) outcomes of DNP education for each student.

Information to be presented in a DNP portfolio differs among programs, but generally the portfolio provides evidence of meeting the overall objectives within the DNP program. The portfolio may demonstrate a student's involvement in health-care policy by containing evidence that the student met with a legislator or health-care policy leaders. The portfolio could also contain an example of the student's work with implementing an electronic medical record or Web site for a particular medical setting or developing a theoretical framework for practice in a specific setting. One DNP program requires a portfolio of sophisticated evidence-based case studies that come from the residency experience (Mundinger, Starck, Hathaway, Shaver, & Fugate Woods, 2009).

Final Capstone Project

Doctoral education in nursing—whether PhD, DNS, or DNP—is distinguished by the completion of a project or portfolio that demonstrates synthesis of the student's work and forms the basis for the student's future scholarship. In the PhD or DNS program, this completion project is a dissertation, which consists of a research project that provides new knowledge to the discipline of nursing. For the DNP student, the final project is often called the *capstone*. A capstone or final project creates a systematic investigation of a problem related to practice. The idea is that completion of the project puts a "capstone" on the student's learning and leads the student from the DNP program into the world of advanced practice nursing at a higher level.

The overall goal of the DNP capstone project is to provide a scholarly experience that implements the principles of evidence-based practice and translation. The project is completed under the guidance of an experienced faculty mentor. The product of the capstone project is in the form of a paper or presentation or both and is reviewed and evaluated by an academic committee. The requirements for the final capstone project, time and credit hours to completion, final product, and method of review differ among academic institutions, and students should pay close attention to the requirements for final capstone topic approval, implementation, and evaluation.

The purpose of the DNP final project is to use best evidence to create a project to improve patient outcomes or improve community health or both or to advance health-care policy and advocacy. Best evidence may be found in scientific literature, scientific studies, systematic reviews, clinical guidelines, expert opinion, consensus panels, and community perspectives. The student may be required to modify and adapt theory or evidence for a particular clinical population or community. For example, evidence may indicate that education and providing information may improve compliance with diabetic medication regimens in older adults; however, in a group of Haitian adults, more behavioral modification is required because of cultural beliefs about disease and diabetes.

Implementation and evaluation of strategies to meet the goals of the final or capstone project include constructing and testing cost-effective, culturally appropriate interventions that are sustainable and that can be disseminated to other advanced practice nurses through journal articles and conference presentations. Final or capstone projects can also focus on health informatics, such as developing data sets or registries or creating Web sites for providing patient information and self-management. Final projects may also focus on health policy issues and patient advocacy in health-care legislative decision making with involvement in the legislative process or work with a legislator on a specific health-related issue.

Because population-based health is an important part of DNP education, students should be encouraged to explore opportunities to collaborate with community groups, consumers, or stakeholders to investigate a mutually agreed on clinical question. Negotiating and collaborating with community members and health professionals are valuable skills and learning experiences. The DNP would use the final or capstone project to focus on integration, application, and teaching of knowledge. DNP final projects could add to the body of nursing research on a more local and practice-oriented basis (Edwardson, 2009).

Final or Capstone Project Research

Some DNP final projects completed to date have been research studies. Loretta Ford, one of the founders of the nurse practitioner movement, suggested that DNPs should participate in and explore clinical phenomena by conducting research (Stanley, 2005). The National Organization of Nurse Practitioner Faculty proposed that DNPs be prepared to use research knowledge and methods to create practice-based questions, identify interventions to answer the questions, implement the interventions or ideas, and evaluate them. The National Organization of Nurse Practitioner Faculty proposed that DNPs be involved in collaborative clinical trial research (Fulton & Lyon, 2005).

It is important that the DNP have a background in finding, evaluating, and implementing evidence-based practice research findings. The DNP student can undertake research projects if the prerequisites exist in the institution to support research. According to the AACN (2006), these prerequisites include a culture supportive of research and scholarship, mentoring for novice researchers, and provision of the necessary infrastructure to support research efforts, such as institutional review boards (IRBs) and research databases. Creating a culture of research and evidence-based practice across the discipline requires supporting research initiatives that are level appropriate from the BSN to the PhD, including the DNP. Advanced practice nurses prepared at the DNP level have the ability to translate research knowledge into practice settings and evaluate the appropriateness and acceptance of practices in larger settings. Advanced practice nurses also have access to large numbers of potential participants and research questions that stem from actual practice-based problems. This is especially true in the areas highlighted by the DNP essentials, including leadership skills, health-care policy, and evidence-based practice.

Final Project or Capstone Proposal

The final project or capstone proposal is usually created by the student in coordination with his or her advisor. To be complete and guide the student through the entire project process, the proposal should include the following:

1. *Identification of the challenges or problems leading to the proposed project:* Why was this project subject chosen, how does it relate to the practice, and what special experience do you have to bring to this project?
2. *Description of the project and how it addresses at least one challenge or problem that influences health care for a significant number of people:* Link the project to one of the essential elements of DNP education, such as population-based health, health promotion, health policy, or evidence-based practice.

3. *Justification of the role of the DNP to address the challenge or problem:* Why is the DNP-prepared advanced practice nurse the appropriate person to investigate this issue and provide a better understanding of how to overcome problems or improve care?
4. *Presentation of current literature regarding the problem or challenge to be addressed:* Completing a review and analysis of the literature is discussed in Chapter 3. It is important to document what is known, what is not known, and where the project fits in terms of extending knowledge and translating research findings.
5. *Timetable including all phases of the project:* Provide a step-by-step outline of all phases and how long each phase is estimated to take.
6. *Citation of resources needed to ensure project completion, including description of budgetary and technologic considerations:* What resources will you need to complete the project? Where will these resources come from? Include what cooperative agreements will be required from agencies where work will take place.
7. *Market analysis; strategic analysis; or product/services, sales/marketing, operations, and financial plan that justifies the need, feasibility, and sustainability of the proposed project:* In other words, can you do what you are planning given the resources available? In some instances, the products of the final project may be able to be sold to other groups or individuals, such as "how-to" manuals or education booklets.
8. *Project evaluation plan including specific measures that will be evaluated during the project:* This evaluation plan includes evidence-based outcomes. Describe how you will evaluate the outcomes of your project. What measurement instruments will you use (e.g., focus groups, scales, surveys, physiologic measures, psychosocial measures)? Are these instruments reliable and valid? How will data be analyzed?

Using a Theoretical Framework for the Final Project or Capstone

As students begin to design their final project or capstone experience, they must identify a theoretical framework. Defining theoretical assumptions and ideas that form the foundation for the project can help guide the student and create assistance with evaluation of the effectiveness for the project. Because theory, research, and practice are linked within the discipline of nursing, all scholarly projects should be constructed using a theoretical framework. Practice-based problems cannot be articulated outside of a conceptual system; the framework chosen by the researcher contributes to new understandings or problem solutions. Theory provides a perspective for identifying and viewing the problem, the approach to solutions, and the effectiveness of solutions. The final project must identify the framework used to articulate the problem, develop solutions, implement solutions, and evaluate findings.

Planning the DNP Final Project

There are six steps in the final project or capstone process. Step 1 is determining what the project is trying to achieve. Step 2 is developing an evaluation plan. Step 3 is determining the population or group to use in the project. Step 4 is implementing the project and collecting the data identified in the evaluation plan. Step 5 is analyzing the data collected. Step 6 is reporting findings. Let us look at each step in depth to provide a complete review of the project planning process.

Step 1

What is the project trying to achieve? What are the primary objectives of the project? The objectives for a project should be *SMART*:

- *S*pecific
- *M*easurable
- *A*chievable
- *R*elevant
- *T*ime limited

Step 2

Developing an evaluation plan requires first determining what the goals and objectives of the project are. The method used to evaluate the project should clearly identify what is being evaluated—people, financial issues, policies, or projects? The evaluation plan measure should be reliable and accurate, easy to understand, relevant to the objectives and purpose of the project, and useful. One difficulty that can arise and make project findings less useful is attributing change to the project alone and not considering all of the other aspects or variables that could have led to the change. For example, if the project is to determine the effect of yoga on migraine headaches, it is important to consider what medications the participants are taking for migraines and the role the medications play in reduced headaches. Another problem can be evaluating change when long periods occur between the implementation of the project and the change itself. If a project to assist in implementing positive health behaviors takes 1 year to effect change and the DNP student wants to complete the project in two semesters and graduate from the DNP program, the evaluation plan may not show improvement yet when the project is completed. One way to overcome this problem is to create short-term evaluation criteria that make inferences about future outcomes possible. It is possible to infer likely outcomes from projects that are well organized and implemented; short-term impacts can be inferred to result in desired longer-term outcomes. Because health projects are often complex and involve numerous activities and participants, it is best to develop an evaluation plan that includes evaluating both the process being used and the outcomes of the process.

Step 3

The selection of participants influences the outcome data in any project. If the project is attempting to determine the effect of yoga on the number of migraine headaches experienced in 1 month, it is less effective for outcome data to recruit patients who have only occasional migraines rather than patients who have frequent migraines. It is important to recruit individuals who are best able to provide the information required rather than simply individuals who more generally fit the population desired.

Step 4

Choosing what data to collect and how to collect the data also affects the outcomes of the project. When considering the final project, questions to ask include: What do you want to find out? What is the best way to do this? Who should collect the data? When determining the type of data you wish to collect and evaluate, participants' cultural beliefs, literacy levels, and individual preferences should be considered. Use standardized data collection tools that have been shown to be valid and reliable for data analysis and inference made from data for the project evaluation.

The most common ways to collect project evaluation data include the following:

- Surveys and questionnaires can be used to obtain a broad understanding for a relatively large population. These tools can be administered face to face or via mail or telephone conversations.
- Interviews are more time-consuming but also more useful for gathering in-depth information. Becoming a competent interviewer using open-ended questions to solicit the essential information usually requires some training. Interviews are best conducted face to face, but they can be completed via the telephone. For data collection, interviews should be taped or video recorded and transcribed so that all of the information gathered can be reviewed and analyzed. Special permission from participants is required for tape or video recording of interviews. A smaller number of participants are generally recruited when using interviews as the main source of evaluation, so it is important to choose participants wisely according to whether they are in a position to provide you with the information you require.
- Focus groups are also useful for gathering in-depth information. Focus-group discussions can enrich the data collected by sharing ideas and thoughts within a group. Some training is required to become a good focus-group facilitator who can manage group interactions effectively.
- Observation is used when the data collector intentionally interacts with the participants to observe changes to people or their environment or both. Observational data methods can record aspects of activities and events, such as the project setting and the way people participate in the project.
- Diaries and logs can be used to record the processes and accomplishments of a project or a particular activity within a project. For example, a diary could be kept of how many yoga sessions a participant attended in a given time period.

Step 5

Step 5 in the process is to analyze, evaluate, and interpret the data collected. The analysis of the data is a way of making sense of what the data reveal to evaluate the outcomes of the practice-based project. Interpreting the data allows for reflection and understanding of what the data reveal.

Step 6

The final step in the process is reporting on or using the findings of the project. Reporting or implementing the findings of the project in practice establishes the difference the project has made and ensures that successes are repeated and mistakes are not repeated. Findings from the project could support and empower a group to move forward with further changes and allow others to learn from the work done on this project.

Advancing Your Knowledge

Refer to the following Advancing Your Knowledge box concerning a hepatitis C clinic pilot project. The student is developing an evaluation plan. The student anticipates about 125 people to be included in the project. The clinic diagnoses approximately 250 cases of hepatitis C each quarter.

1. What would the evaluation goals be for this pilot project?
2. What data will the student want to collect? Discuss what biophysical data, survey data, demographic data, and any other type of data you think would be important.
3. How could information about the outcomes of this project be disseminated?

Human Subjects and the DNP Final Project or Capstone

Whether the DNP final project is research, quality assurance, or implementation and evaluation of a new program, if human subjects are involved, obtaining IRB approval is essential. Human subjects are individuals from whom data have been collected through face-to-face contact (including biophysical data, such as blood pressure or weight), interviews, or surveys or obtained from administrative or program records. An IRB is a group that monitors research designs that include data obtained from human subjects. Members of an IRB come from different academic disciplines and from the community where the research is conducted. Students usually use the IRB at the school they are attending; however, if multiple institutions are involved, IRBs at these institutions must also provide permission.

An IRB ensures that when data are being collected for research, the welfare, rights, privileges, and confidentiality of the participants who agree to be a part of the study are protected (Bronte-Tinkew, Allen, & Joyner, 2008). To obtain a consent from the IRB, researchers must provide a description of the design and method to be used and a description of the recruitment of participants, their ages, and whether they are in a vulnerable population (e.g., older adults, children, or individuals who are mentally ill). The IRB reviews flyers and other material used to recruit participants, informed consent documents to be signed by all participants, and letters of support from any outside organizations from which participants will be recruited or who will provide space or services for the project. For example, if a project will take place using residents from a particular nursing home, a letter of support from the nursing home should be included in the IRB packet. Each IRB has specific requirements, and it is best to contact the committee early in the project process to determine what is needed and whether more than one IRB will be involved.

Advancing Your Knowledge

A DNP student is deciding on a final project that will be a pilot study. The student works in a nephrology clinic where many adults are diagnosed with hepatitis C. The student has found that these newly diagnosed patients are not being provided with information regarding their disease, treatment options, and follow-up; as a result, many patients call the practice several times a week to ask questions. These questions take provider time, and there is no way of knowing how effective the education is. The student plans to develop a formal educational session to which all patients newly diagnosed with hepatitis C will be referred. During the educational session, each patient will receive a booklet with a list of commonly asked questions and answers about hepatitis C. The booklet will include pages where personal information about the patient's treatment plan, laboratory results for follow-up, and other important information about the patient's disease and treatment can be written.

1. What documents will the student need to create or obtain for IRB approval?
2. How would the student describe the participants required for this pilot study?
3. What letters of support will the student need to obtain?
4. Are there any ethical issues that would need special attention for this IRB application?

Evaluating the Final Project or Capstone

One of the most important and often challenging aspects of the final project or capstone is evaluating the outcomes of the project. Project evaluation is a step-by-step process of collecting, recording, and organizing information about project results. Information used to evaluate a project would include meeting the project's objectives; increasing patient satisfaction; changing behavior, practice, or policy; or completing a deliverable product such as a Web site.

Evaluating the outcomes of a project is important because such an evaluation provides accountability for meeting outcome goals and objectives set forth in the project proposal. Other reasons for undertaking evaluation of the DNP final project include the following:

- Demonstration of effective and efficient project outcomes for the population involved
- Recognition of actual changes and progress made
- Identification of successful factors in the project that could be duplicated in other areas
- Need for continued improvement where outcomes were not met
- Identification of unrealistic outcome goals
- Validation for project partners that outcomes were achieved

Evaluating project results provides the answers to key questions such as the following:

- Exactly what progress was made?
- Were desired outcomes achieved?
- What were the most successful aspects of the project?
- What could be done differently to make the project more successful in the future?
- Are there ways to refine activities to achieve better outcomes?
- Are there ways in which new partnerships or collaborations could be formed to make the project more successful if attempted again?
- Do the results obtained from the project justify the effort and input of all project collaborators?

Final Project Product Examples

Following are some exemplars of student final projects. These students volunteered to share their final project experiences, and you will be able to see that each felt the experience to be beneficial and an enhancement of practice knowledge and skills. As you reflect on clinical practice issues that you would like to investigate, these exemplars may guide you in developing your practice question and the final project for your DNP.

Here is a list of final project titles:

1. A Nurse Practitioner–Guided Model for Improving Health Outcomes of Older Adults Transitioning from Hospital to Skilled Nursing Facilities After Coronary Artery Bypass Graft Surgery
2. Collaborative Alternatives for Recovery-Focused Environments in Psychiatric Care
3. Increasing Breast Cancer Screening Among Women of Haitian Descent
4. Using the DASH Diet to Reduce Hypertension in Older African American Adults
5. Nurse Practitioner Home Visits to Assess Parental Coping and Transition Readiness for Families of Adolescents With Autism Spectrum Disorders

6. Sister to Sister Weight Management Program: The Effect of a Culturally Congruent Lifestyle Intervention Using Cognitive Behavioral Therapy on Cardiovascular Risk Factors in a Group of African American Women
7. Pressure Ulcer Prevention (PUP) Program in Nursing Home Settings: Starting the PUP Teams
8. Evaluating an Educational Program Concerning Healthy Eating and Nutrition With Children at the Zoo Summer Camp
9. Understanding Barriers and Support in Asthma Management in School-Age Children: Parent's Perspective
10. Diabetes Self-Management and Nutritional Choices With Adult Hispanics
11. Shared Governance and Professional Nurse Empowerment in Practice
12. Engagement of the Mature Clinical Registered Nurse

The following are examples of capstone projects as described by the students.

Student Capstone Exemplar 1

My name is Dr. Darrell Owens, and I am the founder and current director of the Palliative Medicine Service and Primary Palliative Care Clinic at the University of Washington's Harborview Medical Center. I hold a Bachelor of Science in Nursing from Emory University, a Master of Science in Health Services Administration from St. Mary's College of California, a Master of Science in Nursing as a Palliative Care Clinical Nurse Specialist, a post-master's certification as an adult health and geriatric nurse practitioner from Seattle Pacific University, and a Doctor of Nursing Practice from the University of Alabama at Birmingham. I am also a graduate of the Harvard Medical School's Center for Palliative Care Faculty Scholar Program. My educational path was longer than most, as I first pursued an administrative track before returning to my real passion of clinical work. I now consider myself a recovering administrator.

In 2003, I joined the staff of Harborview Medical Center as part of a Robert Wood Johnson Grant to integrate critical and palliative care. Approximately 1 year later, I founded the inpatient Palliative Care Consult Service. Since then the service has grown significantly and now includes inpatient and outpatient services, as well as the only Primary Palliative Care Clinic in the United States.

Harborview Medical Center is a 415-bed academic medical center located in Seattle, Washington. It is owned by King County and operated under a management contract with the University of Washington School of Medicine. Harborview is the safety-net hospital for the county, having provided over $140 million in charity care in 2008. The hospital's occupancy rate is approximately 98%, and despite performing over 224,000 annual clinic visits, the documented number of patients waiting to establish care with a primary provider exceeds 300.

The inpatient consult service performs approximately 500 new consults and over 2000 follow-up visits annually. In 2006, in response to the need to

Continued on page 430

Student Capstone Exemplar 1 *Continued from page 429*

improve access to palliative care for outpatients, the Palliative Care Clinic (PCC) was launched. During the clinic's first year of operation, oncologists from the Hematology-Oncology Clinic (which operates simultaneously with the PCC) began to request that the palliative care nurse practitioner assume responsibility for management of pain and bothersome symptoms for some of their complex patients. While caring for this group of patients, it was noted that many of them had no primary care provider or 24-hour access to a provider who knew their unique needs. Many of these patients frequently utilized the emergency department for pain and symptom management and were at times admitted to the hospital for crises that could have been effectively managed in the outpatient setting by a palliative care specialist.

Based on the identified need to provide patients with a life-limiting illness with 24-hour access to a palliative care specialist, in 2007 the Primary Palliative Care Clinic (PPCC) was launched. The mission of the PPCC is to provide both primary care and palliative care to patients who have a life-limiting illness and no primary provider within the Harborview system or the greater Seattle/King County community. Although initially developed for oncology patients, the clinic quickly began to receive referrals for patients with noncancer diagnoses, including dementia, heart disease, kidney disease, liver disease, and lung disease. Many of the patients served by the clinic also experience homelessness, mental illness, and active addictive disorders. In 2009, a formal relationship was established with a large regional kidney center to provide primary and consultative care to outpatients receiving hemodialysis. The PPCC receives referrals to assume the role of primary care provider from local hospice programs, skilled nursing facilities, community and university providers, and the King County Jail Health System for terminally ill inmates granted compassionate release for end-of-life care. Clinic care is provided three half-days per week, and through home and nursing home visits up to two additional days per week. Enrollment in a hospice program is not required, with only 30% of clinic patients enrolled in hospice. Continuity of care is provided to patients and families via 24-hour access to their assigned primary care provider with a subspecialty certification in hospice and palliative care and who is familiar with their unique situation and needs. In 2010, recognizing that the Primary Palliative Care Clinic was the only one of its kind in the United States, the Regence Foundation awarded the Clinic a 2-year, $100,000 grant.

A doctoral education, specifically a clinical doctorate such as the Doctor of Nursing Practice, is essential for the ability to develop such a clinic, as well as the ability to provide competent clinical care to this complex population. Essential skills range from understanding health systems and payment structures, to managing physical, emotional, and existential issues. As clinical faculty for nursing, medicine, and pharmacy, the DNP also provides me with a solid foundation for the use of evidence-based nursing and medicine in practice and in education.

Some thoughts about the future. As an autonomous, independent nurse practitioner responsible for the provision of direct patient care and clinical education in both primary and palliative care, my practice is dependent on my ability to apply scientific and philosophical approaches to patient care and education. As I reflect back over my practice, especially at the doctoral level, I am able to see that caring for complicated terminally ill patients and their families requires an extensive scientific knowledge, and a solid philosophical foundation, most of which I learned at the doctoral level.

As a doctorally prepared nurse practitioner, I also see it as my role to advocate for those without a voice, and not just for the protection of my income. I believe we must take a lead in health-care reform, something I am better prepared to do as someone with a DNP. Obtaining my DNP renewed my passion, albeit on a more formalized level, to serving the poor. I have joined the Healthcare Coalition for the Homeless, an organization that I did not know existed prior to conducting research in my DNP program. I have 2 more years to my term as a Commissioner on the Washington State Nursing Commission, and have been asked to chair the Rules Committee for writing the rules for the law regarding chronic pain management that was just passed by the legislature and signed by the Governor. All of these activities clearly support the important role of the DNP-prepared nurse practitioner in advocacy and policy.

The completion of my DNP has renewed my pride in nursing, and in being a nurse practitioner. I am proud to have advanced nursing at my institution, by proving that a nurse practitioner can develop and lead a medical specialty service. Our clinic and practice is improving care for the terminally ill in Seattle and King County, Washington, and demonstrating what advanced practice nurses can accomplish. As the health-care system evolves and care becomes more complicated, doctoral level education for nurse practitioners will be essential.

Student Capstone Exemplar 2

As part of the educational process in my terminal degree of Doctor of Nursing Practice (DNP), a capstone project was required. I began this project in May 2010 after completing the IRB requirements of our institution. Part of the project involved enrolling patients into an educational stroke related intervention while they were still in the hospital. I had no idea what I was getting into, but I quickly learned! I had expected that patients would be willing and eager to participate in this project, but my expectations took a backseat to the reality of working with patients after experiencing the crisis of stroke. An example of my experience follows, and is unfortunate from the standpoint that it is not unusual.

I scanned the role of new stroke patients daily, in an effort to identify those patients I would approach for participation in my study. That is when I entered

Continued on page 432

Student Capstone Exemplar 2 *Continued from page 431*

Cathy's room. I stopped dead in my tracks as I observed a 58-year-old woman who was sitting in her chair and practically in a fetal position. She had her arms crossed over her chest, she was crying, and the anguish on her face and in the room was palpable. Her husband was sitting on her bed. I had the consent form in my hand, ready to hand to her as I entered the room. As I made these observations, I withdrew the consent form and returned it to my bag. I pulled up a chair and sat down. I asked her if I could speak with her, because I knew she had had a stroke, and I was quite concerned about how she was feeling and how upset she was. She looked at me with the most miserable expression on her face, and she began to speak through her tears. She told me about her emotional pain since having the stroke, though she did not use this term. She had recently had stents placed in one of her coronary arteries and felt horrified that she was now facing recovery from a stroke. Additionally, she had already expended all of her sick time due to the stents, and she was in fear of being fired due to this new illness. She told me that she supports her family, and is living from paycheck to paycheck, so she could not afford any more time off. Her husband said little during this encounter, only continued to sit on the bed with his arms crossed over his chest. I asked her to tell me more about her concerns and fears. She told me that she felt out of control with her emotions, and could not stop crying. She was afraid that she would have another stroke, and she "just wanted her life back." She could not afford many of the expensive medications that were being prescribed to her, and felt as if she was being told to "either buy them or you will die."

As I listened to Cathy, my mind was calculating the number of services I needed to mobilize for her so that I could lessen her burdens and improve her outcomes. I started by discussing with her what the definition of stroke, and why we had done all of the testing. Also, I went on to explain what medications would be prescribed based on her history of stents, along with the stroke. I told her that there are patient assistance programs that I would help her enroll in that would help pay for the cost of her medication. I asked her nurse to contact pastoral care and social services immediately to see this patient, and this was done. I discussed her obvious depression, how depressive symptoms are common after a stroke and that an antidepressant medication might be helpful. She agreed with this plan and I went to her chart and wrote an order for the antidepressant. I offered her my card, so that she could contact me whenever she needed me. I knew how much she needed this support. Finally, I had her work fax the FMLA paperwork she would need to secure time off she would need to recover from her stroke. I told her that I had initially come to her room to ask her about a research project, but it was more important to take care of these needs first. If the time came to discuss the project, I would do so then.

I visited Cathy every day thereafter in the hospital as she recovered from stroke and was impressed with her progress. I did not bring up the study again, feeling that she had so much on her mind; my needs to complete my study were minor compared to the problems she was facing. On her day of discharge, I walked into her room, and she was preparing to leave. Her mood was improved; the anxiety and depression were tempered. She clasped my hand and thanked me for being there for her. She told me that she thought she would have lost her mind if she had not had someone who "heard her." Then, she asked me if she could join my research study. I was so surprised, but happy to give her a consent form and continue our working relationship. As it turned out, she was assigned to my "intervention" group, and I was able to continue my teaching and interventions, including smoking cessation.

I recently saw Cathy in clinic for a 3-month follow-up, and I am impressed with her progress. She received medication assistance, and support from her workplace. Her recovery from stroke is not complete, but she has stopped smoking, has started exercise, is controlling her cholesterol, and is following dietary guidelines.

My experience with Cathy reminded me that in this fast-paced society, one of the greatest gifts we utilize in patient care is the ability to listen with our hearts, and to help our patients find solid footing on which to stand while recovering and coping with illness. My DNP program had enabled me to take a broader view of the stroke patient population, to encompass the complete range of care that they require in my treatment plan and to develop an evidence-based approach to post-stroke patients including depressive symptoms and treatments.

Student Capstone Exemplar 3

Many years ago, when I was working as an intern psychiatric nurse practitioner, I remember meeting a quiet, pale, young woman who was hospitalized for depression after the recent death of her father with whom she lived. This woman had been treated with numerous antidepressants but showed little improvement. At the time of her first visit my role was to complete a physical exam in preparation of electric convulsant therapy (ECT), which was used when other less invasive therapies to improve the patient's depression were not successful. When I met the patient in the exam room she was withdrawn and almost catatonic. I asked her to sit on the table for the physical. I began my exam as usual starting from head working to toe. As I began I noticed the woman had patches of missing hair on her scalp. I knew that hair loss could be attributed to depression or "nerve problems," but it was a remarkable finding. I completed the head-to-toe assessment, which was significant for hair loss on her scalp, decreased reflexes, pale skin, and pronounced mental status changes reflective of depression. Her mood and affect were sad; she was soft spoken, bashful, quiet, and had a flat affect. She was not tearful even when talking quietly about the loss of her dad. We finished the work-up and I investigated

Continued on page 434

Student Capstone Exemplar 3 *Continued from page 433*

causes of hair loss. The differential was lengthy but I carefully considered each and every possibility. With each possibility I made note of which lab tests could prove or disprove the diagnosis. I ordered all labs that could explain physical reasons for the bald spots on this woman's scalp. Days were numbered before she would begin ECT treatments and I was anxious to explore all explanations before this treatment began. I waited for results all of which were negative until finally a positive heavy metal screen was returned. The metal detected in the test was arsenic. How could this be? Was it a suicide attempt? The young woman seemed as surprised as I was with the finding. A case worker asked the woman's permission to go to her home and investigate where this heavy metal came from. The case worker wasted no time in finding the cause of the poisoning. Under the sink a bag of garden pesticide had a listing for the arsenic. The woman reported that she and her father used the powder on their vegetable garden and it could have been ingested by eating the vegetables they grew. Now the question that arose was did her father die of this poison? His cause of death was listed as liver disease and kidney failure both which could be caused by arsenic. We began treating her by chelating to remove the arsenic in her system. She improved over time and escaped the need for ECT treatment with the possible side effects that would have impacted her memory still leaving the arsenic.

I learned a lot from this experience, and it propelled me to seek the highest level of education in my field, the DNP. It was early in my career as a nurse practitioner and helped me to realize that as a nurse practitioner I had a lot to offer patients. This experience created the practice knowledge for my capstone project, which was a systematic review of the literature on causes of acute confusion and depression including environmental causes, physical causes, and genetic causes. The second step in my capstone was to create a guideline for assessment of acute onset of depression. Now that I have completed the DNP, I feel even more secure in my ability to search the evidence and find alternative answers to patient's problems. I am proud that as a nurse practitioner I took the opportunity to investigate beyond this young woman's depression. Many physician colleagues remark that with my abilities I "should have been a doctor"; well now I am a doctor of nursing practice, which provides me with the knowledge and ability to be the best that I can be in my field.

Conclusion

To evaluate the knowledge gained in any DNP program, three different methods are used: (1) a residency to demonstrate knowledge in the practice area and fulfill part of the 1000 hours of clinical practice required; (2) a portfolio to document experiences and knowledge gained during DNP course work; and (3) a final project or capstone that allows the DNP student to demonstrate knowledge by developing, implementing, and evaluating a program or project.

As the DNP becomes the entry into advanced practice, the final project will provide evidence that the DNP is prepared to become a leader or collaborator and practice to the full extent of his or her education and training. Improving access to care and adequate care coordination will improve the health of Americans in general and will require the DNP to be ready to step into the role of autonomous health-care provider.

References

Accreditation Counsel for Graduate Medical Education (ACGME). (2006). Introduction to competency based residency education. Retrieved from http://www.acgme.org/acWebsite/home/home.asp

American Association of Colleges of Nursing. (2006). The essentials of doctoral education for advanced nursing practice. Retrieved from http://www.aacn.nche.edu/dnp/pdf/essentials.pdf

Bronte-Tinkew, J., Allen, T., & Joyner, K. (2008). Institutional review boards (IRBs): What are they, and why are they important? Part 7 in a series on practical evaluation methods. *Child Trends: Practitioner Insights, Research-to-Results.* Retrieved from http://www.childtrends.org/Files/Child_Trends-2008_02_19_Evaluation7IRBs.pdf

Brown-Benedict, D. (2008). The doctor of nursing practice degree: Lessons from the history of the professional doctorate in other health disciplines. *Journal of Nursing Education, 47*(10), 448–456.

Edwardson, S. (2009). Doctor of philosophy and doctor of nursing practice as complementary degrees. *Journal of Professional Nursing, 26*(3), 137–140.

Fulton, J. S., & Lyon, B. L. (2005, September 30). The need for some sense making: Doctor of nursing practice. *Online Journal of Issues in Nursing, 10* (3), Article 3. Retrieved from www.nursingworld.org/MainMenuCategories/ANAMarketplace/ANAPeriodicals/OJIN/TableofContents/Volume102005/No3Sept05/tpc28_316027.aspx

Mundinger, M., Starck, P., Hathaway, D., Shaver, J., & Fugate Woods, N. (2009). The ABCs of the doctor of nursing practice: Assessing resources, building a culture of clinical scholarship, curricula models. *Journal of Professional Nursing, 25*(2), 69–74.

Stanley, J. (2005). Evaluating the doctor of nursing practice: Moving toward a new vision of nurse practitioner education. *Nurse Practitioner Journal,* November/December 2005. Retrieved from www.npjournal.org

Index

Page numbers followed by b indicate boxes, page numbers followed by f indicate figures, and page numbers followed by t indicate tables.

A

E

F

I

O

P

Q

R

S

T

U

V

Made in the USA
Lexington, KY
27 August 2012